GIVE US THE CHANCE

SPORT AND PHYSICAL

RECREATION WITH PEOPLE

WITH A MENTAL HANDICAP

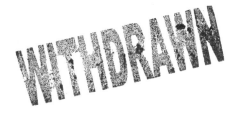

GIVE US THE CHANCE

SPORT AND PHYSICAL RECREATION WITH PEOPLE WITH A MENTAL HANDICAP

KAY LATTO DipPE MCSP

BARBARA NORRICE DipPE

Illustrations by Elaine Batt

Published by the
Disabled Living Foundation
London

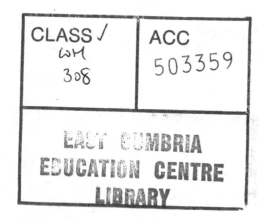
First published 1981
Revised edition 1989

British Library Cataloguing in Publication data
Latto, Kay
   Give us the chance: sport and physical recreation
   with people with a mental handicap. - 2nd. ed./Kay
   Latto and Barbara Norrice.
   1. Physical activities for mentally handicapped
   persons. Teaching Manuals
   I. Title   II. Norrice, Barbara   III. Disabled Living
   Foundation
   790.1'96

ISBN 0-901908-38-X

Printed in Great Britain by BPCC Wheatons Ltd, Exeter

Contents

Preface

Since 1981, physical activities and sport for people with a mental handicap have developed in many ways, showing the need not only to update the original book but also to include four new chapters — 'Physical Activities for People with a Severe or Profound Mental Handicap' — 'Movement and Dance Therapy' — 'Two views on Integration' — 'Riding and Driving'.

Chapters 1 and 2, A Doctor's View and a Psychologist's View, have both been updated by Dr Peter Sylvester and Mr John Clements.

In view of the discussions and research carried out on atlanto-axial dislocation a statement approved by the then Department of Health and Social Security has been included as Appendix 4, and the World Health Organisation's definitions of impairments of intelligence appear in the Introduction.

Basic game skills, movement exercises and dance steps and formations remain in Chapters 7, 11 and 13. Some new games and practices have been added together with details of the Uniplay Sports Awards and games with a parachute (in Chapter 7). Ribbon dancing, Chinese parasol and Morris dancing are included in Chapter 13.

An updated version of 'It's a Knockout' and a new event 'Superstars' with descriptions of the preparation and performance of these events and their value will be found in Chapter 10. Riding and driving has become one of the most popular activities not only for people with a mental handicap but also for those people with many other kinds of disability; it no longer appears in the chapter on Outdoor Pursuits, as it merits a chapter of its own (Chapter 16).

Many outdoor activity centres (see Chapter 15) have opened since 1981, offering a wide choice of aims and activities using the countryside — the sea, rivers, canals, lakes and reservoirs. Guidelines to choosing an outdoor pursuits centre have been added to this chapter to assist leaders to find one appropriate to the needs of their particular group.

Other chapters have been updated with relevant/interesting developments, new awards and training facilities/resources.

This book was originally compiled as a result of visits to hospitals, Adult Training Centres and clubs throughout the United Kingdom. The purpose of these was to see activities being practised and to discover the value, programme content, organisation and future development of physical activities and sports for adults and children (see Appendix 1). Discussions took place with a variety of individuals, organisations, health, social service and local authority personnel. The content was prepared with the following groups in mind:

medical, nursing and other staff in hospitals who may have little technical knowledge about teaching sports and physical activities;

physical education specialists and qualified teachers, instructors and coaches of individual sports and activities who may have little knowledge of the techniques of working with people with a mental handicap;

the parent or volunteer who may lack background and training in both these areas.

The book is designed to assist these groups by including:

the expert knowledge of a doctor and a clinical psychologist (Chapters 1 and 2);

the descriptions of a number of programme activities and examples of projects and events;

general guidelines on organisation, presentation, facilities and resources.

The information is not exhaustive. It is designed to give readers sufficient confidence and impetus to try out new ideas and to extend their own knowledge in physical recreation and sport through experience, training courses and further study.

It is hoped that this publication will inspire all those working with people with a mental handicap, whether in hospital, training centre, club, at home or elsewhere to introduce a wider choice of activitiies in their programmes and to encourage a greater number of individuals to take part in them.

WE SHOULD GIVE PEOPLE WITH A MENTAL HANDICAP THE SAME OPPORTUNITIES TO TAKE PART IN PHYSICAL ACTIVITIES, SPORTS AND OUTDOOR PURSUITS AS THE REST OF US.

Kay Latto (Maskell)
Barbara Norrice

Acknowledgements

In this revised edition we are grateful to all those who updated their former contributions and to those who have given us new ideas.

We are indebted to H J Tohill, Senior Tutor of the Broadlands School of Nursing at Little Plumstead Hospital, Norwich, who made it possible for a pilot project to be organised from 1981-83 involving the regular teaching of students in the theory and practice of physical activities for people with a mental handicap, which was undertaken by Barbara Norrice. Based on the shared experience and evaluation of students, tutors and ward staff, the Unit of Learning was drawn up on the premise that 40 hours could be given to this work during a 3-year nurse training programme.

Our thanks go to Kenneth Pugsley, Nursing Officer (Mental Health) at the Department of Health, for guiding us through the early stages of the negotiations with the English National Board for Nursing, Midwifery and Health Visiting (ENB), which have resulted in the Unit of Learning being accepted by the ENB and in the development of a working relationship between the ENB Education Officers, National Development Officer and ourselves.

We specially mention Mrs M Williams, Education South West Regional Officer, ENB, who has co-ordinated the administration of the regional courses/workshops being held using activities from this book.

We thank Elizabeth Dendy, Executive Officer of the Sports Council, and Mark Southam, National Development Officer, UKSAPMH, for undertaking the task of reading the text and for their suggestions which have been included in the final text.

To Elaine Batt our thanks for once again providing extra illustrations for the new chapters and the new cover, and to Des O'Halloran for the cover design.

We should also like to thank Diana de Deney, Editor, DLF Publications, for her guidance throughout the revision and for editing the script ready for publication; Hilda Wilsker who willingly typed and re-typed the script; and Kay Evans for her inspiration and help with proof reading.

No acknowledgement would be complete without remembering all those who contributed to the original book — the many people who gave us information on the original visits, the members of the DLF Steering Group who have guided us over the years, and Sports Councils of England, Scotland, Northern Ireland and Wales for their continued interest.

Kay Latto (Maskell)
Barbara Norrice

Foreword

Since this textbook was first published in 1981, the opportunities for people with a mental handicap have progressively increased, and the United Kingdom Sports Association for People with a Mental Handicap (UKSAPMH), formed in the same year, has developed steadily. The Association now has a number of regional offices and employs some development officers, both nationally and regionally. Those in the DLF working on this project have done so in close so-operation with UKSAPMH.

It was also in 1981 that a key project worker, Miss Barbara Norrice, DipPE, offered to work voluntarily for the DLF following her retirement as Senior Lecturer in Physical Education from Keswick Hall College of Education. One of her responsibilities there had been the training of teachers to work in special schools. For the past 7 years she has been responsible in the DLF for promoting physical activities for those with severe mental handicap in co-operation with the English National Board for Nursing, Midwifery and Health Visiting (ENB). The Board has now accepted the Unit of Learning on 'Physical Activities for Children/Adults with Mental Handicap' compiled by Miss Barbara Norrice and Mr J H Tohill, Senior Tutor of the Broadland School of Nursing, as part of its syllabus for nurses and students for the RNMS qualification.

In 1983 the film 'Give us the Chance', devised by the DLF Project Workers, was launched by the Lord Mayor of London. The film was aimed at all those concerned with daily living problems of people with a mental handicap whether in hospital or in the community. It had an excellent reception and DLF is grateful for the support of the many funding bodies who grant aided the film and financed the extra copies needed to meet the many requests to hire or purchase. The film won the BLAT (British Life Assurance Trust) Award in 1983 — the quality of its content was commended for use with people with a mental handicap.

This new edition of 'Give us the Chance' contains the original content updated by Kay Latto and Barbara Norrice together with additional material as outlined in the preface.

The DLF Trustees would like to repeat their gratitude to Dr Sylvester and to Mr Clements for their continuing contributions to the work. Additional delightful illustrations and a revised cover drawing to include further activities have been contributed by Mrs Elaine Batt whose continuing interest is also greatly appreciated.

This project has been unique in DLF's history in that during ten years all the principal project workers have been highly qualified volunteers who have undertaken immense work. The DLF Trustees are deeply grateful to Kay Latto, DipPE MCSP (Mrs Dan Maskell) and to Barbara Norrice the authors of 'Give us the Chance', and to Miss Kay Evans MBE DipPE MCSP, for her continuing help and advice. The Second Sidbury Trust has now supported DLF's work in this field for 12 years and has been principal funders throughout. The DLF Trustees thank the Trust sincerely for this continuing and understanding generosity in meeting the other expenses of the work.

This second edition of 'Give us the Chance is offered with the same hope for its practical usefulness as the first. Again comment, contributions and criticisms would be welcomed. In the last years it has become apparent that the majority of activities described in 'Give us the Chance' are, with appropriate adaptation suitable for people with any form of disability and also for the infirm elderly, and comment on ideas on this further use would be received with pleasure as well.

W M Hamilton

Introduction

Before selecting activities or events from the practical chapters (6 to 14) of the book, readers should read chapters 1 to 5. These first chapters contain much background information relevant to the rest of the text, including a description of mental handicap and of problems which arise when teaching people with a mental handicap including those who are severely handicapped, an account of general teaching methods, and guidance on how to choose an activity and on making the most of indoor and outdoor space available.

The illustrations are indicative of activities and skills and are not intended to show accurate technique. Female figures are shown with pigtails or appropriate headdress.

Most of the activities and events describes in the text are those actually seen by the authors.

Activities suitable for people with a severe mental handicap are included in Chapter 14 and those in the remainder of the text are indexed under *mental handicap, severe* (see pages 197-8).

TERMINOLOGY

In recent years the terminology used to describe the problems faced by the people with whom this book is concerned has changed in many ways. There is little agreement. Terms such as intellectual impairment, learning difficulties, learning disabilities, mental impairment and developmental disabilities can all be found in modern texts. It is obviously important to discard terms which have a negative connotation. At the same time it is important to be able to communicate accurately about the problems people face.

The term 'mental handicap' is retained in the present text albeit with some diffidence. Two reasons are thought to justify this usage. The people with whom this book is concerned suffer an underlying impairment to their intellectual functioning which makes ti hard for them to learn (hence the term developmental disability). But this book is about functioning in everyday life — about ways in which people can be helped to participate in activities and enjoy as full and normal a life as possible. It is therefore about the handicaps which may arise when you have an intellectual impairment and learning difficulties but which can sometimes be overcome. Hence it did not seem inappropriate to retain the term handicapped.

The second reason for retaining this usage is that 'mental handicap' and 'people with a mental handicap' are still phrases used and understood by many practitioners (unlike many of the newer terms). Such terminology also remains enshrined in a number of institutions (e.g., MENCAP, BIMH). Undoubtedly some may be offended that a new edition of this text did not alter the basic terminology used, but is is hoped that differences of opinion within an area of common interest can be tolerated.

Similarly, in different areas of the country different terms are used to describe the same group of people, i.e:

i) those who attend Adult Training Centres/Social Education Centres are variously described as trainees, clients or students (in a wider context, the term student refers to those attending open or in-service training courses);

ii) those in hospital are patients or residents;

iii) those teaching in ATCs/SECs, hospitals or Gateway Clubs are teachers, instructors, leaders, recreation officers or coaches;

iv) those who sometimes work in co-operation with members of staff are volunteers, enablers, carers, care-givers.

The terms Sports Centre, Sports Leisure Centre or Recreation Centre denote a large sports complex including facilities for indoor/outdoor sports and swimming on one campus or a centre for indoor/outdoor sports with swimming bath/pool in separate localities.

WHAT IS MENTAL HANDICAP?

The World Health Organisation has classified the categories of intellectual impairment in the following way:

Profound mental retardation	IQ under 20. Individuals who may respond to skill training in the use of legs, hands and jaws.
Severe mental retardation	IQ 20-34. Individuals who can profit from systematic habit training.
Moderate mental retardation	IQ 35-49. Individuals who can learn simple communication, elementary health and safety habits, and simple manual skills, but do not progress in functional reading or arithmetic.
Mild mental retardation	IQ 50-70. Individuals who can acquire practical skills and functional reading and arithmetic abilities with special education, and who can be guided towards social conformity.

ORGANISATION OF THE PROJECT

The Steering Group, representing organisations concerned with the daily living of people with a mental handicap and those who have contributed to the development of sport and physical activities for them, was formed in autumn 1976.

Terms of reference

To prepare a manuscript for publication to serve as guide for parents, families and friends, for staff and helpers, teachers, leaders and coaches responsible for organising fitness training, games and sports, and outdoor activities in hospitals, adult training centres, Gateway Clubs and hostels in the community generally.

Questionnaire

A simple questionnaire was sent to all hospitals for people with a mental handicap and to all directors of social services for distribution to adult training centres and hostels in England, Northern Ireland, Scotland and Wales.

The purpose of the questionnaire was to discover what physical activities and sports were provided for people with a mental handicap, what facilities were available and what personnel were employed to teach these activities. As a result of the information received the author selected various establishments to visit. In making her choice, she took the following factors into consideration:

(i)   the nature and variety of activities being practised, the interesting and constructive comments made on the value, planning and content of the individual programme;

(ii)   the need to give as wide a coverage as possible to the four countries within the limits of time and financial resources;

(iii)   the need to see as many people with a mental handicap as possible taking part in a wide variety of physical activities, sports and outdoor pursuits;

(iv)   the information gathered as a result of the Press Release and information obtained from the Disabled Living Foundation Information Service and from other sources.

Organisation of visits

Arrangements to visit hospitals and adult training centres were made through the hospital administrators and directors of social services and through the latter to managers of the training centres.

All arrangements for visits in Scotland were made by the Development Officer of the Scottish Sports Association for the Disabled, for the visit in Ireland by the Sports Council of Northern Ireland in association with the area health boards and for the visit to Wales by the Sports Council for Wales.

Visits were made to adult training centres, hostels and Gateway Clubs and several events, sports days, swimming sports, inter-hospital matches and sports days, displays and finals days were attended. Many meetings were held with representatives of the medical and ancillary professions, hospital administrators, nursing staff and recreation officers together with managers, staff and helpers of adult training centres. Where possible contact was made with the physical education departments of the training establishments running the 1-year diploma course for instructors of adult training centres.

During the visits small groups of specialists were brought together for discussion and consultations were held with many individuals.

Chapter 1

A Doctor's View

Dr Peter Sylvester

This chapter is mostly concerned with people with a mental handicap. They have special needs but much that applies to them in the field of sport and recreation also applies to other groups of disabled people.

Mental handicap is the failure of a child's mind to develop and mature adequately with the consequent limitation of intelligence. There are many causes.

A child may grow normally but the mind remains behind the level expected of a child of similar age. Thus a child falls behind his peers in achievement. Good physique and healthy looks may lead the child to attend a normal school but failure or slowness in learning to read, write and generally take care of himself draws attention to special needs.

There are different degrees of handicap. Some children are mildly handicapped and able to learn skills in reading and writing, while others are so severely or profoundly handicapped that they are unable to learn to speak and control their bodily functions.

People with a mental handicap often have other problems. Physical handicap (cerebral palsy), blindness, deafness and epilepsy are common. Additional handicaps make it more difficult for a child to cope with living and he therefore needs special help from staff who are acquainted with his problems and specially trained to cope with them. Children may be so handicapped that they require assistance with feeding, washing, dressing and toileting. There are nearly half a million people in England and Wales, of all ages, with varying degrees of mental handicap.

It is important that children with a mental handicap be identified as early as possible so that they can be directed into suitable programmes of education and training. Sometimes the decision is easy; for instance, it is well known that children with Down's Syndrome (Mongolism) can be recognised at birth and a forecast of the child's future development predicted. Other children appear quite normal at birth and start to grow and develop in the normal way. It is only when they reach the age of two, three, or perhaps start school, that their handicap becomes obvious. There are different ways of detecting children with a mental handicap. One is recording 'milestone of development', that is to say, the age at which a child is expected to achieve sitting up, crawling, standing, walking, talking and controlling his toilet habits. If these do not appear at predicted times they may be the first important clues to a child's future mental disability. Fuller assessment requires complicated programmes of observation and testing and takes into account the social and educational aspects of a child's life.

Mental handicap sometimes goes by other names including mental deficiency, mental retardation and subnormality of mind.

It is frequently confused with mental illness or psychosis, but the two conditions are completely different. Mental illness affects the minds of otherwise normal people — thinking processes become disturbed or confused but are amenable to treatment so that cures can be made; mental handicap, on the other hand, is often a symptom of some previous disease process and is a permanent condition which cannot be cured although it can be influenced and the person's mental and physical condition considerably improved. It must be said that the handicapped person can sometimes develop symptoms of mental illness in the same way as ordinary individuals. Legally, both mental handicap and mental illness are grouped together as mental disorder.

GENERAL HEALTH

Every person with a mental handicap is subject to the same type of physical illness and injuries as other people, including coughs, colds, influenza, pneumonia, skin infections, high blood pressure and heart attacks, to name but a few. Some conditions, not strictly speaking illnesses, occur more frequently in the handicapped person than in the intelligent — epilepsy, physical handicap, communication difficulties, blindness, and deafness are common conditions. These complications are secondary to damage of the brain, which may also be the responsible factor for the mental handicap. Clearly, if extra handicaps occur management problems are increased and can be very difficult to handle.

Preventive measures against illness in childhood, including immunisation programmes for diptheria, tetanus, poliomyelitis and tuberculosis, have helped to give a child with a mental handicap a much better chance to enjoy good physical health. In times gone by, tuberculosis, chronic ear disease with offensive discharges, dental sepsis, chronic constipation, and skin conditions were common, but today these conditions are largely controlled and do not constitute the menace they once did to physical well-being.

If sport and recreation are to be enjoyed and result in further improvement in the physical and mental well-being of people with a mental handicap, it is important that life starts with the best possible health. Ambulant handicapped people can have poor posture and gait. It is not always clear why this is so, but in many it is connected with lack of participation in physical activities. Such people are likely to derive great benefit from sport and physical recreation and their posture improves.

Children have always been able to participate in group games and sports because they attend special schools, where such things form part of their educational programme, but in mainstream schools some children do not always have this opportunity. It is important to carry forward opportunities learnt in school into adult life. Fortunately, disabled people are increasingly welcome to attend community sport grounds and leisure centres and enjoy the facilities provided.

PLAY

Play, which is essential to people of all ages, eventually merges with sport and physical recreation. Failure to meet schedules in development is likely to end with some degree of deprivation in emotional, social and even intellectual capacities. The handicappd child is unfortunately exposed to these risks. Nurses, teachers, parents, play leaders, recreation officers and volunteers all have their part to play if children are to take part in play, recreation and sports. Many handicapped children have to be taught how to play. Some years ago it was the fashion to have a 'rumpus room' for children. One was created for a number of handicapped boys from seven to 14 years and equipped with an array of expensive toys including tricycles, swings and climbing equipment. It was thought that these were all that were required and the day came when the children were allowed in to play. Unfortunately, they had no idea of how to use the equipment and within a few hours it was reduced to masses of twisted metal. Clearly, play opportunities have to be supplemented with good sensible tutors to enable the children to make the best use of play material.

COMMUNICATION

Communication for most people means reading, writing and speaking. In fact, there is much more to communication than that. The five senses, smell, taste, touch, vision and hearing, plus numerous skilled motor (muscular) movements, are needed in all aspects of communication. Consider the plight of handicapped people, deprived of one or more of the sensitive input and output systems of the nervous systems, and how they have to adapt to an environment not designed for them? Lack of ability to read, write or to speak does not mean a person is totally incapable of communicating. The most severely handicapped children need and respond to elementary forms of communication through touch, cuddles, caresses, simple sounds and body language, in much the same way as small infants. As they progress, more sophisticated sign systems, borrowed or adopted from the Makaton or Bliss method, may be introduced.

Balls and hoops introduce the child to motion and, eventually, to contact with others, since a ball can move from one individual to another — the elements of communication begin to be established. The ball and hoop theme progresses to more complicated games and eventually to sport. These aid the pattern of permanent memory responses for communication, and will require patient repetitive work on the part of parents and carers. Having a wide variety of disabilities calls for an enormous variety of needs.

Art forms, including music and drama, included with play, sport and other recreational activities, provide environments rich with opportunities for communication, not only between individuals, but between individuals and their communities. There are many outstanding examples of how handicapped people have overcome their communication impediments. The autobiography *Tongue tied* by Joey Deacon, a cerebral palsied man, written in collaboration with three other differently handicapped men, is one of the best known. Adventure playgrounds came late into Joey's life, but when asked his views about them

he said, ruefully, through his interpreter, "I wish they had been around when I was small!"

TREATMENT

Treatment or therapy is a comprehensive term. From the doctor's point of view it is divided into various categories: prevention; specific treatment; treatment of complications; supportive treatment; convalescence.

1. Prevention of diseases has improved the health of populations throughout the world; for instance, control of malaria, eradication of tuberculosis. Amongst disabled people, many conditions can now be prevented, especially those caused by injuries, infections and even some of the complicated genetic disorders.

2. Specific treatment may be either surgical as in obstructive hydrocephalus; or medical, in the case of special diets (Phenylketonuria) and replacement hormone therapy (hypothyroisism).

3. Remedial treatment applies, principally, to complications; it is the management and counteracting of the disease processes which flow from complications and demands the skills of carers of all disciplines for disabled people. Some of the work is preventive — an example being keeping paralysed limbs supple and preventing deformities.

4. Supportive measures, to boost morale and encourage confidence as well as dealing with social implications, are all part of the remedial process.

The remedial aspects of sport can be appreciated from a brief resumé of what is involved including: agreeing to take part, training and practice, being 'kitted out', travelling to the event, meeting other competitors, anticipation of the event, celebration and social happenings, return journey, and recounting experiences to others. Each phase has its own emotional halo.

DIET

A good balanced diet of proteins, carbohydrates, fats, minerals and vitamins is essential for everyone. The total daily intake of food (calories) depends on the type of activity undertaken. Men need a higher intake of calories. Proteins are used for tissue building and repair, whilst carbohydrates and fats supply energy. Sugars, especially glucose, are the simplest form of carbohydrates. They are easily absorbed into the body and are quick sources of energy, before sporting events. Salt is an important mineral. It is lost in perspiration during exercise, and, unless a good reserve is built up before sporting events, its loss results in muscular cramps.

ATTITUDES

If a competitor wishes to succeed it is necessary for him to develop an element of aggression in order to win. The correct spirit will make him do his best. Conversely, if the attitude is one of helplessness and timidity, then failure results. One thing all competitors have to overcome is anxiety and perhaps and element of fear while waiting to compete. Variation in personality types means that people have to face and overcome these problems in their own way. Those that do it best, succeed. Encouragement from team mates and coaches is, naturally, supportive.

Competitive sport for the 'hale and hearty' means there must be winners and losers; the important thing for disabled people is to change the rules so that there are no losers. However, an alternative point of view is that the reward comes with the thrill and satisfaction that flow from having competed which builds up confidence in coping with everyday life. The parents of Kevin, who had taken part in Olympic competition, reported: "It was marvellous to see him running freely with other people and joining in most things. Over the months while in training he gradually came out of his shell. He now has much more confidence in every way and moves more freely with most people". Recreation and pastimes which do not have a strong competitive element still have an important part to play. The quality of life is greatly enhanced by contact with others and the opportunities presented of learning new skills. Great patience and initiative on the part of teachers, nurses, physical instructors and physiotherapists to invent, design and evolve new activities to suit every individual's needs is required. Their efforts influence the attitudes of parents and raise hopes and aspirations. Nothing sustains parents more than seeing their children participating happily in ventures which would have seemed pointless not so long before.

It is reasonable when designing recreational training programmes for handicapped people to match them with competitors having similar handicaps.

SOCIAL BENEFITS

Playing in a team, competing in events and meeting other people both on and off the field inspires loyalty and extends the scope of personal contacts and friendships. Sport provides a topic for conversation and therefore improves the possibilities of communication.

The post-match tea or supper is a common event after many team games. Handicapped people should take part in this activity and be encouraged to bring their own supporters, and to provide hospitality for the opposing team out of their own money. Help and encouragement to lay tables, cut sandwiches and act as hosts are important. In this way handicapped people can be taught to develop confidence in looking after themselves at all times instead of relying on others to provide an ever-ready tea party. The customary 'after the match' drink in a pub should not be ignored.

Most handicapped people take longer than able bodied people to carry out a given task, and allowance for this must therefore be made. For example, then a handicapped person is taken swimming he should be encouraged to undress, put on the swimsuit, dry off and redress by himself; but the person accompanying him must appreciate that these preparations can take a long time; a point which should also be pointed out to those providing facilities.

EPILEPSY

Epilepsy, like mental handicap, is not really a disease but a consequence of some illness, perhaps well-defined, perhaps not, but which has left a persistant periodic manifestation. It can be regarded as a complication and takes many forms, the best known being generalised tonic/clonic seizures (formerly called grand mal) and generalised absenses (formerly called petit mal). During a grand mal seizure the person falls unconscious to the ground and goes through a series of convulsions, recovery taking place after a few minutes. Petit mal sufferers have momentary lapses of consciousness which recur at frequent intervals. A child may have drop attacks during which he falls to the ground suddenly but recovers quickly, or salaam attacks during which he makes a bowing motion. Bizarre disturbances of behaviour may signify psychomotor epilepsy. Jacksonian epilepsy is revealed by local twitching affecting either an arm, leg or part of the face.

Epilepsy is common among handicapped people and afflicts one in four who live in long-stay hospitals. Fortunately there are drugs (anti-convulsants) which control the number of fits and their severity. It is possible that fits can be controlled completely. It is well known that flickering light — similar to that reflected from waves in a swimming pool — can provoke an epileptic seizure. However, only a few epileptic people are likely to have their fits triggered off by this sort of stimulation; nevertheless, it is a point that should be borne in mind for the coach at the poolside. Provided staff and organisers of recreational or sporting facilities are aware of a person's epilepsy and consultation with medical advisers is maintained, there is little reason to eliminate him from taking part in full programmes of sport.

FITTING THE SPORT TO THE INDIVIDUAL

The mildly handicapped person who is physically fit can participate in any sport of recreational activity as he wishes. No limits need be put on his participation and he could even compete with able bodied people. Many handicapped people are very keen competitors.

Looking at this problem from the opposite point of view, sport should be chosen and designed for a particular candidate or group of people. Those with a severe mental handicap or disability may find it difficult to accept competitive games especially those involving a great deal of training and skilled performance. However, they can participate in sports and games which are less demanding or specially designed for them. Well known examples are those for blind people who are capable of playing ball games aided by sighted helpers and sometimes by modified equipment, and those for deaf people who can enjoy dancing since the tempo and rhythm are communicated to them through their feet from vibrations in the floor.

HOW THE BODY WORKS

To understand the bodily requirements for exercise it is useful to know how the body functions.

1. The skeleton is a series of internal splints to which muscles are attached and through which they exert their forces when contracting. Joints are necessary for movements to take place. Limb joints occur as ball and socket, and hinge joints; they act as fulcrums around which muscular action if effective. They are surrounded by ligaments. Joint surfaces are very smooth and lubricated by fluids to reduce friction.

    The smooth surface is lost in arthritis, a common malady affecting disabled as well as non-disabled people. Usually painful, it restricts movements and therefore impairs activity. Dislocation, especially of the hip joint, is reasonably common in handicapped children. The child may either be born with it or acquire it later in childhood in some forms of very severe cerebral palsy. One joint, at the top of the neck spine, just below the junction with the skull, deserves special mention because of its importance in Down's Syndrome. It is called the atlanto-occipital joint. Instability is present in some individuals with Down's Syndrome. The joint is at risk of being dislocated if the sufferer participates in vigorous games and pastimes which might jerk it out of position — rather like a whiplash injury. This weakness can be detected clinically and by special investigation. (See Appendix 4).

2. Muscles have the ability to contract and relax. When contracted they exert a force of pull across a joint. Some act in groups to fix a joint for a particular action, e.g. bracing the bow arm when drawing the bow; others are prime movers, e.g. they flex or bend a joint, or extend or straighten a joint. Many muscular actions are complex and, while some muscles contract vigorously, others have to relax in other to execute a desired movement, e.g. kicking a ball.

   Muscles are controlled by nerves and have a rich blood supply. They can become paralysed through two principal mechanisms. Both forms cause weakness of limb movement but differ in that one causes floppy muscles which waste and the other causes stiff, rigid muscles. The first is known as lower motor neurone paralysis and is seen in poliomyelitis (fortunately rare now); the second is an upper motor neurone paralysis seen in cerebral palsy.

3. To supply muscle in active exercise with nutrients, particularly glucose and oxygen, it is necessary that the blood supply be greatly increased. This happens through dilatation of the blood vessels together with an increase in heart rate to augment blood flow.

4. An important requisite to muscular action is a rich supply of oxygen. To obtain this, breathing increases in rate and depth so that more oxygen can enter the blood. This is further facilitated by an increase in the amount of blood circulation through the lungs. Obviously, diseases of the heart and lungs will impair a person's ability to partake vigorously in sport. Congenital heart disease (blue babies), chronic bronchitis and asthma are examples of such illness.

5. When muscles are contracting they undergo increased chemical activity. More oxygen is used, more carbon dioxide produced and, in severe exercise, acid waste products get into the blood. Unless these are removed quickly during vigorous exercise then accumulation causes painful muscular spasms, cramp or knotting.

6. Smooth muscular actions producing competent athletic movements have complex nerve supplies. Some nerves control the state of the blood vessels, others record the state of muscular contraction while others are concerned with exciting muscular action. All this would be of little avail without the higher centres in the brain. Consider the position of a batsman in cricket: he takes an optimum stance for a strike at the ball; he has to watch the delivery, assess the flight and fall of the ball; judge his stroke, flex his muscles for the appropriate action and then, having struck the ball successfully, listen for his partner's call before taking off for runs. In the fraction of a second, numerous messages have been received and interpreted into appropriate action.

   See also *The moving body* by Pat Kennedy (Further reading).

MEDICATION

Many handicapped people are prescribed anti-convulsants, tranquillisers, anti-physchotics and anti-depressants, but this fact should not in general deter them from taking part in sport. The purpose of medication is basically to help people to lead a full and complete life. People on some medication are told that their reactions may be slowed down and that alcoholic beverages should be avoided. This generalisation applies to handicapped people. However, the only person who can really advise in any particular case is the family practitioner and he should be consulted in all cases where there is any element of doubt.

FURTHER READING

Allen of Hurtwood, Lady. *Planning for play.* London, Thames & Hudson, 1975.

Craft, M *ed. Tredgold's mental retardation,* 12th ed. London, Baillière Tindall, 1979.

Deacon, J J. *Tongue tied.* London, National Society for Mentally Handicapped children, 1974.

Guttman, L. *Textbook of sport for the disabled.* Aylesbury, H M & M Publishers, 1976.

Heaton-Ward, W. *Left behind: a study of mental handicap.* London, Woburn Press, 1978.

Horobin, G and May, D eds. *Living with mental handicap.* London, Jessica Kingsley, 1988.

Jeffree, D M and Cheseldine, S. *Let's join in.* London, Souvenir Press, 1974.

Jeffree, D M, McConkey, R and Hewson, S. *Let me play,* 2nd ed. London, Souvenir Press, 1985.

Kennedy, P. *The moving body.* London, Faber and Faber, 1986.

Leighton, A ed. *Mental handicap in the community.* Cambridge, Woodhead-Faulkner, 1988.

Zarkowska, E and Clements, J. *Problem behaviour in people with severe learning difficulties.* London, Croom Helm, 1988.

Dr Peter Sylvester is a former Consultant Psychiatrist, St Lawrence's Hospital, Caterham.

Chapter 2

A Psychologist's View

John Clements

The present text reflects the growing awareness that people with a mental handicap can lead a richer life given appropriate opportunities and help.

For a long time the handicapped person has suffered from the poor expectations held for him by others, and this in its turn has meant that he has been deprived of many of the opportunities open to other members of society. This book demonstrates that people with a mental handicap can participate in and enjoy every kind of sport and physical activity — the examples given are of work that has actually been done rather than what might be done in theory.

These examples highlight the many benefits which such involvement can bring. It provides the handicapped person with a wider and more normal experience of life. Although much has been done in recent years to show how even the most severely disabled people can be taught greater social competence and independence there has been less emphasis on recreation and leisure. This has left an 'empty' part in the life pattern of many handicapped people, a part which these activities can help fill. Sport is a means whereby people from many walks of life can meet and grow to accept and understand each other. By increasing the involvement of the handicapped person in sport, it becomes easier for him to integrate with the rest of society. The more contact there is between the non-handicapped and handicapped people the greater will be the understanding of and tolerance towards disabled people; many examples in this book, eg the Outward Bound courses, illustrate this process at work.

In Chapter One Dr Sylvester discusses the many benefits which can be fostered by physical activities. These include improvements in general health and muscular co-ordination, encouragement of self care skills and social graces and the stimulation of imagination and communication and problem-solving abilities. These specific benefits can in their turn bring about more general improvements in self confidence and adjustment.

Few would argue about these benefits. And yet there are two groups which are often excluded from this kind of involvement — the multiply, profoundly handicapped, and those with severe disturbance in their behaviour. Whilst these groups present many practical problems, it can be argued that they will especially benefit from participation in organised physical activities.

For multiply handicapped people, the extent of their disabilities prevents them from influencing the environment for themselves — it encourages them to withdraw and become passive. It is therefore essential that they are kept involved in the world around them if they are not to become more dependent than necessary (see How to Choose an Activity, Chapter 5).

The solution to behaviour problems also requires active participation in positive programmes. This is not a question of using up people's energy — a model which attributes bad behaviour to an excess of energy is not appropriate in most cases. The benefit of a programme lies in the extent to which it helps people to behave well by giving them more skills, and by ensuring they receive plenty of attention and encouragement for so behaving. Those with disruptive behaviours often find themselves in situations where there is little to stimulate them and where they receive little attention from others, unless they act in a disruptive manner. A focus on teaching positive skills can break this cycle of events. In some specific cases, problem behaviour arises where an individual becomes very anxious. For these people some physical activities, eg yoga, music and movement, may be particularly helpful in teaching them how to relax and prevent the 'explosions' in their behaviour.

The benefits are therefore very real and wide-ranging. Putting the ideas into practice, however, may not always be easy and it is useful to consider some of the general principles involved, and some of the common difficulties encountered in running such activities (see also Teaching and Training Guidelines, Chapter 4).

BASIC STRATEGIES

1. **Be open-minded.** The whole content of this book highlights how handicapped people can be helped to engage in an enormous range of sports and activities. In selecting an activity it is important not to dismiss certain possibilities as being impractical. If in doubt, try it out; and, if it does not work one way, try it another way. This is not the same as being foolhardy. Throughout the book great emphasis is laid on having the right equipment and involving people skilled in the activity in question (even if they are not specialists in the field of mental handicap). But within these constraints, the horizons for handicapped people can be widened enormously by challenging traditional expectations.

2. **Be specific.** When planning a programme it is important to have a clear idea about what will be the result when the programme is successful. It is not enough to aim to 'develop potential' or 'enhance a sense of well being'. These are worthy aims, but before a programme can begin it is important to visualise what people will be doing after the programme is finished and in what way their behaviour will be different.

3. **Observe first, teach later.** Once an activity has been selected it is tempting to start immediately to teach the skills involved. But it may be very useful to take the handicapped person through the activity and watch how he copes with various phases, given only minimal intervention (to prevent accidents, etc.). This kind of observation saves an enormous amount of time later — it may show that the person already

5

has many of the necessary skills. It is important not to rely solely on what others estimate a person can do — give him the opportunity to demonstrate his capabilities. Conversely, he may show deficiencies in skills which people had assumed were present. For example, some people may have been brought up in an environment without steps and may therefore have no idea how to cope with stairs; therefore, if climbing activities are being planned it may be important to start at this very basic level.

4. **Record the observations.** Anyone closely involved in an activity can easily forget what people were like before teaching and training began. If slow, steady improvement goes unnoticed, this will lead to discouragement. Keeping a record — in the form of a diary — can serve as a reminder. The form it takes is not as important as the content, which should relate to observable behaviour rather than to processes that one guesses are going on inside the person.

5. **Simplify complex tasks.** Any activity can be broken down into a number of component steps. It has been shown many times that a person may fail to learn if a task is presented in too complex a fashion, but will progress when that task is broken down into small steps and he is taught one step at a time. Some of the examples in the sections on swimming and canoeing show how tasks can be split up. These are just examples — many more steps might be needed for one person, many fewer for another. There is no text-book recipe on how to analyse a task. The number of steps depends entirely upon the people involved. If they fail to make progress it may be necessary to split the item which they find difficult into several smaller steps. Progress to the next step should only take place after mastery of the previous one in the sequence.

6. **Demonstrate the necessary response.** It is important for the coach or instructor to continually demonstrate the response required from those with whom he is working. It is not enough just to describe it or to give a single quick demonstration; repeated modelling should rather be incorporated into the process of learning.

7. **Maximise correct performance.** Even with a good task analysis it may be necessary to help the person through the step being worked on. Such additional help may take the form of extra instructions and reminders (verbal or gestural), direct physical guidance, or use of a special aid, eg buoyancy aids in swimming. The section on swimming illustrates two ways in which extra help can be provided either by buoyancy aids or by the physical support of an instructor. It also illustrates an important principle that such aids should be seen as temporary devices, which are gradually removed until the individual becomes independent. If help is removed too quickly performance may deteriorate but, if it is never removed, the person will fail to achieve independence. A balance is needed — not too much help, not too little.

8. **Ensure quick and comprehensible feedback.** Many handicapped people have special difficulties with their language development so that they cannot learn just by instructions. They need to see the activities carried out and practise them in real life so that they can learn by their own experience. They need to try out a skill and judge its success by the feedback they receive, so that they can gradually learn the correct ways of responding and drop the incorrect ways. Providing meaningful consequences for behaviour is therefore an essential part of the development and practise of skills.

Such feedback can be given in many ways and it is essential to find something which gets through to the individual or group with whom you are working. For some, words of praise and social attention may be sufficient. Others may practise better if there are tangible prizes for achievement. Some may like to see a visible record of achievement, such as their improvements filled in on a chart of graph. Younger and more severely disabled people may like certain kinds of physical contact (tickling, vibration) or sensory stimulation (lights, music) or direct material rewards (sweets, drinks). For those lucky enough to possess videotape equipment, video feedback may prove a powerful motivator. The important point is to discover what an individual or group responds to, and to make that contingent upon their performance at the selected activity. It should be something which can be provided immediately and frequently, so that the person is encouraged to keep practising until mastery is achieved. Once an activity is mastered, it may provide its own satisfaction, but during the process of learning extra feedback and encouragement may be required.

SOME COMMON PROBLEMS

1. **You can offer people the chance, but they just don't seem interested in the activity.** It is important to recognise that personal enthusiasm for a particular sport will not automatically be infectious, and that initial response to a new situation should not be taken as a reliable guide to the value of an activity. A handicapped person may become very anxious about new situations because, in the past, these have been associated with confusion and failure. He may therefore seek to avoid such situations unless he is gradually and repeatedly exposed to them. This emphasises the need to structure his experience very carefully in the ways outlined in the section on basic strategies (see p.5). Tasks need to be simplified, help given, and motivating feedback provided. Without this care in planning and presentation, avoidance and resistance may be increased, and the whole exercise will become unpleasant for all concerned. But as the description of It's a Knockout shows (see p.84), interest can develop. A key element that this work also highlights is the need to involve the handicapped person in planning activities. He needs to participate; and participation is not just for those who can articulate their needs. It is valuable even for the most severely disabled people if the activities are structured around and involve their known strengths and preferences.

2. **These activities are fine for the well behaved, but you cannot involve those who are disruptive.** It has already been pointed out that sport and other physical activities may have special benefits for those with disruptive behaviour, but some thought must be given to strategies for managing the problems if they are to be involved. The first step is to recognise that many disruptive behaviours have been learned and persist because they achieve some kind of consequences or feedback for the handicapped person. This must be assessed by specifying the problem behaviour, studying the situations in which it occurs and the consequences which are achieved by it. It is important also not just to focus on the difficult behaviour but to ask the question 'What should the person be doing instead?'. If he was not behaving badly, what would he be doing?

These two approaches lead to positive action to develop appropriate behaviour. It will suggest how the disruption might be 'unlearned' by making sure that it does not achieve the consequences maintaining it and by teaching the individual new and better ways of getting what he wants.

These techniques may be neither appropriate nor feasible in some cases; it is then important to seek guidance on alternative ways of dealing with the problems. However, many problems can be solved by so planning a programme that participants have plenty to occupy and interest them, ie minimal waiting or 'empty' times, and by making sure that all attention is focused on appropriate behaviour. This has sometimes been described as making sure you catch people being good.

3. **All these ideas work well for the more able, but what can you do for multiply, severely handicapped people?** This group of people, with physical and sensory handicaps in addition to their learning difficulties, present some of the greatest challenges to the ingenuity of parents, teachers, nurses and all others who work for them. There is little point in minimising the all too obvious difficulties of getting them to participate, but there is still much that can be done and progress is certainly possible. The first step is to ensure that adequate stimulation is received. This group of people often live in a state of sensory deprivation, both by reason of their own handicap and because of some of the environments offered to them. It is important to ensure that a good general level of stimulation is maintained to prevent withdrawal into a world of self-stimulation. The essence of such stimulation is that it be varied and adapted to the disabilities of the individual. Simply having loud music on, or hanging up coloured objects is not sufficient, because of the speed at which the nervous system adapts. Change and novelty are essential, and the exploration of alternative senses such as touch and smell, is needed. Maintaining stimulation is an important first step, but much more can be done.

The second step is to ensure correct positioning for the activity to be attempted. This positioning is critical in facilitating correct, voluntary movements and inhibiting abnormal, involuntary movements. This may necessitate finding a suitable position for the activity chosen, or choosing an activity which is suitable for the 'best' position of the individual concerned.

Selecting skills to teach and maintaining them requires careful thought. The size of step into which a task must be broken may be infinitesimally small — one may be aiming for the eyes to follow a ball moving horizontally from left to right, or encouraging that half-inch movement of the hand that will move the chime bell. Teaching these basic skills requires great sensitivity in the level of help given. Progress may take the form of a very gradual reduction in the physical help required to grasp an object. The helper must be sensitive to the least movement from the handicapped person and reduce his prompting as he feels independent movement coming into play.

Providing comprehensible feedback may be difficult, and routine forms of social or material encouragement may be meaningless. In some situations vibratory stimulation has been found very useful in reinforcing good performance. In others some individuals show strong preference for particular kinds of music (both classical and modern).

Finally, there may be certain activities which more readily encourage responses from the multiply handicapped person. The sections on swimming, riding and music and movement may be particularly helpful (see also the sections on people with a severe mental handicap in Chapters 5 and 14). Some others which might not usually be called 'sport'

are also worth considering, as is the potential of modern electronics to translate simple responses into complex forms of stimulation, eg modern fruit machines with light touch panels which lead to a range of changing visual and auditory effects and computer based activities.

These are only some examples and hints of avenues to explore. There is much still to be learned about involving this group, but enough is known for a start to be made.

4. **You can teach handicapped people to do something one day, but you come back the next day, and they have forgotten all about it.** Making generalisations about 'handicapped people' is always a dangerous exercise. The term mental handicap covers an enormous variety of learning problems in people who also show large individual differences in personality. Some handicapped people may well be forgetful, as are some non-handicapped people, but this is not a general characteristic of those with a mental handicap. They certainly have difficulty in learning skills initially, and once they have been mastered they may need extra practice to consolidate the learning. But with careful teaching and plenty of practice, skills will be retained without an unusual degree of loss over a period.

There is another problem which may sometimes be interpreted as a memory problem. This arises where skills are taught in an artificial situation that cannot easily be related to the real situation. For example, later in the book (see p.147) an example is given of teaching some people to use photographs as an aid in route-finding. The initial stages of this could have been taught in the classroom using a lot of verbal instructions and models of road junctions, houses, trees. If so, it is possible that when placed in the real situation the handicapped person would be none the wiser. A far better strategy is that actually adopted, of going out into the real environment and teaching there. This is a good general guideline, to work in the real environment, using real equipment, rather than spending a lot of time on elaborate mock-ups of the natural situation, whose relevance may not be apparent to the learner.

5. **These are all marvellous ideas, but you need enormous numbers of staff.** In some situations high staffing is essential. But high staffing is not the only answer and, in some cases, too many staff can be as disruptive as too few.

It may be worth considering a few strategies which are useful in working with groups of people. If only one staff member is present for a group he will need to ensure that he uses activities in which all can participate to some degree, and he will need to rapidly move from person to person giving each one brief amounts of individual attention, rather than concentrating on only a few, or spending long periods with each person individually. if two staff members are available one can work with the group whilst the other focuses on individual work. Roles can be swapped around and in this way each person gets periods of one-to-one work even in a situation where staffing ratios would seem to be low.

It may be useful to draw on other sources of help such as volunteers or handicapped members in the group who are competent at the skill. Sometimes this helping process can be facilitated by sub-dividing a large group into teams, and setting a goal for each team and a prize for achieving the goal. Of course, this situation must be handled carefully but it can be very powerful in releasing capacities for self-help.

6. **You try and get this sort of thing going but you get no support, and in the end you just give up.** Many groups criticise each other for failing to support their new ideas. Parents, nurses, teachers and training centre staff all complain that they start a programme but this it does not get carried on by others, and many staff complain of lack of support from their colleagues, both senior and junior. There is no magical answer to ths, but one key element is to decide, before beginning, who is needed to carry on the work and who can sabotage it successfully. This list can be quite long and may include all sorts of people, not necessarily directly involved, eg supplies or transport officers. Everyone on this list must be consulted and involved before starting out. They need to feel that they have had a say and that the work is 'theirs' to some extent. Without this participative attitude in relation to the handicapped person, good ideas will fail to translate into good practice.

CONCLUSION

Involving people with a mental handicap in sports and physical activities is an exciting and under-developed area. This book highlights how expectations can be shattered and horizons widened by carefully planned determination and ingenuity. In the preceding sections of this chapter only a few general principles which may guide those setting out for the first time have been outlined. Putting these principles into practice requires great flexibility and responsiveness to individual needs, interests and abilities. There are no text-book recipes for action but an enormous reservoir of untapped potential in both those with a mental handicap and those who can help them to a fuller participation in our society.

_____

John Clements is Lecturer in Clinical Psychology, Institute of Psychiatry, London.

Chapter 3

Integration: Two Views

The value of integration is generally recognised, but at the same time, there can be difficulties which make it counter-productive.

This chapter outlines two views which raise many of these issues. They complement each other and give guidance when planning programmes.

THE VIEW OF FRED PARSONS

The preface states that: 'We should give people with a mental handicap the same opportunities to take part in physical activities and outdoor pursuits as the rest of us'. Bearing in mind this statement, the Disabled Persons (Services, Consultation and Representation) Act 1986, and the equal opportunity legislation, it is the right of people with a mental handicap to have access to sporting and recreational activities and facilities.

All sporting pursuits can be enjoyed and contributed to by people with a mental handicap. Sport, by its very nature, is usually competitive, but it is important that participation is achieved before the element of winning or losing is introduced.

Integration should take place in sports centres and educational institutes where the appropriate expertise and equipment is readily available. Access to such establishments can often be a problem, either because the building is physically inaccessible or because of discrimination by the staff who perhaps have little understanding of mental handicap. Integration into a community will only be successful if that community 'receives and accepts'. Difficulties will only be reduced if they are brought to the attention of the people in authority.

With regard to the integration of people who sometimes present anti-social behaviour it is imperative to ensure that enough support is provided to manage the type of behaviour manifested. At a later date other participants in the sport can help to reduce problematic behaviour.

Integration into sports sessions and activities should not mean confrontation. It does, however, mean participation, understanding and co-operation. In addition, the integration must be successful since example teaches, and success breeds success. The way forward is epitomised by the Sports Council's slogan 'Sports for All', including those with a mental handicap.

If adhered to, the following guidelines will encourage integration in sports activities for people with a mental handicap.

Fred Parsons is the former Manager of the Mulberry Adult Centre, London Borough of Lewisham.

The person to be integrated

Consultation with the person hoping to take part must take place from the outset. Integration sometimes fails because the person being integrated has not chosen the activity. A parent or member of staff may have chosen the activity thinking that it 'is good for him'. If the person with a mental handicap finds it difficult to make a choice, someone with understanding should make sure that he or she has the opportunity to experience a range of sports activities so that an informed choice can be made. Virtually everyone can make a decision even if this is based on the display of enjoyment or displeasure.

When considering whether someone should join a specific sports session, concentrate on his abilities, not on his disabilities.

Selecting a sports activity

Apart from consultation, other factors that need to be taken into account are:

that the person has a real and developing interest in the activity;

that the person has the ability to contribute to the activity, game or pursuit;

the necessity for peer support and participant's interaction, i.e. in some sports, team work and team members' roles;

that if the activity is competitive, the integrated person can compete at a level which does not cause humiliation;

that the person providing him with support should also have an interest in the pursuits.

Membership of a group

When trying to integrate someone into an already flourishing group activity, it is important not to flood the class with a large proportion of people with a mental handicap. This is not integration; it is tantamount to taking over a group and can be destructive. Integration should take place, as it does for any other member, in his or her own right, with support if required.

The role of the person providing support

People with a mental handicap need support to help them to integrate. Physical and emotional support can be provided by a brother, sister, voluntary worker or staff member.

The support worker should also have an interest in the chosen activity so that he or she can participate as well. Helping someone to see himself as a member of the group and contributing to the activity is another important aspect, as is the ability to progressively withdraw support as competence and contribution levels increase. A patronising attitude is not what is required.

Public education and preparation of activity leader

Before a programme of integration is begun, all those who will be affected, in particular activity leaders whose support and commitment can be invaluable, should be prepared. They will need to be aware of:

the general aspects of mental handicap and realise that the condition should not lead to alienation;

equal opportunities and discrimination;

the aims and objectives of integration;

the expectations of the person being integrated;

the role of the support worker;

whom to contact if problems are encountered

In addition, all those actively involved will need regular reassurance.

The special class or group

Many special classes or groups of sports activities exist for people with a mental handicap. Those within the Social Education Centres or special schools offer little opportunity for integration to be initiated, apart from an invitation to members of the public to participate. (A more useful first step might be to start using community resources outside the establishment, as other members of society do.)

When a special class or group for people with a mental handicap is created within a community, the sports centre, education institute or community centre should be regarded as a stepping stone to integration, since the aim of these groups should be, in part, to educate the public and to encourage members to enrol into other groups.

THE VIEW OF JOHN BERMINGHAM

All disabilities have one effect in common — they tend to isolate from society the people suffering from them, the degree of isolation depending on the severity of the disability. In the past people with mental handicap tended to be confined in large impersonal institutions — a policy which inevitably led to secondary disabilities in those so institutionalised. Worse still, this policy created a negative and erroneous image of handicapped people. The prejudices engendered by ignorance resulted in further isolation, segregation, rejection and neglect. Since the beginning of this century humanity has made a quantum leap forward in realising that it has obligations to the deprived members of the community. This realisation has resulted in the creation of some form of welfare state in almost all countries.

No longer is it accepted that people with a mental handicap should be excluded from society and swept under the institutional carpet. With intensive and personalised education and training, it has been discovered that handicapped people can achieve a high degree of normal functioning. Previously, they

John Bermingham is Executive Director of the COPE Foundation, Eire, which now specialises in the care of people with a mental handicap throughout the county of Cork.

were regarded as incapable of benefiting by specialised educational methods, with the result that they were left without education or training, which inevitably resulted in retrogressive behaviour and achievement. However, it is now clearly established that the gap between handicapped people and their more able-bodied brothers and sisters can be substantially reduced by special education. Some workers, however, with the new found zeal of the convert, often make sweeping and unrealistic claims that everyone can be integrated. This is not so; there will always be the exceptions; but this does not mean that aspirations should be limited. The application of the term mental handicap to all degrees of disability can cause confusion. Mental handicap is a global term covering all degrees of disability. Irrespective of the degree of handicap the aim must be, without exception, to maximise whatever potential a particular person possesses and to set as an ideal objective the integration of that person into the mainstream community. It must be fully understood that integration is the aim, but that this will not necessarily be achieved. Extensive programmes for the education of people with a mental handicap have been undertaken in most countries but, while academic education has obvious values, the teaching milieu and procedures necessary in the case of people with a mental handicap may differ from those attending ordinary school.

Integration must therefore be thought of in two ways:

- direct integration — where people go out into, and take part in, all community activities — with little or no assistance;

- direct or reverse integration — where the community is persuaded to integrate with handicapped people.

Another fundamentally important point is that integration depends on common or shared interests, eg members of golf clubs, football clubs, bird-watchers, and stamp collectors. All human groupings depend on the shared common interests of their members, and it can readily be appreciated that the development of interests is a *sine qua non* for integration.

The place of physical activities

But what about the place of physical activities in relation to mental handicap? Games, sports and hobbies and other pastimes are, of course, valuable in themselves. Too often the hidden values of physical activities are overlooked or unrealised. Physical activities have enormous value from the point of view of both health and recreation — for handicapped people their *integrative* value is predominant.

In the case of younger or non-handicapped children, games can be tailor made, with a little ingenuity, to teach colours, shapes, sizes, even addition and subtraction. In addition, one of their most valuable aspects is training in integration; this takes place through team games, where co-operation and discipline are demanded.

Many sports can also be used as a vehicle for training people in other aspects of daily living, eg swimming, for which the swimmer must learn to dress and undress, wash and dry himself and comb his hair. Activities such as speech and drama can teach self-confidence and the ability to verbalise, how to react to situations by role playing, while music, song and dance can help to create an atmosphere in which people can integrate.

Outdoor pursuits, in particular, take place in community settings and automatically bring handicapped people out into the open. In addition, with careful planning, a number of club interests and activities can be made available to them.

Unfortunately, the idea of education for people with a mental handicap is too often rooted in the classroom. In the future, to enable them to be fully educated, the whole concept of their education must be totally reviewed; in particular, the place of physical activities as an educational tool must be recognised.

The aura of untouchable sanctity clinging to traditional academic educational methods must be dissipated if integration is to be achieved. All those charged with educating handicapped people must bea r in mind that academic prowess is of no value to them if they fail to integrate with their fellows in the community.

Two major points

Two points of major importance are often overlooked or deliberately ignored:

- some people are so handicapped that they are unable to integrate;

- all handicapped people are not young; integration must not be confined to the young or the mildly handicapped, but must be extended to the old and multi-handicapped.

Too often totally unrealistic sweeping statements are made on the basis of a few exceptional successes; *some* people may be directly integrated into the community, but not *all* can be.

It must also be remembered that bringing handicapped people into contact with the community does not necessarily lead to integration. In order to provide for individuals, who for one reason or another, cannot integrate smoothiy into social activities, it will be necessary to provide special sport and leisure centres.

Such centres should:

1. be set up in an isolated situation;

2. provide a full range of physical and recreational activities, ie running tracks, swimming pool, gymnasium, together with a club-house, bar and restaurant;

3. be open to the public (to provide reverse integration);

4. provide for all ages and degrees of handicap;

5. actively promote direction integration.

It should not be overlooked that handicapped people may feel happier and more at ease with their peers than they would if forced out into the community to fend for themselves or to try to compete in games and sports with those who are not handicapped.

Tendency to over-react

The present reaction against institutions has been so intense that there is a tendency to over-react, not in all cases to the benefit of handicapped people. Perhaps the primary aim should be to consider the happiness of handicapped people, taking care that they are not forced into situations which *others* think suitable and appropriate.

Finally, people with a mental handicap must not be considered an amorphous group. They are all individuals, from the very young to the very old, with their own likes and dislikes. Their responsibilities and needs vary. Each person demands an individual approach and programme.

The development of physical activities for people with a mental handicap represents the biggest single advance in their care and development. As the awareness of their potential for integration increases it may be that in the future, it will be unnecessary to say 'Give us a chance'.

Chapter 4

Teaching and Training Guidelines

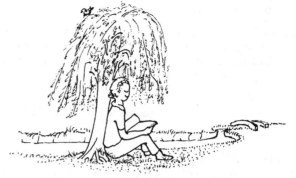

TEACHING GUIDELINES

A teacher/coach in training should, if possible, assist with the coaching of people with a mental handicap particularly of those who are severely/profoundly handicapped in order to become familiar with their problems and the adaptations needed to teach them.

THE TEACHER'S SPECIFIC CONTRIBUTION

1. Keep verbal instructions short and simple. The group will learn through doing rather than listening.

2. A calm controlled voice creates a constructive working relationship. Avoid talking down to the group.

3. The teacher's efficient personal appearance and cheerful facial expression can do much to establish the confidence of those taking part.

4. Choose words carefully and test that instructions have been understood.

5. Rely predominantly on demonstration. Focus attention on what you want the class to look at, eg position of the feet, path of the ball. Be prepared to repeat the demonstration and test the class's understanding of the teaching point made. Demonstration may have to be taken very slowly to focus attention.

6. Reduce each skill to its simplest form so that each individual can achieve some success. Allow plenty of time to learn one skill before progressing to the next.

7. Constantly look for opportunities to praise class members, remembering that effort is as important to encourage as achievement. Create an atmosphere of success.

8. Teacher participation and demonstration are important motivating factors.

9. Discipline must be consistent, firm and clearly understood — 'say what you mean and mean what you say'.

10. Always position yourself where all can see and hear you and where you can see every individual in the group.

11. While thorough preparation of work to be attempted is essential the ability to adapt quickly in response to your observations of their capabilities and motivation is of equal importance.

ORGANISATION AND PRESENTATION

1. All equipment should be ready before the activity starts.

2. Active participation by all may be the ultimate goal, but some will take time to gain confidence and the opportunity to see others enjoying the activity is often a very necessary stage. Even spasmodic participation must be accepted in some circumstances.

3. Involve as many as possible in the preparation and organisation of activities, eg collecting and moving equipment, keeping the score.

4. Practice periods should be short with frequent change of activities to maintain motivation; on the other hand, when success is achieved repeat the activity so that those taking part can experience the joy of accomplishment.

5. Progression is not only measured by making an activity more difficult but also by improved performance, response and memory, eg folk dance sequence (see pp?).

6. Repetition plays a significant part in all stages when teaching people with a mental handicap, eg the importance of routine.

7. Encourage individuals and groups to work at their own variations and adaptations of activities and provide opportunities for them to talk things over with you, eg vary the size of bats and balls or working area, lower the net.

8. Keep rules and adhere to them strictly to ensure good sportsmanship as well as knowing that **they** are also made for the safety and protection of those taking part, eg athletics, swimming, games. Keep up to date with any change in the rules.

9. See that distracting influences are kept to a minimum during the session.

10. A short daily session of physical activity is of greater value than a longer one once a week.

    (NB See Chapter 2 'A Psychologist's View' pp 5-8 for a full discussion of some of the principles involved in teaching and organising physical recreation for people with a mental handicap).

SAFETY

'Nothing venture nothing win', but safety precautions must be taken at all times since some people with a mental handicap seem to have little sense of danger and equally some may suffer from irrational fears. Some safety measures have been included in the main sections of the book; nevertheless, the following points should always be borne in mind when preparing any programme of physical activity and sport.

1. Select the right equipment and ensure its care and maintenance.

2. Try to avoid injury caused by thoughtless organisation, eg running towards glass doors or walls, leaving equipment or

other obstacles 'lying about', playing on uneven, splintery or slippery surfaces.

3. Make sure that suitable and adequate clothing and footwear are worn, eg for indoor work, socks and tights without footwear are always hazardous, but working with bare feet on a clean, non-splintery surface has very specific advantages.

4. Maintain strict discipline and adequate supervision.

5. Choose activities suitable for the group and/or individuals.

6. Have a first aid box. The first aid box need not be a complex one. Most sporting adventures do not result in serious injury. Scratches, abrasions, bruises and occasional cuts are the most frequent types of injury. Anything more serious needs medical attention, The box should include:

   an assortment of bandages, eg 25 mm (1") cotton bandages for fingers, 50mm (2") crepe bandages for sprains and bruises;

   an assortment of different sizes of adhesive of plasters with sterilised dressings to cover cuts and abrasions;

   a roll of cotton wool, useful for padding bruises and sprains and making firm pads to stem bleeding;

   gauze squares 100mm (4") across, for toileting wounds;

   safety pins;

   scissors;

   tweezers for removing splinters;

   a box of tissues;

   plastic incontinence pants;

   sanitary towels - elastic and pins;

   antiseptic cleaning lotion.

TEACHING AIDS

A tape entitled 'Teaching Guidelines' in support of the recommendations in this chapter has been made with illustrations taken from a series of tapes on physical activities with music which are relevant to the presentation of physical activities in general (see Appendix 6).

The series of tapes are listed in the Appendix on page 193.

GUIDELINES FOR TRAINING POTENTIAL TUTORS

Definition of a Tutor

One who prepares 'would-be' teachers/instructors to introduce and to coach physical activities and sport which will be both enjoyable and beneficial to people with a mental handicap.

Who is the tutor?

'Some people are born tutors - others acquire the art'. The tutor may be a person experienced and qualified in training instructors in some aspects of physical education, eg sports, movement and dance, outdoor pursuits.

What makes a successful tutor?

1. An interest in the students (course members) and a knowledge and understanding of people with specific learning difficulties.

2. Being an ongoing learner through study, observation and experience.

3. The ability to

   inspire and help students to train themselves and to enjoy training potential tutors;

   to create a lively group atmosphere where each student can and wants to contribute.

4. The tutor must create the will to learn. She should help students to listen, not just to hear, to see, not just to look, to evaluate, not just to think.

5. Being sensitive to the needs of the potential tutors.

6. She should avoid covering too wide a syllabus - select essentials.

7. Being aware of differing personalities, attitudes and aptitudes and learning the names of students on the course.

Remember:

1. 'I use not only all the brains I have but all I can borrow'.

2. 'No tutor or teacher is ever trained, training is an on-going process'.

3. 'No one can teach anybody anything unless there is a will to learn'.

Points to consider when preparing a syllabus

1. How have the students (potential tutors) been selected - by invitation, from their own choice or in-service requirement?

2. What is the length of the course? How is it divided - eg weekend - sessional - residential?

3. What are the training facilities? The environment should be conducive to learning.

4. Who is responsible for organising the course - business and domestic arrangements, administration, fees and publicity? Those responsible should consult the tutor on syllabus content.

5. What are the aims of the course? These aims should be clearly stated on paper and verbally re-iterated during the first session.

Training guidelines

1. Training should be conducted through practical sessions, talks, discussion groups, tutorials and workshop sessions. Visual/audio aids can be valuable is used wisely.

2. Students learn more by doing than by watching, listening and reading; language and terminology should be as simple as possible; watch the facial expressions of the students: are they confused/bored or intent/relaxed? Aim for the latter.

3. Tutors can generally assess to what degree the students have understood what has been presented to them in group discussion. Equate the time factor with the importance of the issues raised.

4. In any course a client group should be invited to contribute to practical sessions and workshops. Alternatively, arrange to visit a group in it's own environment.

5. Students should be given opportunities for practical work concentrating on training methods.

6. Prepare the content of each session carefully remembering that only so much can be absorbed. Beware of the syndrome or attitude 'I must get through what I've prepared'.

7. The tutor must have courage, confidence and skills in communication in order to be ever ready to adapt the lesson and the method of presentation to any unforeseen changing circumstances.

8. Vary the method or methods of presentation of the course programme with emphasis on the important aspects.

Consider when and how to introduce the following

1. Behavious problems.

2. Use and recruitment of helpers - volunteers.

3. Value of targets - competition, prizes, awards and badges.

4. Safety and precautions - general medical and those relating to physical activities and outdoor pursuits.

5. General knowledge of the resources in the community both statutory and voluntary - see Appendix.

6. The value of 'homework'. Encourage students to make independent visits to activities in an adult training centre or hospital, athletics meetings, swimming galas, Special or Mini Olympics, to increase their awareness of the many opportunities which exist in the community for people with disabilities.

7. Encourage students to make notes (log book), distribute hand-outs when considered appropriate.

8. Emphasise the spin-off value of physical activities in relation to basic education, eg colour recognition, numeracy, verbalisation and social skills.

9. A good tutor should be aware of the differing personalities, attitudes and aptitudes of the students, give encouragement when deserved, avoiding mechanical and meaningless praise.

There is really no 'blue-print' for training tutors. They learn from each other and from their students by listening and seeing and trying out ideas and 'being just human'.

It is never too late to learn!

FURTHER CONSIDERATIONS

1. **Programme.** Offer a varied programme, eg some respond well to physical work with music while others may prefer work with balls. Provision for fitness training should be made, eg jogging, hiking, swimming.

Link sports and physical activities with current sporting events on television, eg World Cup, Olympic Games, 'It's a Knockout', 'Come Dancing'.

2. **Transport.** People with a mental handicap may be denied the opportunity to take part in an activity or even to watch because there is no transport. If public transport is not available or is inappropriate, the provision of transport needs to be considered. In the case of England, Scotland and Wales legislation has given powers for this (see the Chronically Sick and Disabled Persons Act, 1970, section 2, and the Chronically Sick and Disabled Persons (Scotland) Act 1972, section 1).

3. **Integration.** Where their social behaviour is acceptable and they have acquired the necessary skills, individuals with a mental handicap should be encouraged to join with other members of the community to enjoy all sporting activities, particularly those which are non-competitive. It is equally important that members of the general public should realise that some people with a mental handicap are capable of taking part with them in many sports, physical activities and outdoor pursuits (see Snowdon Report: *Integrating the disabled: report of the Snowdon Working Party.* National Fund for Crippling Diseases, Horsham, Sussex, 1976). Remember that people with a mental handicap can only successfully intermingle with the rest of the community if those in the community willingly accept them.

The timing of integration is vital to its success. An unsuccessful attempt at integration is counter-productive. See also Chapter 3.

4. **Resources.** Make the best use of community resources, eg facilities and the people with expertise in sports and physical activities.

5. **Volunteers.** Volunteers can be drawn form many sources, eg parents, friends, voluntary, organisations and students — the volunteers varying in background, experience and age. It is helpful if they can be given some form of advice as to the effective ways of working with people with a mental handicap.

6. **Visual aids.** Make full use of films, film strips, photographs, posters, charts, videotapes and other audio visual materials to reinforce the teacher's expertise. The resourceful teacher can find or improve other aids, eg models, diagrams, blackboard drawings.

7. **Keep up to date.** Continually examine teaching methods and make sure that you keep up to date in your knowledge of people with a mental handicap and the current developments in the world of sport and physical recreation.

COMMUNITY SPORTS LEADERS AWARD SCHEME

In 1974 the Duke of Edinburgh, President of The Central Council of Physical Recreation (CCPR), said: 'The most important people in recreation are the ones who persuade the young to start, to have a go, to try their hand at some form of sport and recreation'.

Bearing these words in mind the CCPR, in conjunction with its member governing bodies, set about developing an award which would provide a quality but low level vocational training, predominantly for volunteers working in sport and recreation with a desire to encourage others to become involved.

Since 1981, when the Community Sports Leaders Award (CSLA) was launched, more than 20,000 people have successfully completed their training. Each participant must complete, as part of his or her training, a minimum of ten hours of supervised voluntary sports leadership. During this time many people have elected to work with disabled people or people with a mental handicap and, upon completing the course, many continue to work in a voluntary capacity.

Both the British Sports Association for the Disabled (BSAD), whose member clubs rely heavily on voluntary assistance, and the United Kingdom Sports Association for People with Mental Handicap (UKSAPMH), have identified the value of the CSLA and have organised courses in conjunction with the CCPR. One strength of the CSLA is that the syllabus is flexible and can be adapted to suit the varying needs of the many organisations it supports.

The success of the CSLA has led to the development of the Higher Award in Community Sports Leadership which will give sports leaders an opportunity to follow their interests not just in sport but in areas of special need.

Two modules of work currently being developed include 'Sport and the Physically Disabled', which has been developed in conjunction with the BSAD, and 'Sport and People with a Mental Handicap', developed in association with the UKSAPMH.

Further modules will include 'Community Dance', 'Sport and the Elderly, 'Sport and Children's Play'. Other Governing Bodies' coaching and leadership awards are in preparation.

The CCPR recognises that if sport and recreation is to succeed in the United Kingdom it must include those who are less able or handicapped. The CSLA Scheme is seen as a means of encouraging greater participation and more effective integration in sport and is available to all people aged 16 years and over, irrespective of their sporting ability.

For further details contact: The Organising Secretary, CCPR Community Sports Leaders Award Scheme, CCPR (see Appendix 2).

SCC's COMMUNITY SPORTS LEADERSHIP COURSES

In 1983 the Scottish Sports Council (SCC) began running Community Sports Leadership Courses at its National Sports Training Centre at Inverclyde, Largs.

The courses provide information on aspects of sports leadership and will be of value to participants whether they come from the professional or voluntary sectors. The participants attending the 1987/88 courses were drawn from several different backgrounds including community education, youth clubs, the YMCA, MSC projects, sports clubs, tenants' associations, and management committees of local facilities.

Although the course at Inverclyde is well established, it represents only an introduction to the highly professional area of leadership in a sporting context. In recent years, a centralised system with a clearly defined vocational orientation has been established by the Scottish Vocational Education Council (SCOTVEC). The SSC considers that this system represents the future for community sports leadership training in Scotland.

16 Plus National Certificate Programme

The SCOTVEC catalogue of modules covers a wide range of disciplines and is extremely comprehensive. The SSC, with SCOTVEC, has designed two levels of community sports leadership modules:

CSL 1 - based on the present SSC theme,
CSL 2 - a more advanced vocationally orientated course which examines key areas in greater depth.

NATIONAL TRAINING ORGANISATIONS

British Sports Association for the Disabled

The British Sports Association for the Disabled (BSAD) has long been recognised as the coordination and development body for sport and physical recreation for people with any disability. BSAD is structured in a similar way to the Sports Council. The National Board is made up of one member from each of its ten Regions and one each from Northern Ireland, Scotland and Wales. There is a Regional Development Officer, and some administrative support, in each region and a small headquarters staff team based in London.

The Association aims to provide opportunities and encouragement for people with any disability to take part in all forms of physical recreation and sport — in a setting, at a level and with a frequency which suits the individual. Through its classification system, BSAD hopes to ensure 'fair' competition on a local, regional, national and international basis for anyone wishing to develop their skills to those levels.

In liaison with the National Governing Bodies of Sport, the National Coaching Foundation, CCPR and the Sports Council it has a development programme that is sports specific. BSAD provides an information service between these bodies and the wide membership. Its strength lies in this regional structure and the ability to bring participative recreation to a broad-based membership, as well as organising championship events in fourteen sports for those members.

Details of the regional offices and information service can be obtained from the headquarters in London: British Sports Association for the Disabled (see Appendix 2).

Central Council of Physical Recreation

The Central Council of Physical Recreation (CCPR) is an independent voluntary organisation comprising about 240 national governing bodies of sport and physical recreation, embracing major spectator sports, outdoor pursuits, water recreation, movement and dance and other specialist bodies from many areas of activity including of course those working in the field of disability.

Although it is not a charity itself, the CCPR has a charitable arm known as the Colson Fellowship Fund, which aims to provide bursaries and scholarships for young handicapped people who wish to take part in sport and recreation.

The highly successful Community Sports Leaders Award, (see above), which trained more than 25,000 sports leaders between 1982 and 1987 and continues to grow in popularity, is considered by the CCPR to be vital to the development of sport at 'grass roots' level and also to promote recreation among those who do not readily participate. Many sports leaders are making a valuable contribution to the lives of the disabled and handicapped and demand from them was instrumental to the development of the Higher Award in Community Sports Leadership which it is hoped will be launched soon. This Award gives sports leaders an opportunity to develop not only their interest in sport but also an opportunity to train and work in areas of special need.

At the Annual General Meeting of the CCPR in June 1988, Prince Philip said, 'I'm all for gold medals but the main priority is to get more people involved in sport, gold medals are the icing on the cake, but they are not the fruit of the business'.

The CCPR believes that all people, irrespective of their ability or disability, should be given an opportunity to enjoy the 'fruit' of sport.

Further information can be obtained from CCPR (see Appendix 2).

English National Board For Nursing, Midwifery and Health Visiting

The DLF and the English National Board (ENB) work together to support tutors who have responsibility for the training of nurses. Following a pilot one-day seminar provided specifically for tutors in the Midlands, plans are now in hand for similar seminars to be held in the north west, north east, south west and south east of England. These seminars, which receive support from UKSAPMH (see below), all stress the development approach and indicate ways in which this work can be integrated into the 1983 syllabus which is being followed by schools of nursing. Wherever it is appropriate this support is readily extended to tutors responsible for the professional training of other staff working with people who have a mental handicap.

National Coaching Foundation

The National Coaching Foundation (NCF) provides a service for anyone wishing to coach, whatever their sport or level of experience. The programmes are designed to supplement and complement the existing National Governing Body schemes and focus on the human aspects of performance rather than on technical competence. There are books, videos, courses and information covering a wide range of topics including coaching/teaching method, safety, fitness and nutrition. The various study units are at four different levels, thus allowing each person to select his/her own programme. Fourteen National Coaching Centres have been established around Britain to provide a network of resource centres at local level. The Foundation believes that with well informed leaders, teachers and coaches, sport can be an exciting and rewarding experience for everyone.

For further details contact: NCF, 4 College Close, Beckett Park, Leeds LS6 3QH.

United Kingdom Sports Association for People with Mental Handicap (UKSAPMH)

UKSAPMH was established in 1979 to act as the co-ordinating body for sport and people with a mental handicap. It also promotes and develops sport and physical activities among the many organisations, both statutory and voluntary, involved in working with people with a mental handicap. The Association is a membership organisation, nationally its members include Gateway, Royal Society MENCAP, Mini Olympics, Special Olympics, the Spastics Society, the British Institute of Mental Handicap and the DLF. Representatives from the DHSS, DOE, DES, the Sports Council and the British Sports Association for the Disabled are actively involved.

The UKSAPMH provides a forum for its members to share information and to discuss areas of need. Individual members have their own programme of events and activities, but collectively stage events as is necessary. Recently, all members worked together towards a Four Nation's Swimming and Athletics Event. For the first time competitors represented their country having undergone a national selection process. A need shared by all members is that of training at all levels. The strength of the UKSAPMH as a co-ordinating body has allowed progress to be made through discussions with other training agencies, the Governing Bodies of Sport and the Central Council of Physical Recreation to develop and implement a wide programme of training courses. Another success of the UKSAPMH has been National Training Conference — a residential weekend offering a wide range activities in practical workshops. The Association hopes to expand the training opportunities available.

The Association is not just a national organisation. Based on the regions of the Sports Council, it has ten Regional and three Home County Associations. Each has its own membership which reflects the national organisation, and promotes a wide range of activities such as 'Come and Try It' festivals, regional sports championships, and coaching and training courses.

Further details about the work of UKSAPMH, both nationally and regionally, or any of the Association's member organisations can be obtained from: The National Officer, UKSAPMH (see Appendix 2).

FURTHER INFORMATION

Information on training courses for those teaching people with a mental handicap can be obtained from: The British Institute of Mental Handicap, Wolverhampton Road, Kidderminster, Worcestershire DY10 3PP, and Castle Priory College, Thames Street, Wallingford, Oxon OX10 OHE. Castle Priory is the Spastics Society's Training College.

For information on dance leaders' training see p. 117.

Training for Special Olympic and Mini Olympic events are arranged by Special Olympics UK and by Mini Olympics in co-operation with the governing bodies of sport.

FURTHER READING

Playtrac. *The Playtrac Handbook*. Playtrac, c/o Harperbury Hospital, Harper Lane, Radlett, Herts WD7 9HW, 1987.

UKSAMPH. *Coaching people with mental handicap*. Leeds, National Coaching Foundation, 1989.

Chapter 5

How to Choose an Activity

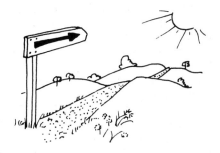

This book provides ideas on how to introduce physical activities and sport into the lives of people with a mental handicap. Whether these ideas are effective or not depends to a great extent on whether the teacher is sensitive to the needs of individuals and to the community in which the work is being done. A good activity can be successfully introduced in one situation, yet fail in another.

Being aware of the varying needs of people with a mental handicap will help the teacher to make a wise choice of activity (see Chapter 1, pp 1-4).

1. DEGREE OF PHYSICAL FITNESS

A group consisting of people with multiple handicaps may have to sit for most of the day. For these, non-weight bearing activities must be provided for body movement (see People with a severe mental handicap below). Others may be ambulant and perhaps over-protected. These would need a more active programme, eg fitness training (see pp 102-107), games (see Chapter 7) or swimming (see Chapter 9).

2. PLAY

Play is essential in the life of the child; through it he learns. In many instances play becomes recreation in adult life. Severely multiply handicapped adults may have missed many of the experiences play can provide and developmentally they may still need 'to play'. A teacher faced with this situation might consider using:

(i)   an adventure playground (see Chapter 17)

(ii) a soft play area (see p 143)

(iii) a good floor for movement activities (see p 18).

Having analysed the needs of the group and having found several suitable activities, the teacher must be practical and relate the choice to the facilities available.

3. MOVEMENT IS A LANGUAGE

Many adults with a mental handicap have severe problems of communication and have difficulty in relating to other people. Activities that involve some physical contact can help to build up relationships between themselves and the teacher and with each other. See, for example:

(i)   Veronica Sherborne's approach to movement (see p 94)

(ii) folk dancing (see p 116)

(iii) Jasmine Pasch's approach (see p 113)

(iv) Morris dancing (see p 137).

4. MOTOR SKILLS

Since these are less dependent on intelligence than many other activities, success which helps to build up confidence can be developed through the learning of specific skills:

(i)   ball skills (see pp 25-31)

(ii) swimming (see Chapter 9)

(iii) gymnastics (see p 63).

(iv) riding (see Chapter 16).

5. OPPORTUNITIES FOR INTEGRATION

To establish the confidence of those coming to help (eg parents, friends, students, coaches) is as important a consideration as the needs of the handicapped people. Dancing is excellent for all ages (see Chapter 13). If the helpers are young it might be:

(i)   games (see Chapter 7)

(ii) gymnastics (see pp 63 and 104)

(iii) swimming (see Chapter 9)

(iv) athletics (see Chapter 8)

(v)   outdoor pursuits (see Chapter 15).

The facilities available are crucial in choosing the activity (see p 175).

6. HELPERS

The leader needs to relate activities chosen to a number of helpers that are available. When many helpers are available new experiences can be given to a client that would be impractical in other situations. Clients will get satisfaction from working with a helper before they need to co-operate with another client as a partner. (See Aides and volunteers p 139).

7. IMPORTANCE OF GROUP MOTIVATION

When summer holidays are a topic of conversation and the weather is good, an interest in camping and other outdoor activities could be encouraging for the more able (see p 144).

8. AGE OF THOSE TAKING PART

This is an important consideration especially if many are elderly. Activities in which music is used could provide the greatest encouragement for these (see p 97).

9. PEOPLE WITH A SEVERE MENTAL HANDICAP

Staff dealing with people with a severe mental handicap should not be 'put off' by the amount of material in this book which obviously relates to the more able.

While most people with a severe mental handicap will never aspire to many of the games, sports and leisure activities described, the text contains a fund of suitable ideas for such people (see **Mental handicap, severe**, in the Index). Any purposeful physical activity often seems to act as a stimulant to mental activity, and may itself be stimulated by the use of music or simple brightly coloured and interesting apparatus.

A first activity could be clapping in time to music — the rhythm being changed frequently in order to maintain interest and prevent a mechanical response. This may be expanded by alternate touching of some part of the body, such as 'Clap — touch head; clap — touch toes' etc. Such simple exercises can be undertaken with those who are also confined to bed or chair.

Adherence to a rhythm provides a kind of discipline which tends to promote more purposeful movements that might otherwise be achieved.

Equipment for people with a very severe mental handicap must be extremely simple: complicated apparatus only leads to confusion. Activities using bean bags, balls of various sizes, hoops, ropes, parachutes and ribbons encourage maximum effort.

Bouncing and catching movements are fairly easy to encourage but throwing creates problems — 'letting go' the ball at the optimum point of the arm swing being the main one. A forceful arm swing is often produced, then — to the player's surprise — he finds he is still holding the ball. With practice this difficulty can be overcome; the aiming practice games described in Chapter 6 (see pp.42-45) could be helpful.

The bold entries in the index should provide ideas for a basic programme of activities from which it may be possible to lead on to more complicated exercises as improvement takes place. Appropriate material must be selected according to individual circumstances and potential. Other activities not specifically picked out in the index need not necessarily be precluded.

(See also Chapter 14, 'Physical activities for people with severe or profound mental handicap').

10. COMMUNITY LIFE

Establishments need to develop their own community life. Carefully chosen physical activities play an important part, eg:

(i) dancing (see Chapter 13)

(ii) 'It's a Knockout' (see pp 84-88)

(iii) potted sports (see pp 80-83).

(iv) Superstars (see pp 88-93)

(v) outdoor pursuits (see pp 144-162).

11. CONTACT WITH NEIGHBOURING ESTABLISHEMENTS

Such contact is not only stimulating for handicapped people but also for the staff. Carefully selected physical activities shared with others can be instrumental in 'building bridges' over a period of time, eg

(i) a shared gymnastic club;

(ii) a folk dance club.

(iii) outdoor pursuits.

Annual events such as a dance evening or a sports day can also play their part in establishing contact with other organisations. This is also a way in which good facilities and teachers can be shared. To create and maintain lines of communication and chose liaison with the health and social services, education and recreation and leisure departments of the local authority is vital.

12. FACILITIES

This book introduces teachers to many activities. It should enable them to select a sport or activity relevant to the facilities. Some need generous indoor or outdoor space, some are dependent on a good floor surface, while others can be practised on a fairly indifferent surface.

A resourceful teacher should be able to introduce some type of physical activity into the programme of residents and trainees even where facilities are comparatively poor, provided the establishment gives the necessary support. As progress is made so further consideration would need to be given to improving facilities (see p 175).

13. SPECTATORS

The interest of the more severely handicapped people in sport and physical activities will mainly consist of watching others, although they should be continuously encouraged to 'move' and to share in some of the experiences, such as riding (if only in a pony trap), kite flying or swimming. The 'watching' can be made more worthwhile by simple explanation and by ensuring an uninterrupted view.

For some spectators 'watching' may be the first stage in gaining confidence to take part, but there will probably be a wide variation in the length of time they take to become involved. The teacher's sensitive reacting to this unpredictable situation is all important if further progress is to be made. It can be useful if a note is made when someone joins in if only for a brief period of time.

Spectators at out-of-door events can become very cold, particularly if they are severely handicapped and the weather is cold and wet. Warm clothing should be worn including wheelchair mackintoshes and body and foot muffs when necessary. Spectators should be encouraged to sit or stand in as sheltered a place as possible.

If people with a mental handicap have the opportunity to watch sporting events on TV, some explanation of the activity being shown by parents or teachers will be invaluable.

Chapter 6

Landscape for Sport, Physical Recreation and Play

Peter R Thoday

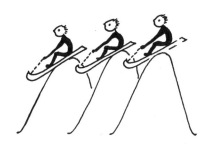

The grounds of schools, day and residential establishments for people with a mental handicap are very often examples of institutional landscapes which, unlike public open spaces, offer a rich opportunity to design specifically for a known group of people.The provision of open air facilities for sport, physical recreation and play should be an essential requirement of any design as it reflects the establishment's imaginative and supportive role in the life of people with a mental handicap.

In addition, sites of suitable size may well offer opportunities to establish road safety training areas, gardening activities, pet keeping projects and such imaginative features as adventure play sites, camp sites, barbecue and picnic areas, quiet gardens and 'wilderness'. Although such items are space demanding, imaginative people have established them in surprisingly small grounds often with little upheaval to an existing design; in fact, run-down Victorian gardens are often excellent starting points.

Few establishments will have ideal sites for every type of outdoor activity but some of the most successful facilities have been developed as a result of drive and initiative in what appeared to be very unpromising locations. If however, no space is available near the building, a weekly trip to a nearby park or playing area can be arranged.

The various sites discussed below are intended to serve the major recreational activities which, in turn, stimulate different group and individual reactions and place different organisational and managerial demands upon the staff.

Anyone siting these activities should bear in mind their accessibility and distance from domestic facilities particularly toilets and stores although the noise generated by a group at play can be disturbing both within and beyond the institution.

Convenient storage is a very important consideration as a 'long haul with the gear' is often the final deterrent or excuse for the faint-hearted. In addition, the safety of the participants must be considered particularly the risk of running on to vehicular roads in moments of excitement. Nearby windows will also be at risk as there will inevitably be the occasional wild throw or kick. Finally, the ease with which such sites can be supervised and maintained must be considered and maximum use should be made of any existing landscape features.

Open air recreational sites are considered here under three headings: 3 sports pitches, 2 tracks and 8 informal play areas.

SPORTS PITCHES

The construction and maintenance of high grade sports pitches, courts and tracks is a specialist subject; the skilled and qualified groundsmen concerned are well supplied with technical literature relating to the needs and problems of supplying outdoor playing surfaces all the year round.

Further useful information is produced by the grass seed companies, the agricultural chemical industry, sports field construction companies, the Sports Council and the Sports Turf Research Institute.

In spite of such an array of technical data, many establishments are faced with adapting old grounds themselves, and the following general advice may be useful.

Most sports demand a pitch of a certain shape and/or size; it must usually be level or near level and have a reasonably true and smooth surface. These common requirements do not demand that the pitch be set in a rigid angular site. The somewhat harsh geometric features of sports pitches can be far more successfully integrated into surrounding leisure grounds if they are marked out from within a larger informal shape. This policy also has the great merit that it ensures that space for spectators is provided.

Pitch marking is a chore; one imaginative aid is to permanently mark out all corner points, etc., by sinking large nails or short metal bars safely below the surface and locating them when required by means of a metal detector. In practice this technique proves to be very straightforward and saves a great deal of time at the beginning of each 'season'.

Sports surfaces are all prone to wear. A grass turf which is cheap to establish and delightful to look at when in good condition must be respected as a living sheet of vegetation; over use, particularly under harsh weather conditions, inevitably results in fundamental, long term problems. The degree of damage varies with the season and is greatly influenced by the weather. Much of the current work on grass type selection, land drainage, the use of fertilisers, irrigation, mowing, and aeration has helped schools and public authorities to increase the use of their pitches. The current literature contains some very useful hints on these topics. Tough hard wearing alternatives to grass have been developed: broadly speaking they are of three types, the bound mineral type, polymer bonded materials and 'plastic grass'. These materials can produce surfaces of excellent quality but they are very expensive to install and are by no means maintenance free. The general public often refer to them as 'all weather' pitches but this claim is rarely made by responsible manufacturers. Small courts with synthetic surfaces have been built are a few caring institutions but asphalt remains by far the most common hard alternative to grass. When carefully laid it can produce a tolerably safe and very hard wearing surface. Concrete is a far more 'vicious' material and should not be used.

TRACKS

Play features such as nature trails, trim tracks, follow-my-leader play — the list of linear or path activities has increased considerably in recent years — are best constructed within, or, more accurately, between existing mature features, since part of their appeal is the visual separation of the 'stations'. Track designers should try to convey the feeling of a journey with a clear start and finish as this encourages participants to keep going to the end. The details of each station will undoubtedly be different but the common basic requirement is for a clear linking path, not necessarily of the same surfacing material throughout. The stations must have ample space for their particluar activity or, where appropriate, house a prominent marker post; they must all have a clear way marker indicating the continuation of the track. Tracks offer the opportunity to use the landscape to provide **attainable** challenges combining physical obstacles with tests of initiative and independence (see p. 106).

INFORMAL PLAY AREAS

These multi-purpose sites serve as everything from kick-about areas to the open air venue for organised games, social events and dance.

The landscape demanded by these activities is far less precise in both size and form than that required by 'formall' sports. Indeed, in contrast to the sports field, there are considerable advantages in developing an informal play site within mature grounds, as slopes, banks, robust trees and shrub masses can add greatly to the range of activities.

Such informal designs are ideal for the 'back gardens' of community homes which are currently replacing institutional accommodation.

The first requirement is for a reasonably level, well drained area of tough turf or hard surface which is free from obstacles. The strongest argument in support of any necesary redesign — the removal of intruding paths, flower beds, shrubs and small trees etc — is to remind objectors that the grounds are an integral part of the caring institution.

The features and the planting that surround the play area must be robust; inevitably people and play equipment stray, and tough shrubs like *Symphoricarpus* 'Hancock' and ground cover such as *Hypericum calycinum* will survive the occasional wanderer while a regiment of tulips will not.

When the site is used for ball games a lot of time can be saved if a retrieval net, possibly in combination with grass banks, is used. Many types of cheap twine and plastic garden net are now obtainable, and are preferable to the cage-like appearance of wire netting or chain link fencing. Temporary nets can be removed when not in use but , if they are to be succesful, they must be easy to assemble and quick to dismantle. Uprights should be designed to slip into permanent sockets and any horizontal cross peices can be linked by the simple devices sold in garden shops for the construction of fruit cages.

If possible, informal play areas should be within reach of mains electricity and water, for special occasions a long length of heavy duty garden hose fitted with a shut off nozzle and a similar length of high quality extension lead with outdoor fittings will suffice, although of course these items require an outdoor tap and a weatherproof socket — facilities which are often absent. It is also important to know how temporary services are going to reach the play area: preferably they should be 'round the back' so that they are out of harms way and cannot trip anybody up.

Such services provide the opportunity for special events, for example music, lights, paddling pools and play fountains.

Permanent water features, no matter how shallow, are not acceptable to some caring authorities while others take great pride in showing off their pools and fish ponds. There is much to be said for **temporary** water which can be made a special play feature in very hot weather. Sand pits and deliberately constructed hollows in the grass can be turned into shallow pools by simply spreading out and flooding a sheet of 500-1000 gauge plastic or, better still, butyl rubber; a spray jet on a hose pipe is all that is necessary to complete some very wet entertainment for suitably clad youngsters. There are a number of play fountain designs which produce either fine spray or foaming water. The water returns below ground level without an exposed basin. These are extremely safe and provide a great deal of pleasure.

The basic movements of running, swinging climbing, sliding and see-sawing can be set into verdant backgrounds, a point often made by the adventure play movement. Both traditional and adventure play use fixed equipment, but the visual impact, interest and safety of such equipment varies enormously. There is little doubt that on all three counts some of the best designs currently available come from Scandinavia, Holland and Germany. However, the most recent British designs show a great improvement. The range is frequently reviewed in landscape architecture journals which also carry trade advertisements.

Unfortunately, fixed play equipment ofter looks as if it has been 'dumped' in the middle of a ten acre field, but it is best to avoid exposed open sites, and shrub screens and shade trees are valuable as they help to tie the apparatus into the landscape. On the other hand small strips and patches of turf easily become mud; they should be dispensed with as they are expensive and awkward to maintain. All fixed equipment should be securely and safely anchored with no exposed footings or protruding bolts; their surrounds should be well drained, mud free and soft enough to cushion accidental falls.

In most European countries fixed equipment is set within loose sand or bark chips such as that marketed as Cambark. If these are inappropriate, fexible tiles may be used. Slides are often built into the side of a play mound while sand pits can be integrated into the landscape by simply constructing them rather like golf bunkers within turf. Alternatively, they are sometimes bounded by a low palisade of vertical logs.

FURTHER READING

Bengtsson, A. *Environmental planning for children's play.* St Albans, Crosby Lockwood, 1972.

Playing fields and hard surface areas. Department of Education and Science. Building Bulletin 28, 1966.

Thoday, P R. *Hospital grounds utilisation.* University of Bath, 1974.

Rowson, N J and Thoday, P R. *Landscape design for disabled people in public open spaces.* University of Bath, 1985.

Thoday, P R, Rowson, J J and Skinner, P. *Landscape in care.* University of Bath, 1983.

Peter Thoday is Senior Lecturer in the Amenity Horticulture School of Biological Sciences, University of Bath.

Chapter 7

Games and Sports

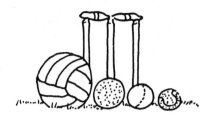

Planning a games session — Adaptations — Scoring — The teaching of skills — Activities using hoops, ropes balls, beanbags and quoits — Uniplay Games Award Scheme — Activities using improvised equipment — Forms of tag — Team races — Team races using various formations and equipment — Group games without equipment — Easy games in circle formation — Fun games without equipment — More difficult games — Skills leading up to minor and major games — Examples of minor games — Games with a difference — Contact sports — Gymnastics.

Practically all the major games and sports can be played with success by some people with a mental handicap, provided the required skills are sufficiently mastered and the appropriate adaptations are made. It is important for the teacher to know the up-to-date rules of any game and sport that is to be taught, since the ultimate aim is to play the game to the official rules, However, players with a mental handicap should never be thrust into an activity or game before they are ready for it - ready mentally as well as physically, socially and emotionally.

The following is a list of games and sports which are played to a greater or lesser degree in adult training centres and/or hospitals and clubs (the list is increasing yearly):

archery	netball
association football	petanque
athletics	quoits
badminton	racket ball
bagatelle	roller skating
batington	rounders
basket ball	rowing
billiards	rugger
boccia	short tennis
bowls	skiing
cricket	snooker
croquet	squash rackets
darts	swimming
frisbee	table tennis
fencing	table skittles
fives	tennis
golf	ten pin bowling
gymnastics	trampolining
handball	tug-of-war
hockey	uniboule
ice skating	unihoc
indoor bowls	unishuffle
jogging	volley ball
judo	weight lifting
karate	weight training
karting	yoga
lacrosse and pop lacrosse	
lawn tennis	
model flying	

Some games and sports require only one or two participants, eg badminton, bowls, table tennis, archery, skating. Since these can become leisure pursuits throughout life, opportunities to play some of these should be encouraged.

Games and sports can be played:

as a session devoted to games;

as recreation in a lunch hour;

at camps and holidays;

at sports leisure centres;

at parties and social evenings;

at sports meetings and tournaments (see Chapter 9);

as an item in displays of physical activity.

National games and sports have not been included. The national governing body of each sport will provide the current rules, coaching manuals, films and charts (see Appendix 3).

The following games and variations are included in some detail because they are less well known but are enjoyed enormously and can be played by people with a wide variety of abilities: batington, petanque, unihoc, play with boomerangs and frisbees, skittles, boccia, unicurl and short tennis.

Games and sports are valuable because they:

1. train dexterity and co-ordination particularly of eye and hand

2. develop the necessary skills which serve as training for all games and sports such as football, netball, unihoc, athletics, badminton, bowls

3. channel excess energy into purposeful skills and provide and outlet for repressed emotions

4. stimulate the less active to move

5. help to develop alertness, perseverance, self-control, optimism, courage and confidence

6. increase the will and the ability to play to the rules, to be a good loser and to co-operate with others

7. create opportunities for competition of varying types

8. give the players responsibilities, eg helping with the organisation and care of equipment, leading a team, training them to take care of their own personal sportswear. (See also Chapter 1, p. 3 and p. 176).

Before planning a games session consider:

1. the physical and mental abilities, likes and dislikes and the difficulties of the group of players;

2. the facilities — indoor and outdoor — the size and type of the surface and the nature of the playing space;

3. what equipment is available, is it safe and in good repair?

4. any hazards, eg low ceiling lights, glass windows; unstacked chairs and out-of-doors obstructions such as trees, posts and broken glass;

5. the play area and the markings within it — the dimensions will naturally influence the number of players taking part and the type of equipment being used;

6. the playing area must be contained and be clear of obstacles if ballgames are to be played, If the ball is lost under obstacles, the game stops and the aim of continuous activity is defeated.

PLANNING A GAMES SESSION

A games session will only prove successful if it is carefully prepared and presented. The number of practices and games will depend on the length of the period and on the number and ability of the players. The presentation will, of course, need to be adapted to the ability and mood of the class.

Select activities, practices and games which provide activity for:

1. everyone rather than those in which the majority of players are quickly 'put out';

2. the less able players.

Organisation (See Teaching and training guidelines p 12).

1. Make sure that equipment is available.

2. Make any floor markings before the session starts (players may well be able to help).

3. Mark the boundaries of the playing space clearly. If it is smaller than the whole space — by chalk lines, 'masking' tape or rope, benches, chairs (even skittles can be used, providing they are sturdy and do not create a hazard).

Suggested plan

A session of half an hour to one hour working time should include:

1. a warming-up activity with or without apparatus (individually with a partner or in small group) (see below and p. 95);

2. one or more skill practices (see pp 23-31);

3. a team race, a group, a minor or a major game.

Presentation (See Teaching and training guidelines p 12)

Game-like activities and games are an important part of the whole programme of recreation. The following are further suggestions to remember when preparing a games session:

1. know how to play the game yourself in order to demonstrate and coach effectively;

2. it is better to start with a small group of 'would be' enthusiasts who, through their enjoyment, naturally encourage others to join in;

3. decide the least numbers of skills the players need to know before they can take part in the game or a modified form of it;

4. practise these skills individually, in pairs or group activities, then 'have a go' at the game;

5. teach the players to understand the meaning of and obey the whistle or the word 'stop';

6. be firm in enforcing the rules and encourage the players to accept the referee's decision with good grace;

7. collect a variety of game-like activities and simple games which can be used in unexpected circumstances;

8. remember the less skilled who are unable or incapable of playing the more complicated team games; modified games, or games invented by yourself, can be successful for these players;

9. introduce one game or one skill at a time.

Adaptations

Adaptation is often necessary. Here are some examples:

1. substitute walking or running;

2. substitute equipment of different size and weight;

3. adapt equipment, eg shorten handle of badminton racquet;

4. reduce or increase the size of the playing area;

5. restrict players to definite zones;

6. hit the ball on the second bounce;

7. allow players to hold the ball for a longer period;

8. use a bounce, roll or underarm throw to replace an overarm throw;

9. simplify scoring.

SCORING

1. 'Beat your own standard' method - useful when practising simple activities, eg increase the distance or height of a throw.

2. Count the number of goals, eg football; points, eg table tennis; games, eg tennis; runs, eg cricket.

3. Count 1 point for achieving a part of a complete rounder, eg in rounders or Danish rounders: 1 point for reaching 2nd base, 2 points for reaching 3rd base, 3 points for reaching 4th base, 4 points for a rounder - without being out.

Only adapt the scoring when necessary, eg badminton, volleyball and lawn tennis scoring can be difficult to understand; a simplified method such as the points system in table tennis might be used at first. It is essential that the players understand the method of scoring at every stage.

WARMING UP

It is vitally important that the body is warmed up and prepared for more vigorous activities — games and sports.

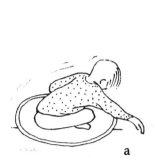 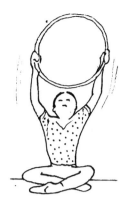 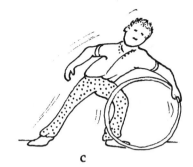

Figure 7.1 Activities using hoops

Different ways of achieving this are:

1. easy jogging;

2. general body exercises (see pp 95-97);

3. carefully selected games of tag (see p 33);

4. activities using various equipment — practised individually or in pairs.

The warming-up period should be short and at the beginning of any games session; it should start easily, building up to more vigorous movement, eg before going outside to play football or netball, a short warm-up session might be taken in the hall/gym.

THE TEACHING OF SKILLS

First and foremost, players must be taught to play with, for example, balls bats and hoops of different sizes, weights and types, so that they feel at ease with them. By degrees the skills of throwing, catching, kicking, fielding, intercepting, dodging, aiming and hitting - which are common to all games - can be introduced. These skills are based on certain fundamentals learnt largely through experience, practising and playing, and once reasonably well mastered, players will be able to grasp new games more quickly. Sometimes, at an earlier stage, it is advisable to play the games with the least possible number of rules.

When practising players can work individually, in twos or small groups. As the fundamentals of the various techniques and skills are understood and mastered, competition can be introduced on an individual, partner or team basis. The teacher, by experimenting with such apparatus as beach-balls, balloons, old shuttle-cocks, beanbags, quoits and improvised apparatus, and later balls and bats, can discover many enjoyable and interesting ways of using them, thereby inventing an endless variety of activities. Often the players themselves will offer ideas.

ACTIVITIES USING HOOPS, ROPES, BALLS, BEANBAGS AND QUOITS

1. Sit in the hoop with one part of the body touching the floor outside it, eg foot – elbow; change to another part, eg hand, knee (Fig 7.1a).

2. Sit outside the hoop with one or more parts of the body touching the floor inside it.

3. Hold the hoop up like a mirror 'look through'. Repeat holding the hoop high – move it high, low and side to side (Fig 7.1b).

4. Sit with hoop on the floor in front, touch the hoop in different places, one hand, then the other, then alternately – make the touch light, touch near, touch the far side.

   Variations: (i) clap after each tap – touch and clap – clap high; **(ii)** move hoop further away and to one side, then the other. Stretch as much as possible in all directions.

5. Stand with the hoop on the floor. Step in and out of the hoop in different directions, Right in, left in - left out, right out — forwards sideways and backwards.

   Variation: jump with and without a rebound — hop in and out of hoop.

6. Stand with feet apart, hoop in front, one edge resting on the floor, hold the hoop loosely with both hands on top — 15 - 22.5 cm (6-9") — apart. Roll the hoop from side to side keeping hold of it, gradually increase the movement — rolling it from one hand to the other and swaying from foot to foot (Fig 7.1c).

7. Bowl the hoop, keeping close to it.

8. Bowl the hoop forwards — move to catch it before it drops.

   Variation: roll the hoop to a partner who catches it and rolls it back.

9. Stand, spin the hoop, let it nearly 'die', then pick it up.

   Variation: spin the hoop, run to a line or run round the hoop, catch it before it drops.

With partners

10. Stand with feet apart, one hoop between two partners facing each other, holding the hoop loosely with both hands at waist level (hoop parallel to the floor). Swing the hoop from side to side letting the body weight sway from foot to foot (easy knees) — gradually increase the width and height of the swing.

    Variation: look through the hoop as it swings high — develop it into a 'pancake turn'.

11. One partner holds the hoop at right angles to the floor; the other partner gets through the hoop without touching it; change over.

    Variation: one partner holds the hoop parallel to the floor between knee and hip height, other partner gets through by stepping over the hoop — curling up and coming out from underneath; repeat from underneath coming out over the top; change over.

12. Spread hoops out on the floor — use the hoops as stepping stones — step from hoop to hoop, leap from hoop to hoop. Many other ways of using hoops will be discovered. Hoops, beanbags or balls can be used together bouncing and throwing through a hoop from varying distances, in pairs or threes — one holding the hoop when necessary.

Long ropes — 6-8m (20-26') long

Two ropes stretched across room, held at knee height (hold the ropes lightly).

1. Two or three at a time step forward over the rope, moving on to next rope; repeat, turn and run back to place.

2. Step sideways over the rope and back again and over again, along the rope - move on to the next rope.

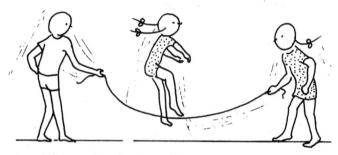

Figure 7.2 Activities using ropes

3. Rope on the floor, spring over it; gradually raise the height.

4. Swing rope from side to side, jump over low swinging rope. Jump as the rope swings towards you (Fig.7.2).

5. Hold ropes at hip height, move forwards under the first rope and sideways under the second. Move under the rope with a turn or backwards. Try not to touch the rope. Gradually increase the speed.

6. As (5) in pairs, one guiding the other with a twist — one moving forwards the other moving backwards. Vary the speed.

7. Turn the ropes in unison slowly and quickly.

8. One rope turned across the centre of the room, with the rope turning towards them, the players run under the turning rope — one at a time at first, later two at the same time.

   Progress to 'keeping the pot boiling'.

   Progress to skipping.

   Remember to change the 'rope turners'.

Skipping individually

9. People with a mental handicap can learn to skip individually. Skipping ropes should be long enough to touch the ankles when the arms are fully stretched sideways.(Fig 7.3a). If handles are available, they should have ball bearings to allow the rope to turn freely without twisting - if ropes are provided without handles, then the ends should be bound. Practise -

   (i) skipping on the spot with a rebound;

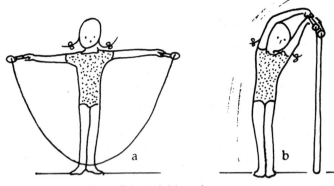

Figure 7.3 Activities using ropes

   (ii) skipping on the spot without a rebound;

   (iii) combine (i) and (ii) 4 skips with a rebound followed by 8 skips without a rebound;

   (iv) skip moving forwards and backwards;

   (v) stand, turn the rope overhead to one side followed by the other (Fig 7.3b).

   Rope turn 4 turns on left, 4 on right. Rope turn 2 turns on left, 2 turns on right. Alternate turns left, right, left, right.

Dance steps, eg, polka, step and hop, pas de basques, can all be performed in a skipping rope. The rope can be turned either forwards or backwards, (practise both). To change from backwards to forwards skipping, practise 7 skips with a rebound, 'check' the rope by dropping the handles downwards. This checks the rope in front as the 8th skip is performed. The next 7 skips are then performed with the rope turning forwards, check the rope on 8 and skip backwards again.

Skipping with short or long ropes

10. Two turning — 1 skipping; using skipping rhymes. Here are some examples:

   (i) I am (Edward) dressed in (blue)
       These are the things he can do,
       Clap his hands, touch his toes,
       Skip one more and out he goes.
       Increase the number of skips 2 - 3 - 4 etc.

   (ii) Sally's in the garden,
        Doing some skipping
        Along comes Peter,
        And out goes Sally.
        (Use individual skipper's names when possible.)

   (iii) Two little sausages frying in a pan,
         one went pop (clap) and one went bang.
         (Jump with feet astride the rope.)

   (iv) House to let
        Apply within
        When you go out
        I come in.

   (v) Keep the kettle boiling *(running under a turning rope)*
       Miss the beat - you're out
       next in.

   (vi) All in together
        This fine weather
        When it's your birthday please jump out,

January, February, March, April, May .etc.
(Skipper runs out when the birthday month is called.)

(vii) Using 'name of person skipping' twice to give two skips between each action.
Rosemary, Rosemary touch the ground
Rosemary, Rosemary turn right round,
Rosemary, Rosemary climb upstairs,
Rosemary, Rosemary say your prayers.
Rosemary, Rosemary switch out the light,
Rosemary, Rosemary say goodnight.
Run out.
(Many other actions could be substituted.)

(viii) Salt, Mustard, Vinegar, Pepper — 4 slow skips with rebound — 8 quick skips without a rebound.
Make up your own rhymes.

THE BALL

Playing with a ball fascinates people of all ages; the ball is 'alive'. Even before any specific skills have been mastered a ball can be used to stimulate movement. At the same time the properties of the ball are being explored and demands on concentration are being made. At this stage it is preferable to use larger size balls. The teacher initiates activities and works with the group. Variety of task is more important than the developing of specific motor skills.

Example of an activity session

Each with own ball including the teacher.

1. Hold it with both hands, roll it from right to left hand etc. Feel its shape and texture. Hold it as high up as possible — look at it.

2. Put it very carefully on the floor. Creep round it very quietly, jump round it, etc.

3. Sit with the ball; use hands to roll ball across or round you, under knees etc — make patterns.

4. Stand with ball in hands. In contrast to previous activity use the ball to make a noise, ie big bounces which encourage vigorous body movement; do not be too concerned with catching the ball.

5. Throw and catch — encourage carefulness and quietness in contrast to 4.

6. Place the ball on the floor, dribble it using the inside of the feet, then try using other parts of the body — hand, and from siting, elbow, seat, head, etc. Notice the range of body movement, the effort involved.

7. Stand, make up a game keeping the ball off the floor as much as possible; regard effort to do so as success.

8. Roll the ball and run after it to retrieve it.

9. Use flat of hand to pat-bounce downwards or upwards.

Climax: Free choice, alone or with partner.

Observe the capacity to play without specific direction. This will help the teacher to plan the next session. This approach can be adapted to the use of other small apparatus, eg hoops, ropes, quoits, beanbags.

Activities can be adapted to suit indoor or outdoor activities, eg if working on asphalt the players cannot be asked to sit or crawl on the ground.

Getting the feel of it

In the early stages, let each member of the group choose from a box of balls of different sizes, weights and colours. Help them to feel the weight and shape of the ball, also its texture. Talk about its shape and texture. Let them discover what can be done with a ball.

Ball practices for specific skills

The skills can be devised with:

1 ball for each person; 1 ball between two; in small groups.

Players can develop skill with a ball if they are given the opportunity to learn the technique of: rolling — throwing — bouncing — controlling and stopping — passing — catching — dribbling — kicking — batting (hitting) — heading — trapping — with all kinds of balls, large, small, heavy, light, hard, soft.

As players become familiar with the ball and can perform most of the skills, more difficult activities can be taught involving more than one skill, eg bouncing and throwing, hitting, catching and throwing.

Rolling the ball

1. Roll a ball between partners (Fig 7.4).

2. Roll a ball to the side of a partner to pick up and return.

3. Roll different size balls between skittles.

4. Roll balls through the legs of a chair placed between two players. Count the number of balls which go through — which couple can get 2 - 4 - 6 balls through in the shortest time — which pair can roll two or more balls through consecutively.

5. Sit with knees bent — hold the ball in both hands, resting on knees — let it roll down to the ankles — kick it up with feet

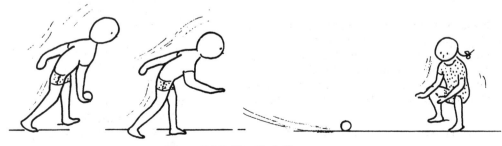

Figure 7.4 Rolling the ball

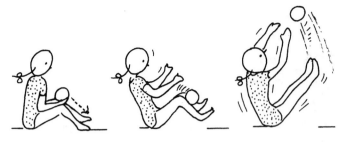

Figure 7.5 Roll and throw

and catch it (Fig 7.5).

Variation: kick the ball up to a partner.

Bouncing the ball (different sizes of ball)

- Hold the ball in both hands with fingers spread at the sides (hands take the shape of the ball);

- press with the hands to make it bounce;

- watch where the ball bounces and move to catch it.

1. Bounce the ball

    (a) with both hands — catch after each bounce (Fig 7.6a);

    (b) at waist level continuously;

    (c) as high as possible;

    (d) as low as possible

    (e) right hand only;

    (f) left hand only;

    (g) alternate hands;

    (h) as (g) travelling;

    (i) 3 times with right hand, 3 with left;

    (j) as (i) travelling;

    (k) to a partner (vary the distance apart);

    (l) into a chalk circle to partner (vary the distance apart).

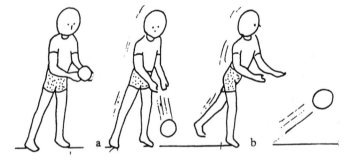

Figure 7.6 Bouncing the ball

When bouncing a ball and travelling bounce the ball forward (ahead) (Fig 7.6b).

2. Bounce the ball with either hand walking round a circle (5 m (6 ½') diameter); repeat running.

3. Bounce the ball on the floor and catch it as it rebounds off a wall.

4. Bounce the ball with a two-handed bounce to partner. Start the bounce high overhead. Start as 4, aiming to bounce ball

in a circle (1m (3'3") diameter).

Bounce pass

Stand with feet slightly apart —

- hold ball between waist and hip with both hands;

- spread fingers at each side of ball, thumbs behind ball;

- extend elbows and wrists and push ball to the floor to bounce about 1m (3'3") in front of team-mate or partner (Fig 7.7),

- follow through with hands, thumbs pushing the ball and elbows close to sides.

Dribbling (as in Basket Ball)

Stand with one foot slightly in front of the other; hold ball in hands (as in bounce pass), push forward and downward, bouncing the ball; keep ball close to the hand in a continuous bounce movement on the spot. The fingers controlling the direction of the bounce and the wrist supplying the force; move along a straight line dribbling the ball, keeping the body erect; move along in a crouched position guarding the ball with your body (Fig 7.8).

Throwing

A good throw depends on a number of points such as the size and weight of the ball, the accuracy of the direction in which it is thrown, the distance and speed. The whole body weight must go into the throw. The right stance is important to enable the weight of the whole body to supplement the arm movement in a forceful throw (Fig 7.9). The underarm throw is valuable when only a short distance is to be covered.

Single underarm throw (right-handed) (small ball)

Step onto the left foot towards the target; swing the right arm backward transferring the weight on to the right foot; swing the right arm downward and forward towards the target, transferring the weight to the left foot; follow through, stepping onto the right foot in line with the ball, and extending the wrist and elbow in the direction of the throw. Let each player find out which hand is easiest to use but practise with both.

Overarm throw (right handed)

Hold the ball in the fingers, step onto the left foot with the left shoulder pointing towards the target; extend the right elbow backward behind the shoulder (away from the body) transferring the weight to the right foot; with the elbow leading, release the ball in front of the shoulder (transferring the weight from right to left foot during the throw); follow through with the whole body extending the arm, wrist and fingers and stepping onto the right foot in line with the ball (Fig 7.10).

Quoit throw (right handed)

Hold the quoit flat, thumb on top of the quoit; bend the wrist and elbow towards the body; step forward onto the right foot at the same time as the elbow and wrist are extended in the direction of the throw; the quoit should travel through the air 'flat'(fig 7.11). Rubber quoits are smooth and easier to handle than rope quoits.

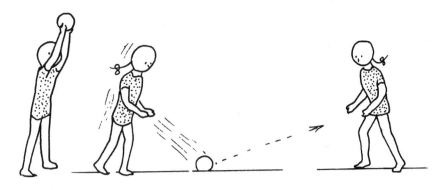

Figure 7.7 Bounce pass

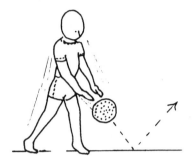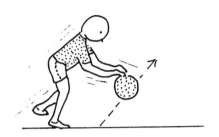

Figure 7.8 Dribbling the ball

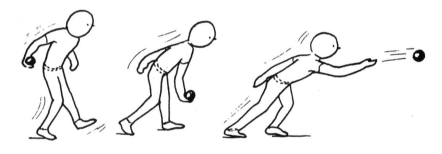

Figure 7.9 Single under-arm throw

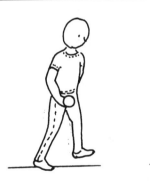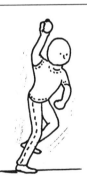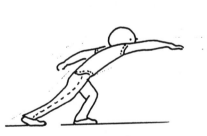

Figure 7.10 Over-arm throw

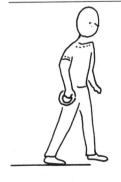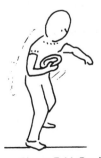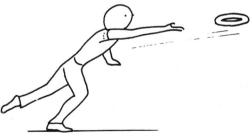

Figure 7.11 Quoit throw

Practices

Practise —

(i) throwing and catching in twos, catching with both hands at first;

(ii) throwing quoits over an object — cricket stump, skittle — or stick held in the air.

Catching

Watch the ball carefully, note its rise and fall and move towards it; extend the arms and hands to meet the ball, spread the fingers in the direction of the ball; close the fingers round the ball and pull it towards the body as it is caught; the whole body, particularly the arms, must 'give' so that the ball is caught softly in the hands.

Catch with both hands at first, then with alternate hands. Beanbags are easier to catch particularly for older people. If they are made of bright colours they are often more easily seen than a ball.

The basic principles of throwing and catching are the same as for small balls. One advantage of a beanbag is that it drops rather than rolls away if it is not caught.

Practices

1. Throw the beanbag up and catch it — increase the height;

2. throw the beanbag up and clap once and catch it; repeat increasing the number of claps;

3. throw the beanbag ahead, run and catch it.

A beanbag can be substituted for a ball in all activities except bouncing, batting and kicking.

Throwing, passing and catching practices

Examples — beanbags, beach balls, balloons or quoits can be used when appropriate (Fig 7.12). Use both underarm and overarm throws according to the players' ability.

Individual

1. Standing throw the ball up with:

   (a) two hands and catch it (Fig 7.13a);

   (b) right hand, catch in two hands;

   (c) left hand, catch in two hands;

   (d) right hand, catch with right hand;

   (e) left hand, catch with left hand;

   (f) right hand, catch with left hand (Fig 7.13b);

   (g) left hand, catch with right hand (Fig 7.13c).

   Variation: (a) — (g) against a wall with a bounce between the throw and the catch (Fig 7.14).

2. Throw ball against a wall and catch before bouncing, with right, left, or both hands. As players improve, introduce a bounce back.

3. Throw ball upward and forward and catch it on the run with right, left or both hands (Fig 7.15).

4. Throw and catch over measured distances; A holds the ball, B stands at a stump or mark 3m (10') away; 3 or 4 other stumps are placed in a line behind B at intervals of 1.5 - 2m (5'- 6'6"). A throw overarm to B, B returns it to A, moves back to next stump and so on. The aim being to increase the length of throw and to return the ball accurately.

With partners

5. Throw to a partner, vary the height and distance of throw. Three beanbags or other objects are put on the ground in triangular formation, 3-4m (10-13') apart. A stands at one beanbag and B at another. A throws a ball to B; B returns it to A and immediately runs towards the third beanbag trying to catch the ball thrown in that direction by A, before it touches the ground.

   A practice for passing ahead of a player and running forward to catch as in netball and basketball.

6. Throw a ball to a partner over a rope or net at different heights.

In small groups

7. Circles of 4 to 6 players, 1 ball to each player. Instructor or helper stands in the centre. The instructor throws the ball to each player in turn who returns the ball. Count the number of catches and accurate throws. Change direction. This practice gives the instructor a chance to correct the throwing and catching technique of the players.

8. As 7 but throw to players anywhere round the circle.

Kicking, trapping and heading

1. *Kicking with inside of foot(right foot).* Place ball in front of the feet. The left foot should be to one side and slightly behind the ball as a supporting foot. The kicking leg is brought back with the knee slightly bent and toes extended pointing down. The leg is brought forward with the toes close to the ground and turned outward to make contact with the ball when the knee is straightened. The direction of the ball can be controlled by changing the direction of the toes. To increase the distance of the kick point the toes downward, this will keep the ball low and fast. The further the leg follows through the higher the ball will go. The ball can also be kicked by the inside of the foot by making sure the foot gets well under the ball when making contact (Fig 7.16).

2. *Kicking with outside of foot(right foot).* The kick is similar to the previous one, but the ball is kicked with the outside of the foot. The ball will travel to the right when flicked or kicked by the outside of the foot: to the left when kicked with the inside of the foot. Pointing the toe and keeping the foot straight and making contact with the ball on the top of the foot keeps the ball low and fast — strongest kick. The non-kick foot should be ahead of the ball

3. *Dribbling.* The ball is pushed along the ground in front of the player by kicking it gently with the either foot, inside or outside of foot. The ball can be dibbled by one foot and then the other to keep it moving or just by one foot. The body should be crouched slightly over the ball, but remember to lift the head at times to see where you are going. Ball should be kept close to feet when dribbling. Practise dribbling along a straight line and then a crooked line or circle, changing

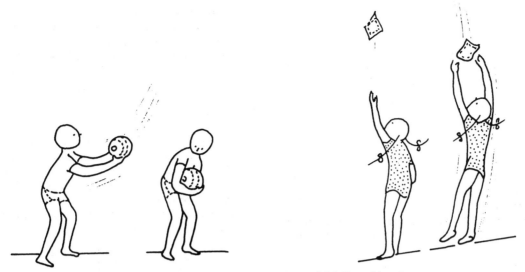

Figure 7.12 Throwing and catching with balls and beanbags

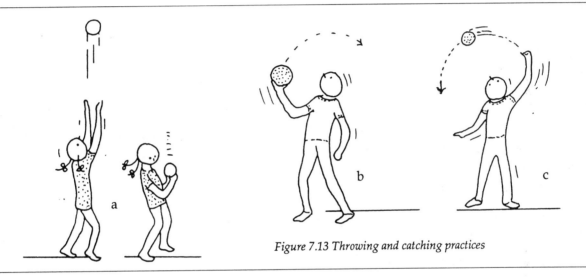

a   b   c

Figure 7.13 Throwing and catching practices

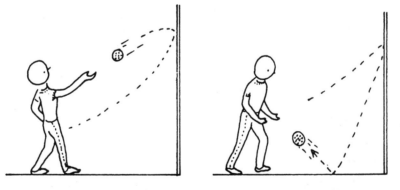

Figure 7.14 Throwing and catching practices against a wall

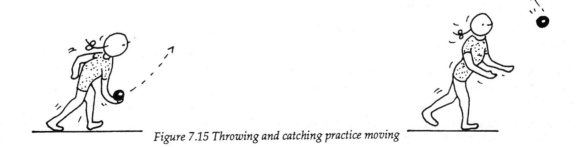

Figure 7.15 Throwing and catching practice moving

speed and direction — stopping, slowing down and turning (Fig 7.17).

4. *Trapping with the sole of foot:*

   (a) throw the ball up slightly in the air to a partner;

   (b) keep the eye on flight of ball;

   (c) move forwards as the ball descends;

   (d) lift the foot slightly to make contact with ball as it strikes the ground;

   (e) the sole of foot traps the ball by placing it on top of the ball (Fig 7.18).

Trapping with outside of foot (right foot):

   (a) throw the ball up into the air;

   (b) keep the eye on the flight of ball at all times;

   (c) move forwards and to the side as the ball descends;

   (d) lift the right foot slightly off the ground;

   (e) right foot is bent over at the ankle, knee moving outwards when making contact with the ball as it strikes the ground;

   (f) body should be moving to the right in a slightly crouched position. Hands to be used for balance.

Trapping with other parts of the body:

   (a) *Calf or thigh.* When the ball is descending or bouncing high the leg contacting the ball must remain limp and give with the ball so that it will drop immediately in front of the player. Pull the thigh back and inwards, cushioning the momentum of the ball as it makes contact with the thigh.

   (b) *Chest or stomach.* Balls coming at you quickly or slowly above waist height are usually trapped by the chest and sometimes the stomach. To cushion the ball, the body must move back with back arched, arms by sides or slightly in front bent position. This reduces the ball's momentum and, therefore, helps direct the ball to the ground near the feet of the player. Body should be wrapped well round the ball, arms and hands should not touch the ball.

5. *Heading*

The ball should be contacted at all times with the front of the forehead at the hairline. The neck and spine are held rigid and feet should be off the ground although at the start this is not necessary. Eyes follow the flight of the ball until contact is made between the head and the ball. Greater distance can be obtained by using the neck muscles and driving the ball away. It is good practice to try and place the ball by heading it in different directions and also to get above it and head it down to a partner's feet.

Dribbling practices

1. Dribble a ball with right foot and then left foot for a distance of 8m(26') round an obstacle and back — walking.

2. Dribble, on the trot, as above.

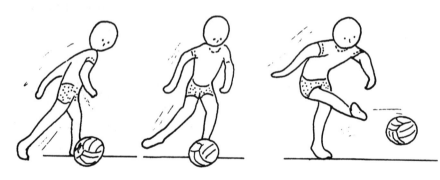

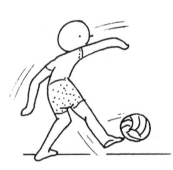

Figure 7.16 Kicking (with inside of foot)

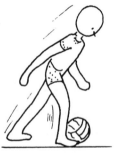

Figure 7.17 Dribbling the ball

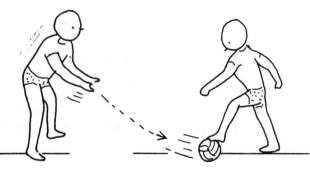

Figure 7.18 Trapping the ball

3. Dribble, using both feet, continuous passing, round an obstacle at 8m(26') distance and back.

4. Dribble a ball out and in and around four skittles in a line each about 600mm(2') apart without touching them with the ball. Inside and outside of foot to be used.

It is difficult to dribble or control the ball while running. If possible, therefore, this should be done out-of-doors on a grass surface. The ball should never be passed so far ahead as to be out of control.

Kicking practices

1. Kick ball against a wall while standing and stopping it on the return.

2. Kick ball at an angle to a wall and run on to ball on return and stop it.

3. Kick ball against a wall and move on to the return and kick it back against the wall. Use alternate feet.

4. Kick ball to partner and receive it back.

5. Kick ball between two skittles about 600mm (2') apart.

6. Kick ball inside circle or hoop on the wall.

7. Kick ball a distance of 10m (32'6").

8. Kick ball a distance of 15m (48'9") two times out of four.

9. Distance is measured to the point where the ball stops rolling.

10. Kick ball continuously with either foot as it rebounds off a marked area on a wall. Try to do this ten times without stopping the ball.

11. Practise kicking ball from penalty spot on football pitch between the goalposts. Then introduce a partner to act as goalkeeper.

Heading practices

1. Head ball back to partner using the forehead.

2. Head ball with side of the head to partner.

3. Head ball on forehead down to feet of partner.

4. Head ball on forehead against a wall.

UNIPLAY GAMES AWARD SCHEME

This non-profit-making scheme is sponsored by the Uniplay company of Coventry and organised by a lecturer at Trent Polytechnic in Nottingham.

It aims to:

1. facilitate the presentation of games skills activities from basic to advanced;

2. offer instructors/teachers/helpers a definite framework for the progressive development of abilities;

3. motivate the participants to practise the various skills in order to achieve the basic tasks necessary for a Badge level.

The scheme provides variations for ATC/GATEWAY centres/

clubs, ESN(S) schools, ESN(M) Primary level and a version for physically handicapped pupils. There are three levels - Bronze, Silver and Gold, all requiring a consistent level of performance in three areas - Skills, Skills and Basic Games, Recreational/Social Tasks. The tasks progress from simple manipulative and ballistic closed skills which require a sound body alignment and basic reach, contact grasp manipulation release/propulsion. The more advanced ones concentrate on the adaptive-type tasks demanding body co-ordination, perception and social co-operation. Each Centre using the scheme 'sets' its particular level of criteria for the tasks. Some Centres ask outside people to test, after they have been adequately briefed, eg physical education teachers.

Two positive effects of the scheme are that:

1. it has provided a logical framework for instructors to follow (some Centres have used it for staff development);

2. the notional levels of Bronze, Silver and Gold performance can then be used for matching teams for ball skill competitions between clubs or centres. (This way of clarifying ball skills was suggested by Tony Burroughs of Nottingham.) It has since been verified, with significant correlations being shown between a person's Badge level and his/her straw points scores in a potted sports competition, for example. One Centre can therefore invite another to bring a minibus contingent of only Bronze level participants to their Centre for a friendly contest. In other words, it is not always the 'best' who are picked to represent their club, centre, or school.

Further information can be obtained from: D C Williamson, Co-ordinator, 64 Whitworth Drive, Radcliffe-on-Trent, Nottingham, NG12 2ER.

ACTIVITIES USING IMPROVISED EQUIPMENT

NOTE: The games described on pp   are only a selection, many more can be devised by the teacher.

1. Tyre stepping

Equipment: 10 car tyres 500mm (20") apart.

Rules:

1. Players step from tyre to tyre without stepping anywhere else other than within the tyres.

2. The course runs from point A to B and back again to A as illustrated (Fig. 7.19).

3. The player completing the course in the shortest time is the winner.

2. Drums

Equipment: 5 car tyres 500mm (20") apart, drums.

Game: Start line is 20m (4") wide. Player rolls tyres and endeavours to knock down drum or drums. Each drum has a point score. If a drum is knocked it is immediately reset in position. Each competitor has five tyres and two attempts (Fig 7.20).

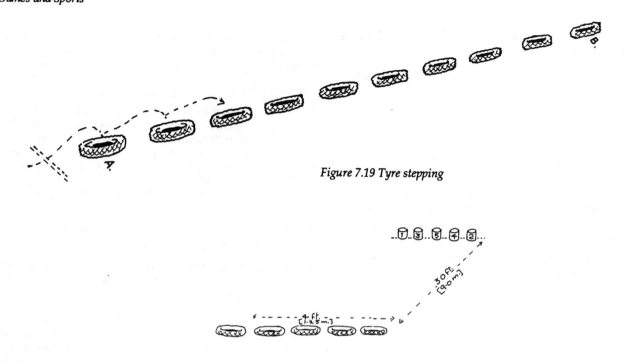

Figure 7.19 Tyre stepping

Figure 7.20 Drums

3. Horse shoe throwing

Equipment: Five pieces of 25mm (1") dowelling (broomstick handle), 300mm (12") high and 500mm (20") apart set into a base board 12mm ($^{1}/_{2}$") thick. Five horse shoes, 300mm (12") high and 200mm (8") wide, made from hardboard.

Game: The player tries to score as many points as possible by throwing onto the peg or landing between lines (Fig 21).

Rules:

1. Each peg and square carry a score rating.
2. Each shoe must land within the designated playing area. Shoes outside are out of bounds (see diagram).
3. One foul throw, ie out of bounds, is allowed.
4. The player with the highest number of points is the winner.
5. If a shoe is more than halfway on the peg but not the full way, the full peg value is scored.
6. In the event of a draw a throw off will take place.

4. Skittles variation

Equipment: 10 painted coke tins (empty), circle marked on ground, medium sized plastic ball.

Game: Each tin has a given value of 1 - 10 points. The competitor endeavours to knock as many tins as possible from the circle.

Rules:

1. The tins are placed in a triangle shape — within the circle.
2. Only tins knocked completely outside the circle score.
3. The radius of the circle is 450mm (18").
4. The throwing distance is 300mm (12").
5. Each competitor has three attempts at the full set of skittles each time, the total number of points being the final score.
6. The competitor with the greatest number of points is deemed the winner.

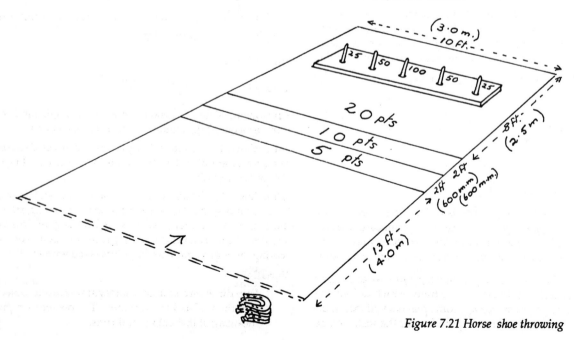

Figure 7.21 Horse shoe throwing

7. In the event of a tie, a throw off will take place until a winner is found.

FORMS OF TAG

1. Tag

Equipment and formation: A coloured band for each player — one, the catcher, wearing her band, the remainder holding theirs.
Game: The catcher tags a player who puts on and becomes a catcher. The game continues until everyone has been caught.

Variation: All players tuck their band loosely in the back of the skirt or shorts.

Game: Everyone tries to take the others' bands. The winner is the player who has taken the most bands.

2. Release

Equipment: None.
Formation: Free.

Game: One or more catchers. When caught a player bobs down. Continue until all are caught.

Variation: Other players can 'release' a 'caught' player by touching them. They then rejoin the game.

3. Arches

Formation: Players in pairs round the room. One couple hold hands forming an arch.

Directions: On a signal the players run under the arch and round the room. They try not to be caught under the arch when the whistle goes. Any couple caught under it stands by the first arch and makes another one. This continues until only one couple is left running under the arches. When the whistle goes any number of couples can be caught under the arches. The last couple to be caught are the winners.

4. Chain tag

Formation: Players run freely in the play area. One catcher.

Game: The first player caught joins hands with the catcher and they chase the rest. When another player is tagged the catchers join hands to make a chain of three. When the next player is tagged the chain divides into two pairs and so on, until all the players are caught.

TEAM RACES

Presentation

1. The race should be simple.

2. Be sure there are the same number of players in each team; arrange for a player to run twice if the teams are uneven, rather than have one standing out. If some players are unable to take part, make use of them as scorers or markers.

3. Teams should never be longer than 6 players — long teams mean long waits and very little activity which defeats the purpose of the race; moreover, some players will lose interest and be a nuisance, spoiling the fun for the rest. Where helpers are available, the numbers of players in a team can be reduced (more teams).

4. The course should be clearly indicated and conditions must be fair for all.

5. Players must play to the rules, eg (i) feet behind the line before being touched off; (ii) finish as directed; (iii) lines to be straight and the players in the right order.

6. In races in files make it clear on which side of their teams the players run — remember it is easier to run round an object such as a chair or skittle rather than round a ground marking.

7. Explain exactly how the race starts and finishes and the method of scoring. Check that the players understand.

8. Indicate teams either by names or colours, but in group games, minor or major games, teams should be marked by coloured bibs or bands.

9. Demonstrate the pathway of the race and what specific skill is used, eg running to pick up an object. Let No 1 in each team walk it through while you prompt, then No 2 and so on until each player has had a practice turn. Repeat this if necessary, then let them 'have a go', increasing the speed as they improve. Announce the winner.

Scoring

1. The team as a unit scores at the end of the race.

2. The individual players may score on behalf of the team, eg score a point for the winner each time Nos 1, 2, 3 or 4 has run. Each player needs to remember his number.

TEAM RACES USING VARIOUS FORMATIONS AND EQUIPMENT

Formations

For team races a variety of formations can be used, eg circles, files (one behind the other), files divided into two, triangular, ranks (side by side), one formation v another (circle, line etc), star, free formation.

The following are some simple team races using these formations.

Small circles

'Shopping'

Equipment: Four or less objects of any suitable kind for each team, eg a beanbag, a quoit, a ball, a coloured band.

Formations: Each team of 4 - 6 players sits in a circle formation. The objects are placed in the centre of the circle. Players are numbered (Fig 7.22).

Directions: The instructor calls out a number and an object, eg No 2 - beanbag. No 2 gets up, picks up the beanbag, runs round the outside of the circle, replaces the beanbag, returns to place and sits. The first player to be sitting receives a point and the team scoring the highest number of points is the winner.

Variations:

1. Four different coloured beanbags replace the 4 objects. The call then is No 3 and a colour. The player then picks the beanbag of that colour and runs.

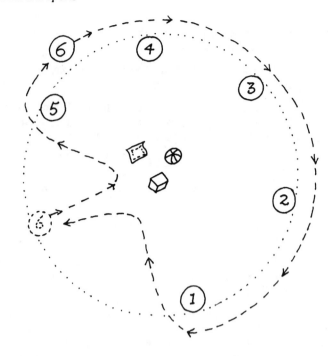

Figure 7.22 'Shopping'

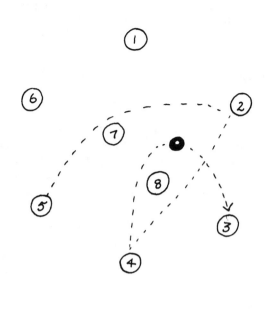

Figure 7.23 Wandering ball

2. Two objects replace 4, each one represents a shop, eg grocer, greengrocer or butcher. The call is No 1 plus some article purchased in either of the two shops. This can be built up to 3 shops.

3. One object representing a shop. The call is No 4 plus a commodity which may or may not be purchased in that shop. If it is, the player picks the object up and runs as before. If not, the player sits still.

This game has many possibilities and can be used to help colour identification, shopping knowledge. Start with a small number of objects and build up.

Large circles

Wandering ball

Equipment: 1 beanbag or ball.

Formation: The players form a circle with one or more in the middle.

Directions: A beanbag is thrown from player to player while those in the centre try to intercept (Fig 7.23). The beanbag should be thrown quickly and passes vary in height. When one of the middle players intercepts the beanbag he changes with the player who threw it. Other ball passing and bouncing games can be played in this formation, eg Circle Dodge Ball.

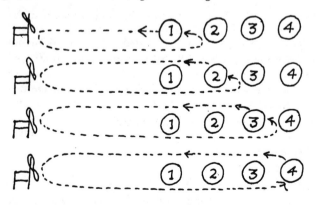

Figure 7.24 Band relay

Files

Band relay

Equipment: 1 coloured band for each player. 1 suitable for each team.

Formation: Each team of 4 - 6 players stands in a file behind a marked line. A chair is placed 8 - 10m (26 -33') in front of each team.

Directions:

1. No 1 runs to the chair and loops (ties) the band onto the chair (on most chairs there is a place where this can be done; it may have to be upside down). No 1 runs back and touches off No 2. Continue until all players have tied the band onto the chair and are back in place (Fig 7.24). The first team to be sitting in a straight line is the winner.

2. Repeat the running, but untying the band, the first team sitting with their bands on is the winner.

Variation: Complete 1. and 2. in one race.

Files divided into two

Roll and run relay

Equipment: One ball for each team.

Formation: Each team of 8 - 12 players is divided into two sections which face each other. No 1 holds the ball.

Team of 8

Directions: No 1 rolls the ball to No 2 and runs across to stand behind No 8. No 5 rolls the ball to No 6 and runs across to stand behind No 1. The game continues until all are back in their correct order but on the opposite side to which they started. The ball is thrown to No 1 who holds it up (Fig 7.25).

NB. If there is an odd player, Nos 1 - 4 facing Nos 5 - 7 at the finish, No 1 will be in possession of the ball and no extra throw will be needed.

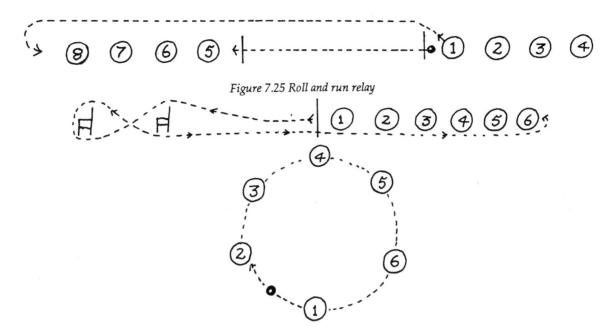

Figure 7.25 Roll and run relay

Figure 7.26 Circle passing v team running

Variations:

1. throw the ball;
2. bounce the ball;
3. roll the ball through the legs of a chair placed between the two half files.

Free formation

Pat and Bounce

Equipment: One tennis, plastic or sponge ball for each player. A number of obstacles, eg chairs, skittles.

Formation: Each team of any number of players stands in free formation and the obstacles are placed anywhere in the room.

Directions: Each player bounces the ball 5 times on the spot and then runs completely round 2 obstacles holding the ball in his hand. Repeat the bouncing and runs round two more obstacles, excluding the last obstacle used. Repeat the bouncing again and sit. The Instructor calls 'Stop!' at the end of a given time and each player who is sitting scores one point for the team. The team scoring the greatest number of points is the winner.

Variations: Vary the size of ball, the number of bounces and the number of obstacles to run round.

One formation v another

Circle passing v team running

Equipment: 1 large ball or beanbag, 1 chair or more chairs.

Formation: Two teams of 6 - 8 players. 1 team stands in a file behind a marked line, the other round a large marked circle (Fig 7.26).

Directions: The team in the circle pass the ball anti-clockwise from one to another counting each pass, while the other team run a set course one after another, No 1 running first. When No 6 has completed the course he calls 'Stop!' The centre players stop and announce the number of passes made.

If the ball is dropped:

1. the counting is continuous, dropped passes **not** being scored, or

2. counting must start at 1 again.

Teams change over and the game is repeated. The team with the highest number of passes is the winner.

Variations:

1. Vary the shape of the course.
2. Vary the direction of the running and throwing.
3. Bounce the ball instead of throwing.

Ranks

Quoit Passing

Equipment: 1 quoit (beanbag or ball can be used).

Formation: Each team of 6-8 players stands in a rank (players stand side by side in a line).

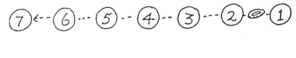

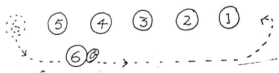

Figure 7.27 Quoit passing

Directions: No1 has the quoit. Pass the quoit from one to the other to the end of the rank. Each player must handle it, the end player runs up behind the rank to No 1's place, all move down 1 place. Continue passing the object down the line until each player has had a turn, and they are all in their original places. To finish, No 1 runs up to the top and holds the object up. The first team to finish is the winner(Fig 7.27).

Variation: Pass the quoit behind the back.

Star or wheel

Star Trek

Equipment: 1 ball for each team.

Formation: Each team of 4-8 players stands side by side in a rank forming 1 spoke of the star. No 1 in each team is at the centre of the star.

Directions: No 1 bounces the ball to No 2 who catches it and bounces it to No 3 and so on until it reaches the last player. The last player catches it and runs round the star in the direction in which the teams are facing, back to the end of the team, up in front of the team and takes No 1's place. The game is repeated until No 1, back in place, holds up the ball (Fig 7.28).

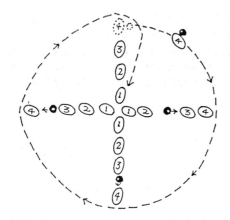

Figure 7.28 Star trek

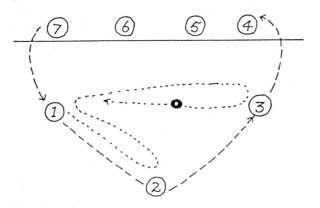

Figure 7.29 Triangular throw

Variations:

1. Pat bounce the ball from one to another instead of catching between each bounce.

2. Spread out (more distance between players). Throw the ball from one to another.

Triangular

Triangular Throw

Equipment: 1 ball for each team (beanbag or quoit can be used).

Formation: Each team of 6-8 players is arranged as in diagram (Fig 7.29), Nos 1, 2, and 3 standing in small circles and the rest of the team behind a marked line parallel to the base of the triangle formed by the circles. No 1 holds the ball.

Directions: No 1 throws to No 2 who returns it to No 1. No 1 throws to No 3 who returns it to No 1. No 1 puts the ball on the ground and calls 'Change!' No 1 runs to No 2 circle. On 'Change' No 2 runs to No 3's circle. No 3 runs behind the line by No 4. No 6 runs to No 1's circle, picks up the ball and throws to No 1. The team to finish with No 1 back in the original position with the ball held up is the winner.

TEAM RACES WITH EQUIPMENT

Belisha Beacon

No in team: 4-6 players.

Equipment: Cardboard tubes 300mm (12") long, some black, some white, 1 orange ball for each team.

Formation: Teams stand behind the starting line, each player has a white or black tube alternately— the last player has the ball.

Directions: The leader runs to a given mark and stands the tube on end. Each member of the team runs and builds the tube on the one before (alternate black and white). The last player puts the ball on top. The team with the Belisha Beacon built and standing is the winner (Figure 7.30).

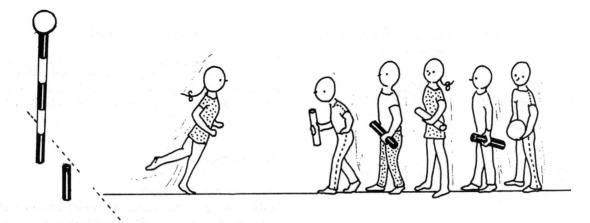

Figure 7.30 Belisha Beacon

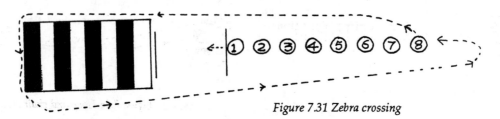

Figure 7.31 Zebra crossing

Zebra Crossing

Using black and white strips of hardboard a Zebra crossing can be built as in Belisha Beacon (Fig 7.31)

Building Bricks

No in team: 4-6 players.

Equipment: Plastic building bricks which fit into each other, 1 for each player.

Formation: teams line up behind the starting line. The leader runs and puts the brick on a given mark and returns to place. Each player runs in turn and builds on the previous bricks until the 'tower' is built. The team completing the tower first wins.

Variations:

1. Build on a table (Fig 7.32).
2. Crawl under the table and then build, crawl back under table and run to touch off the next player.
3. Build on a chair placed on the table. Players may have to step on to another chair to reach the top. Make it a little more difficult each time.

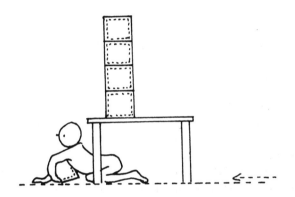

Figure 7.32 Building bricks on a table

Bricks and Balls

No in team: 4-6 players.

Equipment: 2 bricks and 1 ball for each team.

Formation: Put 2 bricks 10-15 m (33'-50') apart on the floor in front of each team. 1 ball 150mm (6") diameter is placed on 1 brick.

Directions: Each member of the team runs in turn to move the ball from one brick to the other as directed (Fig 7.33).

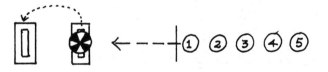

Figure 7.33 Bricks and balls

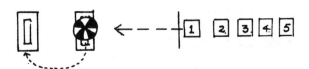

Variations:

1. Move 2 balls between 3 bricks.
2. Increase the number of bricks.
3. Increase the number of balls.
4. Vary the way the balls are moved on the bricks.

Bean Bag Relay

No in each team: 4-6 players.

Equipment: One beanbag for each team.

Formation: Teams sit on floor. Two circles are marked on the floor, one at the top and the other half way between the first circle and the team. The beanbag is in first circle (Fig 7.34)

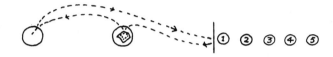

Figure 7.34 Bean bag relay

Directions: The leader runs, picks up the beanbag and puts it in the circle at the top, returns and sits down. The next player runs and changes the beanbag to the other circle. Continue until the whole team has moved the beanbag in turn. The team sitting in a straight line first is the winner (Fig 7.34)

Bucket and Ball Relay

No in each team: 4-6 players.

Equipment: Buckets, 1 for each team. Tennis balls and other soft balls which bounce, **1 for each player.**

Formation: Teams stand behind the starting line with a bucket at the other end of the room.

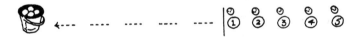

Figure 7.35 Bucket and ball relay

Direction: The leader bounces a tennis ball up to and into the bucket and returns to place. Each player repeats this in turn. The last player brings the bucket of tennis balls back to the front of the team. The first team to be in line with the bucket of balls in front is the winner (Fig 7.35).

Hoop and Chair Relay

No in each team: 4-6 players.

Equipment: Teams sit in a line. A chair is placed in front of each team some distance away. Each player has a hoop on the floor at the side.

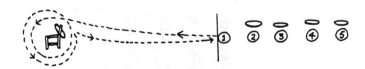

Figure 7.36 Hoop and chair relay

Directions: The leader lifts up the hoop, runs up and round the chair, stops and puts the hoop over the chair and returns to place. Each player repeats this until all the hoops are on the chair. The first team to have all the hoops on the chair and be sitting down in place. wins (Fig 7.36).

Repeat Collecting each hoop in turn.

Variation: Bowl the hoop to the chair.

Run and Throw Back Relay

No in each team: 4-6 players.

Equipment: 1 ball for each team.

Formation: Teams line up behind starting line, the leader of each team has the ball.

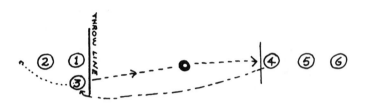

Figure 7.37 Run and throw back relay

Directions: The leader with the ball runs to a mark or line a short distance away, stops, turns and throws the ball to the next player who catches it and runs up to the line and throws it the next player–then stands behind the leader. Play continues until all the team are lined up behind the leader who has the ball. Each player must go to the **end** of the line **after** throwing. Repeat the relay until team is back in the original place (Fig 7.37).

Basket Ball Relay

No in each team: 4 - 6 players.

Equipment: Plastic footballs, 1 for each team, 1 set of uprights (4) for each team (skittles).

Formation: Teams stand in a line; uprights are set up in pairs — the course is 15-16m (approx. 50-55') long.

Directions: The leader bounces the ball (basket ball style) — passing between the uprights and runs back to give the ball to the next player. The team finishing first wins (Fig 7.38).

TEAM RACES WITHOUT EQUIPMENT

Circle Weave

No in team: 4-6 players.

Formation: Each team stands in a circle. Each team member is numbered.

Directions: The leader runs and weaves in and out through the team members to the right, the leader touches off No 2 and stands in No 2's place. No 2 does the same and this is repeated by each player until the last player finishes in No 1's place. The first team to finish and sit down in the circle wins.

Leap Frog Relay

No in team 4-6 players.

Formation: Teams stand in a file at least 'two arms' length apart. All players except the last in each team bend over in leap frog position (keep heads tucked in).

Directions: The last player leaps over the 'frogs' in the team to the front and takes up the leap frog position — the rest of the team repeat this from the back of the line. The first team to finish and sit down wins.

Numbers Relay

No in team: 4-6 players.

Formation: Teams stand in a line — numbered.

Directions: The teacher calls a number. The player in each team with the number called runs up round a marker (chair) and back to his place. The first runner back in place scores 1 point for the team (see that all the numbers are called). The team scoring the greatest number of points wins.

Variations: The action may take various forms, eg walking, skipping, hopping, crab walking, jumping with two feet together.

Trains

No in team: 3-4 players.

Formation: Team stands in a line facing a marker (chair) 8-10m (26-33') from line.

Directions: The leader runs round the marker, back round the end of the team and picks up the next player who holds hands (round waist), both run, pick up the next. The 'train' to finish back in line without losing the 'trucks' wins.

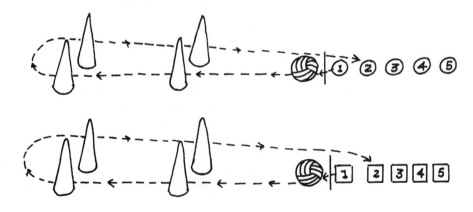

Figure 7.38 Basket ball relay

GROUP GAMES WITHOUT EQUIPMENT

Quick Formation

Formation: The players are divided into two teams of equal numbers.

Directions: The two teams skip round the room following their leaders. On the signal from the teacher who may shout the words 'file', 'straight line', 'circle', 'sit down', each team makes such a formation. The first team to do so gains a point. The team gaining most points at the end of the designated time is the winner.

Simon Says

Formation: Free.

Directions: The teacher, or player chosen by the players to be leader, stands in front of the rest. Commands are given such as 'jump', 'sit', 'turn round', 'clap hands', 'stamp feet'. If the command is preceded by 'Simon says', then the players must obey. If 'Simon says' is omitted the command must be ignored. If the player makes 3 mistakes he is either eliminated or takes the place of the leader. The winner is the last one out.

Grandmother's Steps

Formation: Free

Directions: The teacher or 1 player chosen to be leader stands at one end of the play area — the rest at the other end, standing behind a line. The aim is to creep up to tag the leader without being seen. The leader turns round from time to time and anyone seen moving is sent back to the start. The player who tags the leader without being seen becomes the leader.

The Fish in the Sea

Formation: All players sit in a circle on the floor or chairs. Each player is given the name of a fish, kipper, haddock, cod, mackerel etc, several players to each fish.

Directions: The teacher says 'The cod is swimming in the sea' (all the cods jump up and move round the circle anti-clockwise). 'The sea is calm' — players walk. 'The sea is choppy' — players run. 'The sea is rough' — players leap and spring. At any stage the words can bring other fish into the sea, send some back or have all in the sea together. The condition of the sea can also change.

The Animal Farm

Formation: All players sit in a circle on the floor or chairs. Each player represents something found on a farm. The farmer, the farmer's wife, the children, the cockerel, hens, sheep, goats, cows, dogs, cats, horses, ponies, a plough, combine harvester, barn, etc.

Directions: The teacher tells a story about a farm bringing in all the words. The players, when their word is said, run round the outside of the circle and back to their place. Make the story as realistic as possible and have more than one sheep, goat, cow etc. It may be necessary for some players to represent two words.

Variations:

1. Marketing — players represent different kinds of shops — grocer — baker — butcher — chemist etc. The teacher calls out a commodity and the 'shop' which sells it stands up and runs round.

2. Substitute the Zoo or Circus for the farm.

Noughts and Crosses

This is a very popular quiet game based on its namesake. With nine chairs in the centre of the hall (Fig 7.39).

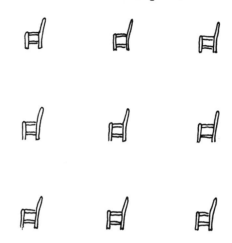

Figure 7.39 Noughts and crosses

Two teams stand on each side of the hall identified either by sex or a band. The teams in turn are asked a question suitable to the ability of the player on any subject, ie general knowledge, local knowledge, hygiene, sport, etc. If the correct answer is given the player sits on one of the nine chairs; if the answer is wrong the question is then given to the other team and so the game proceeds until one team or the other has completed a line of three as in the paper and pencil version .

EASY GAMES IN CIRCLE FORMATION

The following games can be used as practices in one circle or one circle and another. This depends on the number and skill of the players.

Circle Pass Ball

Equipment: Football or smaller ball.

Formation: Circle.

Directions: Pass ball round circle in various ways:

1. Clockwise - anti-clockwise.
2. Bounce round circle.
3. Throw and catch with one hand.
4. Throw high and low.
5. Throw to alternate players (miss one player).

Centre Pass Ball

Equipment: Football or smaller ball.

Formation: Circle. 1 player in centre.

Directions: The centre player passes the ball in various ways to each player who returns it in the same way.

1. Throw underarm - overarm.
2. Bounce.
3. High, low.
4. On the move.

Circle Gap

Equipment: Football or smaller ball.

Formation: Circle. 1 player in the centre.

Directions: The centre player passes the ball to No 1 on the outside of the circle. No 1 returns it and runs to a new position between Nos 2 and 3 where he again receives the ball from the player in the centre. He returns it and moves to a position between Nos 3 and 4 and so on until he reaches his own place.

Wide Legs

Equipment: Football.

Formation: Circle(s). 1 player in the centre.

Directions: Players on the outside of the circle. Stand with legs apart. The player in the centre tries to roll the ball through the legs. The ball can be stopped with hands or arms.

Variation: No player in the centre — try to roll the ball through other players' legs.

Call Ball

Equipment: Football or smaller ball.

Formation: Circle with teacher or player in the centre.

Directions: Teacher or player in the centre throws the ball up in the air and simultaneously calls out the name of a player on the outside of the circle who runs in and tries to catch the ball before it touches the ground.

FUN GAMES WITHOUT EQUIPMENT (competitive and non-competitive)

Stand Up

Start with pairs sitting on the ground, back to back, and arms linked. Stand up together (push against each other's back) next time add a friend and all three stand up together. See how many you can add. . .

Line Tug of War

Two teams line up facing each other on either side of a centre line; each member of the opposing team grasps the hand of the player opposite and tries to pull him over the line. The team which has the most players on its side of the line at the end is the winner.

Crusts and Crumbs

Two teams stand in files facing the teacher.

X	0
X	0
X	0
X	0
X	0
CRUSTS	CRUMBS

The teacher calls c-r-r-r-ust or c-r-r-r-umbs rolling the r's — when the crusts or crumbs are called, the players run to the wall. If a player fails to run or a player of the wrong team runs — that team loses a point.

Knots

Form a circle with everyone facing inward, shoulder to shoulder. Everyone puts their hands out and grasps two other hands. Do not grasp the hands of a person next to you, or two hands of the same person. Now unravel yourselves, without letting go of any hands. (You may pivot on your handholds, but do not let go.) Another version is to make one break before you start, especially if your group is younger.

Spirals

Form a circle, with everyone facing inward, holding hands. Ask one person to break his right hand hold, and start to walk around the person he just broke with, in a large circle, with everyone holding hands and following him. Thus, a spiral is formed, with people being wrapped around the person who stands still. When everyone is wrapped around, the innermost person, still holding hands with the others, ducks down and comes out through the group until the spiral is totally unravelled.

Slip and Through

Formation: 2 circles.

Directions: Each player faces a partner holding hands and forming two circles (inside and outside circles). All the couples slip step round the room. On a signal the players in the inside circle stand still, with their feet apart. Those on the outside run round the circle and through their partner's legs. They finish by sitting, cross-legged, behind their partners (who have now formed the outer circle).

MORE DIFFICULT GAMES

The Devil's in the Middle

Equipment: 5 beanbags.

Formation: Place the 5 beanbags equidistant across the playing area. Two teams – numbered. Try to ensure that the players with the same number are of equal ability. Teams stand — as in diagram.

Directions: On 'go' the first player in each team runs and picks up bag No 1, runs back with it and puts it in a circle in front of his team. The same player repeats this with bag No 2. He then runs for bag No 3 but as this is the only remaining bag, the first player to pick this bag and put it in the circle wins a point for the team. To make the competition even keener, replace No 3 bag with a wrapped sweet! Repeat until all players have had a turn (Fig 7.40).

Variation: Place circles in a different position.

Balloon Tennis

No in team: Any number.

Equipment: A balloon or beach ball, a net or tape fixed at 'reach' height or slightly lower.

Formation: 2 teams, one on either side of the net.

Directions: Toss for 'Service'. The aim is to 'ground' the ball on the opponent's side of the net. The server bats the ball over the net with a flat hand. It is batted with one or two hands back and

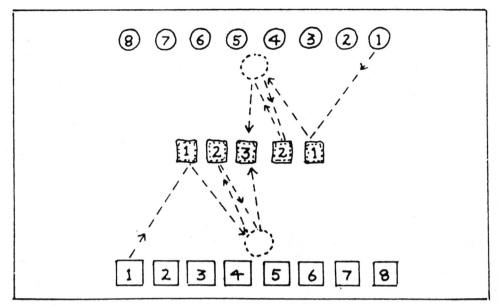

Figure 7.40
Devil's in the middle

forward over the net until it is 'grounded' when one point is scored (Fig 7.41).

Serving: The server continues to serve from alternate sides at the back of the court until a point is lost; then the other side serves. Give everyone a chance to serve. Decide how many points make up a game, 7 - 11- 15- 21.

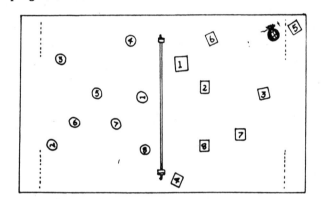

Figure 7.41 Balloon tennis

Practices: 1. Practise batting, throwing and catching a balloon or ball in pairs. 2. As 1. over a net at 'reach' height.

NB. As the players improve the game can be played to Volley Ball rules.

Awkward Hockey

Equipment: 2 broom handles — 2 wood blocks approximately

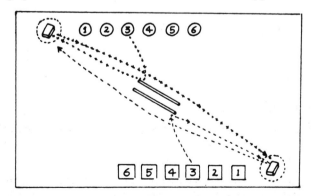

Figure 7.42 Awkward hockey

100 x 50 x 25mm (4 x 2 x 1").

Formation: Two teams are numbered. Wood blocks are placed in the centre of a drawn circle in front of each team. The broom handles are placed in the centre of the playing area.

Directions: The players whose numbers are called run to the centre, pick up the broom handle, run back to the wooden block and propel it across the floor to place it in the opposite circle. The first player to put the block in the circle wins a point (Fig 7.42)

Count Down

Equipment: Frido Ball — baton.

Formation: Two teams. One team forms a circle in the centre of the play area – the second team stand in line with baton (Fig 7.43).

Directions: On the word 'go' the player in the centre of the circle throws the ball in turn to each member of the team who returns it. Each catch is called and counted. The team with the baton run round a planned course, one at a time, handing the baton to the next in line (relay fashion) until the whole team has run. When the last player gets home 'stop' is called. The teams change places and proceed as before. The team with the highest number of catches is the winner.

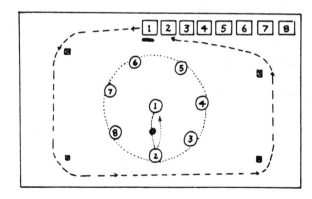

Figure 7.43 Count down

Grand Prix

Equipment: 4 tin plates or old trays — 4 broom handles.

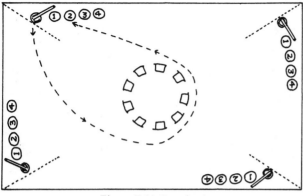

Figure 7.44 Grand prix

Formation: 4 equal teams based in 4 corners of the play area, each team with a plate/tray and broom handle. Make a circle of chairs in the centre to mark the track, seats turned inward. Chalk a line as start line.

Directions: No 1 in each team lines up for 'the off' with tray/plate on floor with broom handles in 'dished' side. On 'go' 'drivers' go round the circle of chairs trying to pass each other. On reaching team pit, the driver hands over the broom handle to the next player who carries on the race. The first team to have raced all team members, wins (Fig 7.44).

Rope Pull

Equipment: Approximately 2m (6'6") of rope, 37mm (1.5") diameter, ends tied together to form circle. Two beanbags.

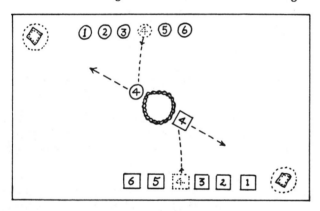

Figure 7.45 Rope pull

Formation: Two teams numbered — ensure that players with the same number are of equal strength. Put rope in a circle in the middle of the playing area and beanbags in chalk circles diagonally opposite to each other.

Directions: When a number is called both players with that number run, take hold of the rope and try to pull each other back to their own team and pick up the beanbag while still holding the rope. The team with the most successes wins (Fig 7.45).

SKILLS LEADING UP TO MINOR AND MAJOR GAMES

Aiming Practices

Aiming at targets of various kinds and with different types of apparatus can be fun. Accurate aiming depends upon quick observation, controlled action, good footwork and co-ordinated movement. The eye should be kept on the target rather than on

the object being kicked, thrown, rolled, hit or pitched, while the follow-through of the kicking leg or throwing arm and the body should also be directed towards the target. Progress can be measured easily and the degree of skill required easily adapted by increasing the distance and decreasing the size of the target.

Many indoor games involve aiming, eg darts, quoits, billiards, skittles, as well as games like bowls, croquet, netball, basketball, football, cricket and ten pin bowling. With imagination many practices can be set up which are valuable as a preparation for these games and sports.

The following are some examples.

1. Roll, throw or pitch a ball towards a small circle drawn at ground level on a wall; field the ball as it rebounds and roll, throw or pitch again. Increase distances (Fig 7.46).

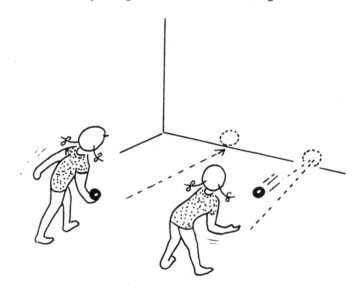

Figure 7.46 Aiming practices at circle on wall

2. Pitch a ball at a skittle 1m (3'3") in front of the wall, field as it rebounds.

3. Throw a ball at a target of several concentric circles painted on a wall - the highest to lowest score from the centre point to the outer circle (Fig 7.47).

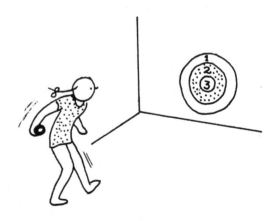

Figure 7.47 Aiming practices at target on wall

4. Draw circles on the floor and throw or slide beanbages or quoits or shuttlecocks onto them (Fig 7.48). Score as for 3.

5. Hang a piece of wood with hooks on it on the wall and throw

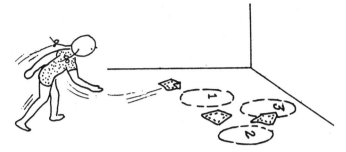

Figure 7.48 Aiming practices at circles on floor

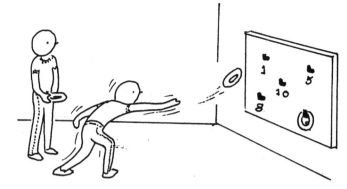

Figure 7.49a Aiming practices at hooks on wall

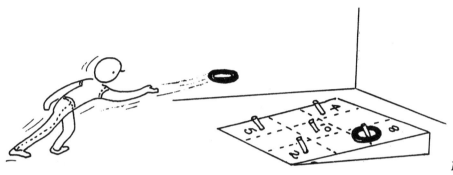

Figure 7.49b Aiming practices at pegs on floor

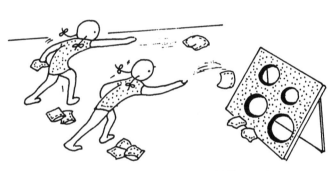

Figure 7.50 Aiming practices at holes of different sizes

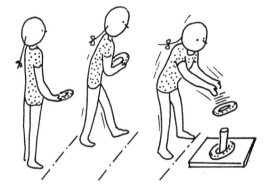

Figure 7.51 Aiming practices over a stump

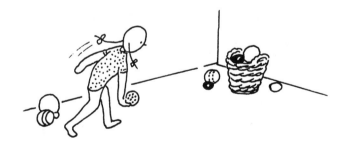

Figure 7.52 Aiming practices at box or basket

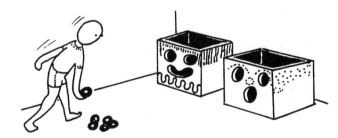

Figure 7.53 Aiming practices at holes in boxes

quoits onto them. Each hook has a different score (Fig 7.49a).

6. As 3 on the floor at an angle (Fig 7.49b).

7. Strong piece of wood 1m (3'3") square, with 5 or 6 holes of different diameter. Each player throws 6 beanbags from a given distance.

Score according to difficulty (size of hole).

Variation: use balls of different size, eg tennis or table tennis.

8. Throw a quoit over a stump from various distances, start by dropping the quoit over the top and gradually moving back step by step (Fig 7.51).

Targets of different colours could be introduced (a) to increase difficulty; (b) in place of number.

9. Throw balls of the same size or of different sizes into a box or basket (Fig 7.52).

10. As 9 but paint faces on the boxes, eg clowns, cowboys, Red

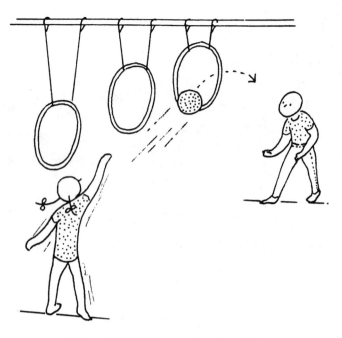

Figure 7.54 Aiming practices through hoop

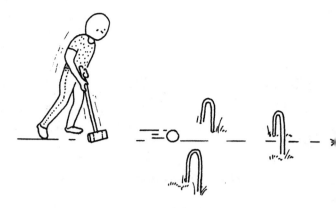

Figure 7.56 Aiming practices with croquet ball

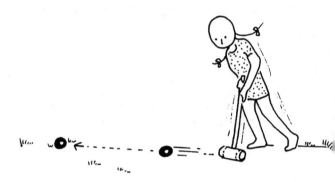

Figure 7.57 Aiming practices with two croquet balls

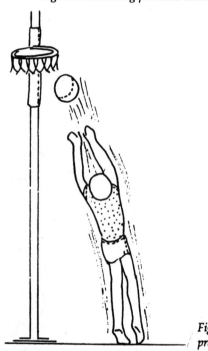

Figure 7.55 Aiming practices into net

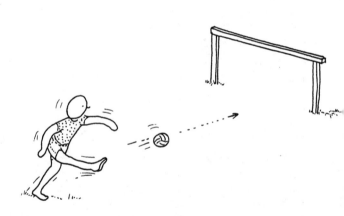

Figure 7.58 Aiming practices with ball through goal posts

Indians, ducks cats, dogs etc. Cut out the mouth and/or eye holes large enough for the size of ball to go through easily. Aim to throw through the mouth or eye holes (Fig 7.53).

11. Throw a ball through a hoop fixed at various heights with a partner (Fig 7.54).

12. Throw a ball into a basketball or netball net (shooting action), from different distances within the shooting area. It is an advantage if the net can be lowered on the post in the early stages of practice (Fig 7.55).

13. Throw or roll a large ball to hit a skittle from 2m (6'6"): gradually increase the distance and decrease the size of the ball.

14. Throw or roll a ball between two skittles at different distances — gradually increase the throwing distance and decrease the distance between the two skittles.

15. Hit a croquet ball with a mallet through a hoop at different distances (Fig 7.56).

16. Hit a croquet ball to hit another croquet ball at different distances (Fig 7.57).

17. Kick a ball through goal posts or marked area the same width from different distances and angles within the football goal area (Fig 7.58).

In pairs

18. A and B face each other with a small chalk circle drawn between them. A pitches ball to B aiming to make it bounce in the circle. B repeats. When 2 or 4 consecutive balls have bounced in the circle, both players move 1 pace backwards. The couple which has successfully pitched at the greatest distance from one another at the finish of the practice is the

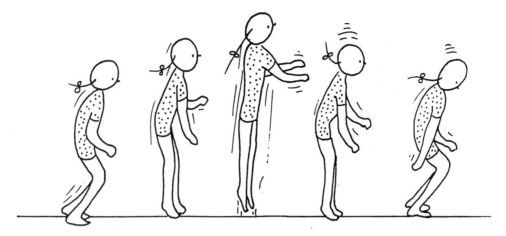

Figure 7.59 Footwork practices - for mobilising and strengthening feet and ankles

winner or scores 1 point each time the ball bounces in the circle.

19. A and B face each other some distance apart, each behind a line, with a skittle between them. A rolls or pitches the ball at the skittle, B fields it and repeats. The couple gaining the greatest number of hits is the winner.

In small groups

20. 4-6 players stand outside a large marked circle. A skittle is placed in the middle of the circle. A ball is thrown across the circle from player to player, on the signal, the player with the ball aims at the skittle. The game continues without a break. The team scoring the highest number of hits is the winner. Alternatively, the throw at the skittle may be made after each 2 or 3 consecutive passes.

21. One basketball or netball ring and 1 football for 4 players. From a given mark or on the run each player shoots in turn, while the other 3 stand round the post ready to jump for the ball if the shot is unsuccessful. Players score 2 points for each goal they shoot and 1 point each time they succeed in holding the ball after having jumped for it.

22. Each team of 4-8 players stand in a circle round a box or basket. Three chalk circles of increasing diameter are marked round the basket at an appropriate distance from it. Each player has 3 beanbags or other small objects. Working at the same time, each player aims to throw the beanbags into the box, one from each circle. If the beanbag misses, it must be collected and thrown again from outside the circle until successful. The team first having all the objects in their basket is the winner.

Footwork Practices

Practically every game involves some movement of the feet - hence the importance of footwork. When waiting to move, whether to catch, field, bat or run a course the player should be alert, ready to move in any direction, eg the sprinter, tennis player or footballer. The feet should be mobile and strong.

For mobilising and strengthening the feet and ankles, with bare feet

1. Small lilting movements both feet together and toes on the ground, gradually increasing to high springs with a rebound. The strong extension in the ankle joint should

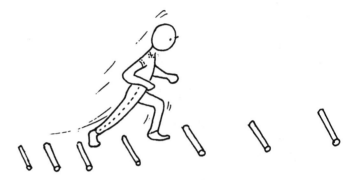

Figure 7.60 Footwork practices - training spring over marked distances

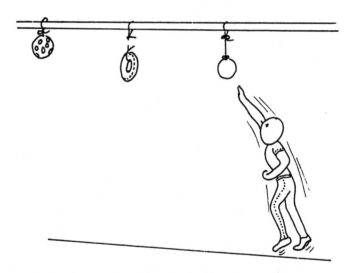

Figure 7.61 Footwork practices - training spring by jumping to touch hanging articles

alternate with relaxation, heels being lowered as far as possible between each rebound (Fig 7.59). (For other footwork exercises see Chapter 11).

For training quick response

1. Spring forward with long strides aiming to cover the ground with a few strides as possible.

2. Run forward on signal, turn and run in the opposite direction or sideways as directed.

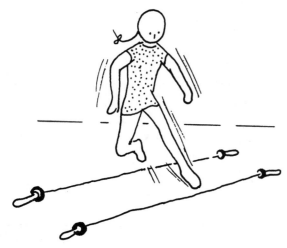

Figure 7.62 Footwork practices - training spring over a widening 'brook'

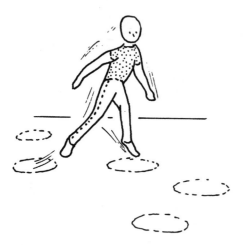

Figure 7.63 Footwork practices - training spring from circle to circle

3. Run forward on signal, jump and land on both feet or one foot followed by the other.

For training spring

1. One the run, spring over marked spaces each wider than the last (Fig 7.60).

2. On the run, jump to touch 3 hanging articles each suspended at a greater height than the last (Fig 7.61).

3. Run and jump a widening 'brook'. Later, spring off alternate feet (Fig 7.62).

4. Step quickly from 1 small chalk circle to another, 6-8 being drawn (not in a straight line). Later, run and jump a set obstacle course, eg spring over 2 chalk lines, step from circle or circle, jump over a rope, run along a form and end with a high spring (Fig 7.63).

Fielding Practices

A good fielder must anticipate when and where to move in order to field a ball. Watch the batsman's movements which will indicate in what direction the ball is likely to be hit. If going for

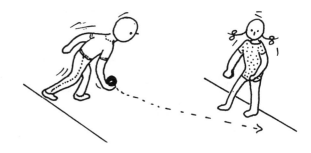

Figure 7.64 Fielding practices in pairs

a catch, fielders should move with arms stretched towards the ball; if going for a low ground drive, they should bend low, hands curved to gather if up to 'throw in'. Later, when more experienced, wide balls, whether they be in the air or on the ground, may be fielded with one hand. The skilful player will learn to gather in or catch and return the ball in one action.

In pairs

1. A pitches or rolls a ball to B and then to either left or right. B moves to cover the ball and returns it with an accurate throw without any break in the action. Later B runs forward or sideways to meet the ball, fielding it on the run.

2. Partners face each other, both with their backs to a wall or marked line. A throws a ball to bounce between them: if the ball passes B and hits the wall or passes over the chalk line, A scores a point. B aims to field the ball so as to prevent it from passing over the line or hitting the wall. Immediately B has fielded it, B pitches it trying to make it pass A. Each player counts his own score (Fig 7.64).

In small groups

3. 4-10 players round a garden roller or other curved surface. One pitches the ball onto the roller, as it will rebound in any direction, all players must be ready and 'on their toes' to receive it. The one who has caught it then pitches it (Fig 7.65).

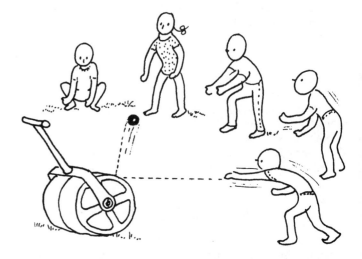

Figure 7.65 Fielding practices in small groups

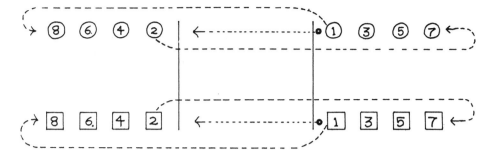

Figure 7.66 Fielding practices - pitch and roll relay

4. Pitch and Roll Relay

Each team 6-8 players divides into 2 files which stand facing each other, some distance apart. No 1 holds a small ball, No 1 pitches or throws the ball to No 2 and then runs forward to stand behind No 8. No 2 keeping the feet behind the line, fields the ball, rolls it to No 3 and runs forward to stand behind No 7. The game continues until all are back in their original places. The ball is always pitched or thrown from one side and rolled from the other. The team to finish first is the winner (Fig 7.66).

Dodging and Marking Practices

Dodging and marking are difficult techniques both to teach and to master; nevertheless, attempts should be made to teach them since they are important skills for many games. Good footwork makes quick adjustment of balance possible while concentration and observation enable the player to observe the position of the ball and the whereabouts and actions of other players (Fig 7.67). Effective dodging and marking can be achieved if:

the marker keeps close to the opponent and anticipates every move;

the dodger makes every effort to outwit the marker;

both are always ready to change from defence to attack.

In addition to the practices given below, those suggested under Footwork and any form of Tag are useful.

For individuals

1. Run fast from side to side of the room or ground; on signal, stop and dodge quickly from side to side once and then continue running.

In pairs

2. B in front of and slightly to one side of A. A moves, at first slowly and then more quickly , in any direction and B tries to keep close to A.

3. A dodges to get away from B. On signal, both players stand still. A scores one point if B cannot touch A. B scores one point if A can be touched. Repeat, B dodging.

In small groups

4. 3-6 players facing the teacher. The teacher dodges in any direction — the group shadow him.

5. 5 players in a space 3 x 3 m (10 x 10'). A and B mark C and D respectively and E is the 'odd' one. E tries to tag. C or D and A and B mark closely to prevent this. When a dodger is tagged, he becomes the 'odd' one and dodgers and markers change place.

6. As (5) E holding ball. E tries to pass to C or D (no overhead passing allowed). When A or B intercept a pass, all change places and the practice continues.

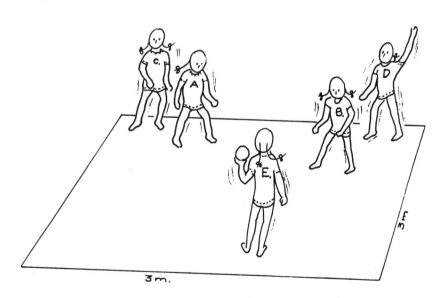

Figure 7.67 Dodging and marking practice

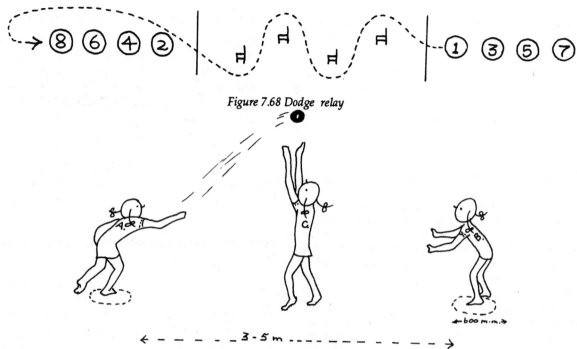

Figure 7.68 Dodge relay

Figure 7.69 Interception practices in chalk circles

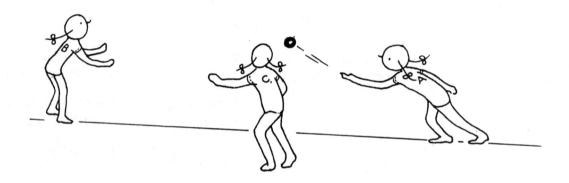

Figure 7.70 Interception practices running forward

7. **Dodge relay.** Each team of 4-8 players divides into 2 half files — odd numbers face even; 3 or 4 chairs are placed in the space between them fairly close together.

    No 1 runs the course dodging the chairs, touches No 2 and runs on to stand behind No 8. Each player has two runs. When No 2 is touched by No 8 after the second turn, No 2 holds up a hand. If any player touches a chair the whole course must be run again (Fig 7.68).

8. **Touch and hand over.** Two teams, red and blue, of 4-10 players in free formation - one football. Reds make as many passes as possible. Blues try to touch Reds. If a Red, whilst holding a ball, is touched by a Blue, the Red hands over the ball to the Blue and the Blue team then passes. Running with the ball is allowed but players should pass the ball as quickly as possible, otherwise they run the risk of being touched. Team leaders count their score aloud and the team making the greater number of consecutive passes is the winner; if the ball is dropped, counting has to re-start at one.

    The area of play must be adapted to the number of players. It should not be too large.

Interception Practices

When intercepting, ie preventing a moving object arriving to a player for whom it is intended, a fielder must anticipate the direction of its flight and accurately judge when to move, so as to outwit the opponent; try looking at the player with the ball or object you want to intercept.

In small groups

1. In threes — A and B standing in chalk circles 600 mm (2') in diameter and 3-5m (10'-16'3") apart, and C at mid-point. A and B pass a ball or beanbag to each other — they may use any type of throw but must have one foot in the circle when receiving the ball. C tries to intercept; if successful, C changes places with the player who threw the ball (Fig 7.69).

2. Four players stand some distance apart, A and B being partners, C and D being partners. A holding a quoit tries to throw it over a short stick held by B. C and D try to intercept the throw. If B catches the quoit, it is thrown back to A. When the quoit is intercepted the couples change over.

3. A and B stand 3-5m (10'-16'3") apart, C between them. A and B throw the object one to the other — C tries to intercept. If successful, change places as in (1).

4. As (3), but C stands back from A and B. C runs forward to intercept as the object is passed from A to B (Fig 7.70).

    If successful, change places as in (1).

Hitting Practices (Bat, Racquet or Stick)

Keep the eye on the ball from the moment it has started on its flight towards the hitter until it is actually hit. Feet easily apart. Hit with the centre of the bat, racquet or stick. Keep the bat away from the body (no tucked in elbows). Stand sideways with left shoulder pointing in the direction in which the ball is to travel (right-handed hitter). Grip the hitting implement lightly at first, but firmly as contact is made with the ball; the hitting implement should be regarded and felt as an extension of the arm. With a preparatory swing backward, the arm slightly bent, the weight is transferred onto the back foot, so that the weight of the body may be put into the hit, the arm and body following through in the direction in which the ball is to travel.

For training the ability to watch the ball onto the hand, bat, racquet or stick

1. Pat bounce a small ball downwards with stick or bat, left and right hands alternately: vary the height of the bounce.

2. As (1) pat ball upwards.

3. As (1) pat ball alternately upwards and downwards.

4. (1-3) on the move walking — running.

5. Bat ball against a wall, let it bounce and bat it back against wall.

6. As (5) without letting the ball bounce.

7. Pat bouncing between two players, at first allow ball to bounce twice and later one bounce — see which couple has the highest score of consecutive single bounces.

8. Hit ball to a partner across a net, rope or bench.

9. One ball and one bat or stick between three players. A fieldsman stands behind the hitter, the bowler 3m (10') away. The bowler bowls underarm — the batsman stops (not hits) the ball with the bat, stick or hand — the aim being to watch the ball right onto it. After 6 balls players change places.

10. As (9) but batsman hits the ball.

It is sometimes an advantage to hit a ball back and forward over a low net or against a wall with the hand before using an implement.

For training the adjustment of the stance so that the ball may be hit in any direction

Stand sideways, left shoulder towards wall. Throw ball up with left hand and hit with right hand. Practise hitting the ball in different directions by altering the stance so that the left shoulder points towards the direction in which you want the ball to travel. Let ball bounce, on its rebound hit it again: progress to use a stick, bat or racquet. Aim to hit the ball accurately rather than strongly.

For training the specific batting action of the game to be played

1. Practise the swing the follow through of the batting section with the appropriate implement — racquet, bat or stick.

2. In small groups 4 or 5 — 1 bowler, 1 batsman, I fielder (back-stop) behind the batsman and 2 or more deep fielders. The backstops of each group stand in the circumference of a circle — backs to the centre some distance away from each other (Fig 7.71).

Batting practice

The batsman varies the stance in order to place the hits in different directions.

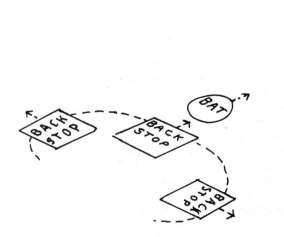

Figure 7.71 Organisation of batting practices

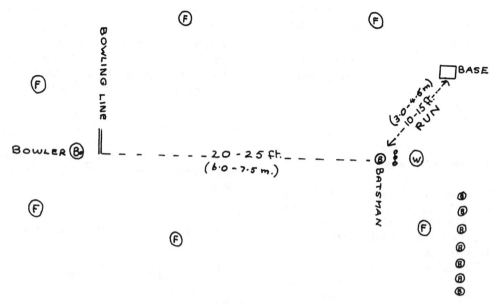

Figure 7.72 Non-stop cricket

SAFETY

During any hitting practice, consider the positioning of the players in relation to the flight of the ball. All practices must be carefully organised and controlled.

EXAMPLES OF MINOR GAMES

Non-stop Cricket

Equipment: One rounders or stoolball bat, one ball (tennis, rounders or stoolball), one wicket approximately 305mm (1') high and 229mm (9") wide, and one base (chalk mark or object).

Formation: Two teams of 6-11 players. The base is marked or placed 3-4.5m (10-15') obliquely behind the wicket, and a bowling line is drawn 6-7.5m (20-25') in front of the wicket. The batsmen line up at the side of the playing area. No 1 ready in front of the wicket; of the fielding team, the bowler stands toeing the bowling line, the wicket-keeper stands behind the wicket, and the remainder position themselves over the pitch (Fig 7.72).

Game: The bowler bowls the ball underarm, close to the ground. The batsman, guarding the wicket with the bat, hits at the ball; if the ball is not hit, the bowler re-bowls. When the ball is hit, the batsman turns and runs to touch the base behind the wicket and returns to the wicket, thus scoring one run. Meanwhile, the ball having been fielded is returned to the bowler who immediately bowls again, whether or not the batsman has got back to the wicket.

The batsman is 'out' by being:

1. bowled or caught;

2. playing on (knocks down the wicket);

3. obstructs a fielder;

4. hit on the leg by a bowled ball while defending the wicket — lbw.

When out the player immediately drops the bat and the No 2 of the batting team takes over.

Whilst this change is being made, the bowler may continue to bowl at the wicket; if it is hit the new batsman is 'out'. The games continues until all players of the batting team are 'out', when the teams change over. The team making the most runs is the winner.

NB. Leave out the lbw rule until it is understood.

Coaching points:

1. The batsmen should place their hits between the fields; backward hits are allowed.

2. Fielders should return the ball quickly to the bowler, who should bowl immediately it is received.

3. To prevent the slowing up of the game, the following rule can be made: if a batsman fails to hit the third ball bowled the batsman is out and the next batsman runs in.

Change Hockey

Equipment: 2 Unihoc sticks, 1 air flow ball.

Formation: Two teams of 8-12 players. Two goal lines are drawn,

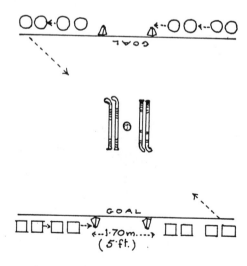

Figure 7.73 Change hockey

one at each end of the playing area, and a goal 1.70m (6') wide is marked by chairs/skittles in the middle of each. The players stand in twos behind their own goal line and the ball and the four sticks are placed in the centre of the pitch.

Game: The right hand couple of each team run out, pick up the sticks and try to hit the ball through their opponents' goal. When the umpire calls 'change' the playing couples drop their sticks and return to the left-hand end of their own teams, whilst couples then standing at the right-hand ends run to the pitch and continue the game without waiting for a further signal. If, after the word 'change' has been called, the ball continues rolling of its own accord and passes between the goal posts before the new defending couple can prevent it, a goal is allowed. After a goal has been scored the game is re-started with the sticks and ball in the centre of the pitch. When all the players have had one (or two) turns, the teams change ends. The team scoring most number of goals is the winner (Fig 7.73).

Rules:

1. Dangerous play must not be allowed.

   Penalty: A free shot at goal taken by one of the opposing couples from where the offence occurrred.

2. On the word 'change!' the playing couples must stop at once, dropping their sticks exactly where they stand.

3. Kicking is not allowed.

   Penalty: A free pass taken by one of the opposing couples from where the offence occurred. This hit may not be taken at goal.

4. Players standing behind the base line must not interfere with play.

NB. Too strict adherence to hockey rules will slow up the game and spoil its spirit.

Change Mat Ball

No of players: 2 teams of 6-11 players.

Equipment: 1 football and 2 fibre mats: if mats are not available, 2 circles, 1.20m (4') in diameter, can be used.

Formation: The play area is a rectangle 21 x 12m (70 x 40') divided into two equal parts, A smaller area should be used for teams smaller in number, 18 x 9m (60 x 30'). The mats (circles) are placed at each end. One player, the catcher, stands on the mat (or in the circle). Teams play towards their own catcher. The players position themselves as for hockey or football (Fig 7.74).

Game: The ball is thrown vertically between the two centre players. Each team then passes the ball between their players until it can be thrown to their own catcher by means of a clear pass, ie the ball must not strike the floor in flight between the thrower and the catcher, thus scoring one point. Immediately the catcher receives the ball, he bounces it out into the field of play. Once it has touched the ground it is deemed to be in play, but it may not be touched by any player until it has bounced. The catcher, having thrown the ball into the field of play, immediately changes place with the thrower and the game continues without a break.

Rules:

1. No player other than the catcher may step on to the mat (or into the circle).

   Penalty: For an offence by (i) an attacker, a free pass to the defending team, taken from the edge of the mat; (ii) a defender, a free pass taken by the catcher of the opposing team.

2. No player may run more than three steps whilst holding the ball, or hold it for longer than three seconds.

   Penalty: A free pass to the opposing team taken from where the foul occurred. This free pass may not be made direct to the catcher.

3. No rough play, eg barging or kicking is allowed.

   Penalty: A free pass to the opposing team from where the offence occurred. This pass may, if desired, by made direct to the catcher and a point scored from it.

Coaching points:

1. Players should mark their own opponents and should use the whole space available.

2. Encourage players to pass and run into a space.

Danish Rounders

Equipment: 1 rounders or tennis ball and a rounders stick or small bat (hand may be used in place of bat).

Formation: 2 teams of 6-15 players. The playing area is a square (or rectangle) with sides of approximately 12-15m (40-50')

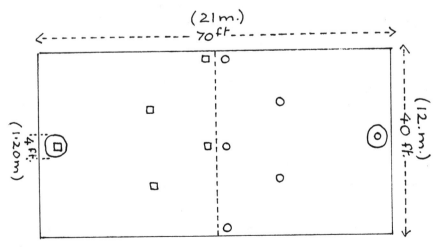

Figure 7.74 Change mat ball

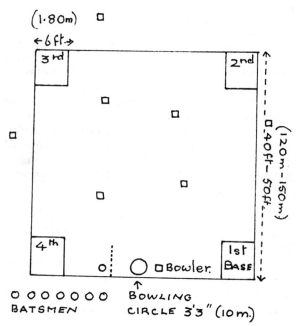

Figure 7.75 Danish rounders

(boundary lines need not be drawn), a base 1.80 x 1.80m (6 x 6') being marked at each corner: a bowling circle 1m (3'3") in diameter is drawn between first and fourth bases, and the batting line 1m (3'3") from the bowling circle is at right angles to the side line. The batsmen line up behind fourth base; the fielders position themselves in the square and in the deep field, the bowler standing on the side of the bowling circle further from the batting line (Fig 7.75).

Game: The bowler bowls by throwing the ball almost vertically upwards between himself and the batsman, to a height of approximately 1.80m (6'). No 1 of the batting team, standing on the batting line, hits at the ball with his hand or closed fist and, whether or not he hits it, immediately runs to first base: he may continue running onto the other bases unless the bowler, holding the ball, touches the ground in the bowling circle and calls 'stop'. If he is between two bases when 'stop' is called, he is out. Batsman No 2 takes his turn as soon as the bowler has the ball, and the game continues until all the batsmen are 'out'. The two teams then change over.

A batsman scores a rounder each time he gets to fourth base having hit the ball, and a half-rounder if he completes the course without having hit the ball. Any number of batsmen may be in the same base at one time; batsmen may also pass one another when running between the bases. The team scoring the greater number of rounders is the winner.

Rules:

1. If, from a hit, the ball is caught by a fielder, the batsman who made the hit and any other batsman running between the bases when the catch is made are 'out'.

2. All batsmen who are between the bases when the bowler shouts 'Stop' are 'out'.

3. The ball may not be hit behind the line forming fourth and first bases.

   Penalty: the batsman who made the hit is 'out'.

4. If there is no batsman waiting for his turn, the bowler throws the ball vertically upwards to a height not less than 1.80m (6') to give one of the batsmen in the field of play a chance to get to fourth base before the ball falls to the ground: if no batsman succeeds the whole side is 'out'.

5. One ball only is bowled to a batsman unless a 'no ball' be given: a good ball is one which, if it fell to the ground, would land within the bowling circle.

Coaching points:

1. In a beginners' game, batsmen may be allowed to get to first base without being put 'out'.

2. The bowler should remain close to the bowling circle so that he is ready to receive the ball from the fielders. When players are quite new to the game, it is helpful if the teacher bowls, as he can then control the game.

3. The batsman must run outside the bowler on his way to first base.

4. Batsmen should be coached to place their hits, and fielders to make a quick return of the ball to the bowler.

Variation: The game can be adapted for use indoors. If the space is long and narrow, first and third bases only may be marked, chairs being placed where the other two bases would normally be; the runners must run round the chairs on their way to the bases, but may only stop at the bases proper. For this variation, two teams of 6 or 7 players make a good game.

Floor Handball

Equipment: 1 football and coloured bands (a lighter ball can be used).

Formation: 2 teams of 6-10 players. The playing area is a rectangle, with a goal line 1m (3'3") inside each of the end boundaries; the side walls may be used as side boundaries. If the playing space is very wide, or if there are not sufficient players to have more than one goalkeeper, goals of approximately 2.7m (9') in width should be marked off in the centre of each goal line. One player from each team stands in the centre of the pitch with the left shoulder towards the opponents' goal; one, two or three, according to the size of the area and the number of players, serve as goalkeepers and stand between the goal line and the end boundary; and the remainder position themselves in their own half of the pitch (Fig 7.76).

Game: The game is started by a 'bully off' between the two centre players, each using her right hand. The players of each team then

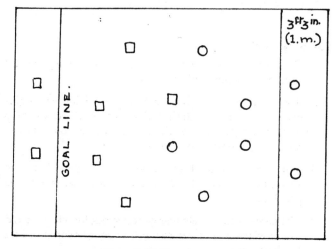

Figure 7.76 Floor handball

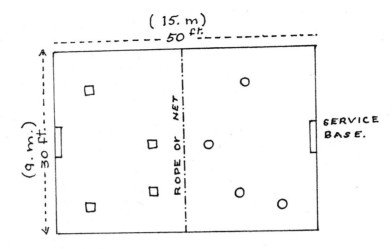

Figure 7.77 Team hand tennis

aim to pass and dribble the ball towards their opponents' goal line. The ball must be kept on the floor; both hands may be used to stop it, but, when hitting, players may use only one hand at a time. After a goal is scored, ie when the ball passes over the goal line or between the goal posts, if marked, the game is re-started from the centre. After a given time, the two teams change ends. The team scoring the most goals is the winner.

Rules:

1. The ball may not be kicked, nor may it be propelled by any part of the body except one hand.

2. No player may pick up the ball or raise it off the ground when hitting.

3. Rough play is not permitted.

   Penalty: For an infringement of any of the above rules, a free hit is taken by a player of the opposing team from where the offence occurrence. This hit may not be made direct at goal.

4. No player, except the goalkeeper, may cross the goal line (the goalkeeper is allowed to move forward into the field of play).

   Penalty: For any offence by: (i) a defender, a free shot at goal, taken by one of the attacking team., standing 3.65m (12') from the goal line; (ii) an attacker, a free hit by one of the opposing goalkeepers, from where the offence occurred.

5. No goal is allowed if the ball, when it passes over the line or between the posts, is off the ground.

Coaching points:

1. Players in the field may move anywhere on the pitch and should be encouraged to combine.

2. The goalkeeper may pick up the ball when it is behind his own line and place it at the point from which he wishes to hit it out into the field of play; it must be hit from between the end boundary and the goal line.

3. When there is more than one goalkeeper, they should be encouraged to interchange and work together behind the goal line.

4. The game is extremely energetic, especially when played in a small space, and should not, therefore, be continued for too long a period.

Team Hand Tennis

Equipment: 1 small ball and 1 rope or badminton net.

Formation: 4-6 players. The maximum size of the court, which should be adapted to suit the play area available and the number and skill of the players, is 15 x 9m (50x30'); the side and back lines may be marked with chalk, or the natural boundaries of the hall may be used. A small serving base is marked on each of the back lines and the rope or net is stretched across the centre of the court 1.20m -1.50m (4-5') from the ground. The players divide themselves equally between the two sides of the court (Fig 7.77).

Game: The server bounces the ball within the service base and then, with the palm of the hand, hits it over the net and into his opponents, court or, alternatively, to one of his partners who may be standing nearer to the net. After the first server has served 5 times consecutively, the service is taken by a player on the opposite side; when the first team regains the service, another player acts as server.

Rules:

1. The ball is in play and may be returned over the next as long as it is still bouncing. It is 'dead' only when it has rolled along the ground or has been hit into or under the net.

2. The ball may be batted with the palm of the hand, but must not be fisted or knocked. It is permissible to bat the ball up into the air to control it and then to allow another player who is better placed to bat is across the net.

3. Only one service is allowed; if it is faulty the server's opponents score one point, if scoring method (ii) is being followed.

Scoring: (two alternative methods)

1. As in lawn tennis.

2. The first team to reach a certain number of points, or the team making the higher score after five minutes' play on both sides of the net, is the winner.

GAMES WITH A DIFFERENCE

Batington

General description of the game. Batington is a combination between the games of badminton and tennis, using a large table tennis or beach ball type of bat, and a badminton shuttlecock. It is played in an area similar to that of a badminton court by two or more players.

Equipment: A bat approx. 305mm (12") long and circular in shape, a shuttlecock, a badminton net with two posts to support the net, a previously marked out course.

Game: The game can be played by severely handicapped and more able people, consequently the rules of the game can be varied and the equipment can be made smaller or larger. The game can be played competitively or as a general fitness exercise. Two or any number can play as long as the size of the area allows enough space for the players to move safely and easily.

The game is started by the toss of a coin, the winner serves, if he misses he does not have a second try — opponents serve. If the shuttlecock falls out of the playing area or does not fall in the opponent's area, the service is lost.

In doubles, the same rules and scoring apply, apart from the service which is taken alternatively by the team. A game can consist of 11 or more points. Scoring as for table tennis is recommended in the early stages.

Coaching points:

1. Discuss the game with the players. Let them handle the equipment.
2. Introduce bat and shuttlecock and begin to practise. Develop co-ordination between bat and shuttlecock.
3. Introduce partner and then practise hitting over the net.
4. Gradually introduce the rules and scoring.

It is a game for all players and is easy to learn. It helps to build up speed and can be played competitively or just as a fun game.

It can be played with simplified rules, inside or out, and can be played with two or any number of players depending on the size of the area.

Boccia

Boccia (pronouced as the slang English term 'gotcha') is a favourite Italian pastime. It is descended from the Greek ball-tossing games. A game similar to Boccia was played throughout the Roman Empire and later developed into such variants as lawn bowling, nine pins and boules.

Boccia is played in a bordered area. Each player tries to position his balls as close as possible to the target ball (jack). The game can be played by two people or teams of three players. Before the game begins, one of the players flips a coin to see which player bowls the target ball. If the first shot does not qualify, players or teams take turns to bowl the target ball until it lands in the proper area. The player who makes the successful shot begins the game. After all balls have been played the score is tallied. All balls closer to the target ball than the opponents' best ball score one point apiece. Opposing balls that are equidistant from the target ball cancel each other from the scoring.

The ball being of solid but pliable nature, with a kinetic and rolling quality, often allows those with a more severe functional disability the opportunity to grip the ball more easily. It also has the effect of reducing the advantage of physical strength, so that

skill becomes a more important factor than pure brute force. However, a player can also propel the ball into court by any manner he or she desires, as long as they are in control at the movement of release. Some players throw or kick the ball, others may use specifically designed devices, such as ramps.

Equipment: Twelve leather covered balls, six of one colour and six of another colour, and one white target ball are used. All balls must weigh between 273 and 277 grams and be 26.3 - 26.7cms ($10\,^{3}/_{8}$ -$10\,^{1}/_{2}$) in circumference.

Game: Before anyone begins to learn how to play Boccia it is imperative that they, either through self experimentation or with the assistance of a teacher, coach or parent, discover the most suitable method for them to propel the ball, be this via hand, foot or other device. Often the first discovered method can be improved upon with experimentation.

Having discovered the best method of ball delivery, the game must be introduced to groups at an appropriate level for that particular person or group.

Skill practices: When learning to play Boccia or considering how to introduce it to players, it is essential to think about enjoyment. Skill development can be enjoyable so, as well as aiming at the target ball, other practices can be used to add variety, which also have a direct relationship to skill development. Bean bags are good alternatives to Boccia balls for initial practices. Players can graduate to Boccia balls, which are fairly expensive, when they have developed some expertise in target practice and in experimenting in various ways of projecting their bean bag — underarm, overarm or by using their feet. These activities may be undertaken standing or sitting but all must sit if one player needs to do it sitting because of disability.

Specific practices:

1. Many of the target practices on pages 42-45 are appropriate in developing concentration and eye/hand co-ordination.
2. Project the beanbag/Boccia ball within the target area. Adapt the size of the target area and the distance from which players aim according to their ability (Fig 7.78).

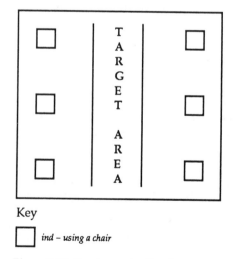

Key

☐ *ind – using a chair*

Figure 7.78 Boccia — adapting the target area

3. Progress from the previous practice to projecting the bean bag/ball on to a specific *line*

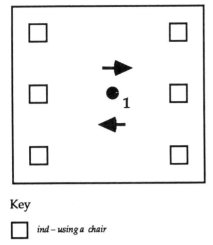

Key

☐ *ind – using a chair*

Figure 7.79 Boccia — hitting the target ball

4. Aim: to hit target ball (1) past the line made by the castors of the oppositions' wheelchairs (see Fig 7.79). Members of the group who are not playing act as feeders to return Boccia balls to their own team as quickly as possible.

Variations:

1. Variations of size and weight of target balls, ie beach ball — soccer ball — volley ball — Boccia jack.

2. Restrict number of Boccia balls on either side.

3. Increase number of target balls.

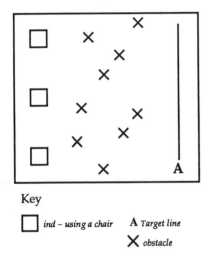

Key

☐ *ind – using a chair*   A *Target line*
✕ *obstacle*

Figure 7.80 Boccia— specific practice with obstacles

4. Aim: To get Boccia balls to line marked A without knocking over obstacles (x). A points system can be devised if appropriate (see Fig 7.80)

Information on Boccia has been supplied by the Spastics Society from whom further information can be obtained: c/o Leisure Services Department, Stephenson House, Brunel Centre, Bletchley, Milton Keynes. MK2 2EW.

Equipment with rules book can be purchased from: the Spastics Society, c/o Newton Products, Meadway Works, Garrets Green Lane, Birmingham B33 0SQ.

The Game of Petanque

Petanque has been played for many centuries in various forms and is now popular in Britain. The joy of petanque is that it can be played by anyone, anywhere and almost at any time. The game can be played by men, women, children, young and old. It can be played on gravel (ideal), grass, tarmac, smooth or rough ground.

No of players: Two teams of two or three players. In teams of two, each player has three boules; in teams of three, each player has two boules.

Equipment: Metal or plastic boules, diameter between 70-80mm ($2^3/4$-$3^1/4$"), weight not to exceed 800gm. ($1^3/4$ lb). The marker ball (cochonet) is wooden, diameter between 25mm (*1*") and 30mm ($1^1/5$ ").

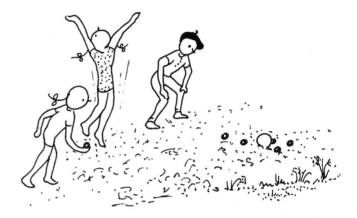

Figure 7.81 Petanque

Game: The starting team is decided by the toss of a coin (Fig 7.81).

1. The first thrower throws the cochonnet between 6m (20') and 10m(33') away, not nearer than 2m (6") from any obstacle (wall tree etc).

2. He then throws his first boule trying to place it as near as possible to the cochonnet.

3. A player in the other team then comes into the circle and tries to throw his boule nearer to the cochonnet, or knock away the leading boule. The boule nearest to the cochonnet leads.

4. It is then up to a player in the team not leading to throw until his team gets a leading boule, and so on.

5. When a team has no more boules the players of the other team throw theirs and try to place them as close as possible to the cochonnet.

6. When both teams have no more boules the points are counted. The winning team gets as many points as it has boules nearer to the cochonnet than the best of the losing team.

7. A player of the winning team throws the cochonnet from where it is, and the game starts again until one team reaches 13 points.

Unihoc

Among others, unihoc is a game which can be easily adapted to the mental and physical ability of people with a mental handicap.

Members of the Alton Adult Training Centre (among others) have played unihoc since 1977. The manager says: 'When asked to enumerate the pros and cons of unihoc, I have found it all

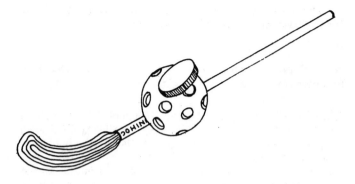

Figure 7.82 Unihoc stick, ball and puck

advantages. At a cost of £30.00 unihoc is the least expensive of the games introduced into the Centre'.

Alton found that more trainees could play unihoc successfully, but that teams must be carefully balanced. Space is not a limiting factor and the game can be played on any surface, indoors or outdoors. The sticks are not rigid and neither they, nor the ball, can hurt anyone struck accidentally.

Unihoc is not a formal game and therefore can be played 'instantly'. As it is easily set up and has immediate impact (it gets going quickly) less active and/or older staff members are just as able to organise and participate.

Presentation: Trainees who have played team games like football and netball can be talked through the rules and be taught to apply them as the game progresses. At the same time the teacher can explain how they should help the less able who may eventually be part of their team.

For the less able trainees at Alton, unihoc was broken down into its component parts:

1. hitting and stopping the ball;
2. passing the ball;
3. tackling;
4. scoring goals;
5. team and competitive play.

This method of presentation has proved successful and there

have been no injury or fear problems providing the less mobile are not indiscriminately mixed with the over active.

Several methods of play have been devised: these range from six-a-side games in the dining hall with upturned tables used as barriers (with all non-players cheering behind them) through use of a larger space at the Sports Centre to twelve-a-side games on the sports field.

The Manager concludes: 'There are innumerable combinations and adaptions of size, abilities, speeds and settings. Such has been the spread of the game since Alton started playing, that we feel it is the most complete game available, especially in the field of physical education, for people with a mental handicap'.

Many other centres, hospitals and clubs are playing unihoc.

No of players: Two teams of six players.

Equipment: 1 set of unihoc, 12 sticks. Air flow balls or standard size, or pucks (Fig 7.82).

Formation: Any size play area from a small gymnasium to a hockey pitch, eg 40 x 20m, 60 x 30m (123 x 66', 200 x 100'). The game can be played on both smaller or larger. The goals should be placed 1.5m (5') from the walls allowing play to continue behind the goal as in ice hockey (Fig 7.83).

Scoring: As in ice hockey or hockey each goal counts one. The team scoring the most goals is the winner.

Game: To start bully off or a 'centre stroke'. All players must be standing in their own half.

> *Bully off:* The referee drops the ball between the stick heads of each team centre forward. Each player must endeavour to hit the ball into their opponents' half. Play then continues as normal.
>
> *Centre stroke:* The centre forward passes the ball to a team member. Opponents should be 3m (10') from the centre spot.

Rules:

A player may

1. Pass and accept a pass irrespective of his own, his team mates' and his opponents' positions.

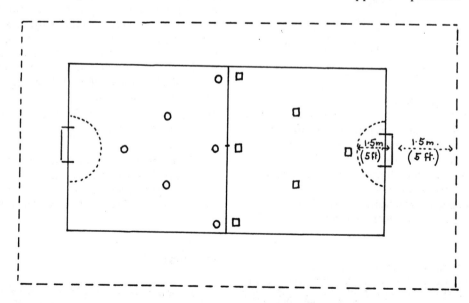

Figure 7.83 Unihoc - plan of court

2. Stop or intercept the ball with any part of the body provided that the manoeuvre is to himself.

3. Shield the ball from opponents with the body and/or stick.

4. Play against the side or back walls as in ice hockey or 5-a-side football.

A player may not

1. Kick, trip, tackle, push or charge with any part of the body or stick.

2. Pass or move the ball in any way with anything other than the stick.

3. Raise the stick above the knee, nor use it to trip an opponent or throw it at either an opponent or the ball.

4. Kneel or lie on the floor in such a way that he prevents an opponent from passing or shooting.

When the rules are broken, the referee may award a free shot (or if possible play to the advantage rule).

Free shot: Where a free shot is awarded, the members of the opposing team must be 3m (10') away from the ball. When the rules are broken within a 3m (10') radius of the goal, a penalty should be awarded.

Penalty shot: Must be taken from a distance not less than 7m (23') from the goal. The goal must be unguarded. All players other than the player taking the penalty must be at least 2m (6'6'') behind the ball.

It is recommended that unihoc be played without a goal-keeper but for those who wish to play with one — the following rules are added.

1. The goal should be larger — a small size 5-a-side soccer goal.

2. The goalkeeper plays with a stick and is allowed to stop and catch the ball within the goal area using his stick or any part of his body.

3. The goalkeeper may throw the ball to the members of his team, but it must bounce at least once in his own half. Alternatively, the goalkeeper may not pass the ball out of the goal by any other means than using the unihoc stick.

4. In the event of a penalty, the goalkeeper must remain on the line until the ball has been hit. The penalty is taken from a minimum distance of 4m (13') from the goal line.

Unihoc equipment can be purchased from; CG Davies & Son, The Sports People, 17 Ludlow Hill Road, West Bridgford, Nottingham NG2 6HD.

Unicurl

Unicurl and short tennis (see below) and their respective equipment have been developed by the same manufacturers that developed unihoc. The benefits are similar. First and foremost they provide very quickly achievable activities.

Unicurl is a form of carpet curling — with a target as in the iced version. There are two sizes of 'stone' so that players need not be muscular in order to play the game. Whilst the equipment is relatively expensive, it has a 20-year guarantee!

Short tennis

The rules of short tennis can be adapted easily to suit the abilities of the players. Very skilled players who began with the unitennis light-weight plastic rackets and soft sponge balls have progressed to the full scale Wimbledon variety.

The rules of short tennis can be obtained from: the Lawn Tennis Association, Palliser Road, London W14 9EG.

Boomerangs

Whilst playing with boomerangs may seem to be rather a novel activity it does have three main advantages when viewed from the point of view of the adult person with a mental handicap. Firstly, boomerangs can be made cheaply from plywood in a workshop or craft centre. This of course creates an initital interest and also provides a great deal of satisfaction — irrespective of the level of craftsmanship — when the varnished boomerang is ready to throw. Secondly, everyone learning to throw a boomerang will have to learn to judge distances, the amount of effort needed for the throw and learn the right 'feel' of the release. The third benefit is that throwing a bommerang will probably involve a considerable amount of additional physical activity in chasing and 'running away' from the curling boomerangs.

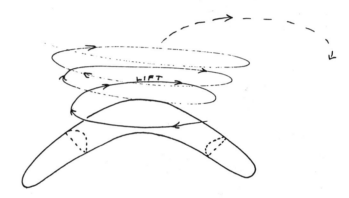

Figure 7.84 Boomerang

Throwing techniques: Throwing is best attempted in a large space like a park or field as bommerangs can get carried considerable distances by the wind. The thrower should be positioned so that he faces into the wind/breeze with the throwing direction at approximately 30°-45° to the right (for right handers). The best grip is the first-club grip, all fingers wrapped around one lower end of the boomerang. It can be launched with the hand forwards or backwards. Perhaps one of the best ways of launching the boomerang after the best throwing arm and grip has been sorted out is to tell the thrower to throw the boomerang straight at the top of a 1.8m (6') high stake placed in the ground about 20m (66') from the thrower. The result should be that the boomerang on nearing the upright post will turn sharply leftwards and upwards high in an arc before descending and turning and thus back towards the left side. All very theoretical of course! However, by trial and error the right angle of throw and effort can very soon be worked out (Fig 7.84).

Construction: The best way is to obtain a proto-type and copy it exactly — especially the angles on the surfaces so that the right aerodynamics will result. Also, B Ruhe's *The boomerang book* (see Further Reading p 64 has excellent illustrations and ideas.

Frisbees

Once a new craze in the USA and now a feature of any English park scene, these colourful plastic 'saucer top' objects are par-

particuarly suitable for use in a physical education/recreation session with people with a mental handicap (Fig 7.85). They are cheap, easy to store and do not break windows! Whilst they can be thrown very hard and over considerable distances their big asset is that they can also be launched with very little effort into a 10m (33') flight to a friend. On such occasions their relatively slow hovering speed makes them easy to monitor for the catching /fielding partner. For this reason many pairs find it a very satisfying activity for a short period — twenty minutes or so.

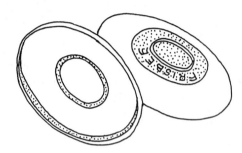

Figure 7.85 Frisbees

After a degree of ability has been developed throwing a frisbee can be made into a game by:

1. trying to throw it so that your partner doesn't have to move to catch or touch it;

2. trying to get it to land or skim through your partner's outstretched legs;

3. aiming at a wall target or hoop on the floor;

4. or just going for distance.

Most of these games with boomerangs and frisbees can be played in a small gym or hall, but any institution or club could help those interested in the games to develop their skill by providing opportunities for them to be used in the break times throughout the day. In addition this interest could be fostered at home if a member of the family was prepared to take part in a fifteen minute activity session in the evening in the garden.

Coaching points:

1. Hold the frisbee with the index finger along the outer edge, thumb on top, other fingers supporting underneath.

2. Make sure the frisbee is level with the floor or ground before, and **as**, it is thrown.

3. Bend the arm and push (to start off with) the frisbee in the direction you want it to go.

4. Follow through so your wrist and fingers point to where the frisbee is to go.

5. Do not swing the arm too vigorously right across the body during the throwing action.

Frisbee golf

Equipment: Frisbees.

Formation: Design a course, according to space available. Map out the holes, including dog legs, hazards etc.

Directions: Using standard golf rules, each player tries to reach the hole in the least number of frisbee throws.

Circle frisbee

No of players 3-12.

Formation: Circle

Directions: Players throw their frisbees to anyone in the circle trying to catch the other player 'off guard'. Start with one or two frisbees and gradually increase the number.

GAMES WITH A PARACHUTE

The parachute is a most versatile piece of apparatus which can give endless pleasure to a group of any ability whether it is used indoors or out-of-doors. It generates fun as much for the helpers as for the players.

Care and safety

1. Only the canopy is used. Construction of parachutes varies. Some parachutes have nylon cords crossing over at the centre. It is usually best to remove them so that when heads pop through the central hole there is no risk of cords constricting the neck.

2. When the parachute is resting on the floor indoors the surface can be very slippery. Do not let people walk on it; they may already lack confidence in balance and need protecting from that kind of hazard.

3. Like all synthetic materials, parachute material can give rise to friction burns. The popular tag game called Japs is the one where leaders need to be sure that the elbow/hand/head, if in direct contact, is covered before moving fast under the canopy.

4. *Never* toss a child up and down on the parachute.

5. Store the parachute in a bag away from direct sunlight.

How to get a parachute

1. Contact the 'Services' eg a local RAF base. Any enquiry should always provide evidence that it is being made on behalf of an organisation caring for people with a handicap. Let them know you would be grateful for an old parachute. The Services are very willing to help the community if they have the resources to do so, but do not be discouraged if there is some delay in getting a response.

2. Some good Army and Navy Stores can obtain a second-hand parachute.

3. Parachutes can be obtained commercially through some education suppliers.

4. If these contacts fail, try New Games UK, 18 Elmthorpe Road, Wolvercote, Oxford, which sometimes has ex Ministry of Defence parachutes.

General guidelines

Initially, spread the parachute out on the floor — most are circular in shape. Then invite the group to sit on the floor/chairs or stand round the edge and pick up the chute. This circle formation helps the group to feel they are a family and many find it easier to relate to each other through holding the parachute than by having direct hand contact with each other.

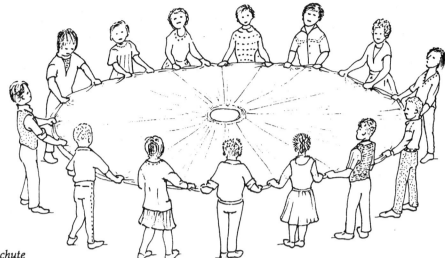

Figure 7.86 Over-grasping the parachute

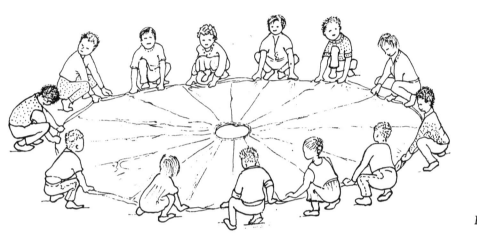

Figure 7.87 Sealing the parachute

Encourage an overgrasp from the start because, when lifting the parachute high up, this is essential (Fig 7.86).

The number that can play at any one time depends on the size of the parachute and the type of activities being undertaken. To ensure the maximum inflation of the parachute, numbers need to be limited to prevent too much tension on the nylon; tension can be lessened if the players take a few steps towards the centre when lifting.

For convenience, games can be grouped under three headings; but classification soon becomes irrelevant as leaders learn to invent their own games and activities appropriate to their particularly circumstances.

Games of co-operation and 'getting to know'

Introductory activities

All face the centre holding the parachute in both hands with waist height overgrasp grip.

1. On command, shake the parachute vigorously - 'stop'.

2. In contrast, quieten the group by creating gentle waves.

3. Walk round in the circle with changes of direction.

4. Run round in the circle with changes of direction holding the parachute with the nearest hand only.

5. All face the centre, pull the parachute taut.

6. Lift the parachute as high as possible 'Who is on the opposite side?'

7. Lift the parachute, call out one person by name to go under the canopy, popping their head through the centre hole as the parachute comes down.

8. Lift — call out the names of two people who exchange places crossing under the canopy.

When this idea has been well established, many variations can develop according to the participants' ability to understand. For example:

Lift — All wearing glasses cross over

— All wearing red cross over

— Visitors cross over

— Men cross over.

Numeracy activities

1. Give everyone a number 1 to 5. Cross under the canopy according to the number called.

2. Numbers race — the group is divided into two equal teams and each team member is given a number. The person in each team whose number is called must move round the outside of the circle and return to his place before the chute

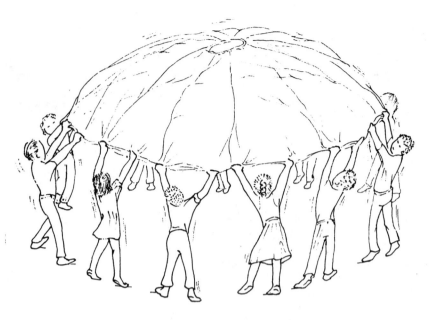

Figure 7.88 Lifting and stretching the parachute

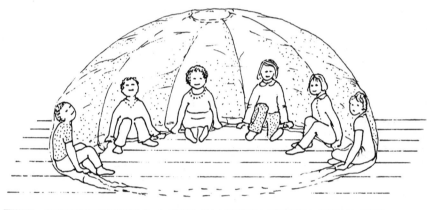

Figure 7.89 Hide-away

touches the ground. The leader chooses the method of moving round.

(NB. Running can be very slippery on some surfaces.)

Group stunt patterns

1. **Inflation.** The basic pattern on which all other stunts are based. When the full range of movement is taught it is not only an excellent chest, back and arm exercise, but also a good therapy for the legs which so often lack strength and stability.

   All face the centre holding the canopy at waist height. On the signal, all squat to seal the parachute flat on the ground so that there is no air underneath (Fig 7.87). The leader cannot proceed to the next stage until this has been achieved. He/she then gives the final signal — 'ready lift stretch' (Fig 7.88). The aim is to get as much air as possible under the canopy. Taking two or three steps into the centre helps to increase the height. Gradually members of the group can become leaders. It is a responsibility they usually enjoy.

2. **Mushroom.** Inflate the parachute as above, then quickly pull the edges down to the floor sealing off the rapid escape of air. (NB. Arms have to work hard against resistance.)

3. **Hide-away.** In this stunt the participants seal themselves inside the canopy.

   a) The chute is inflated and the group take a few steps into the centre. Then they bring the chute over their heads behind their backs and sit down on it (Fig 7.89). In this position they can make up games until the dome comes down, eg stamping their feet as they sit, rolling a ball across the circle.

   b) There is another variation. The parachute is inflated and the group walk in a little way. They quickly turn and regrasp the parachute on the inside edge and then kneel down holding the edge against the ground. There is a progression. Students can be numbered in twos. Number 1 seals the chute from inside while Number 2 seals it from the outside.

4. **Fly away.** Inflate and all release (Fig 7.90). Check first that there is sufficient clearance so that light fixtures are not damaged.

Tag Games

Steal the bacon

A bean bag or other small object is placed under the chute at approximately the middle or centre of the canopy. The class is divided into two equal teams and each player has a team number.

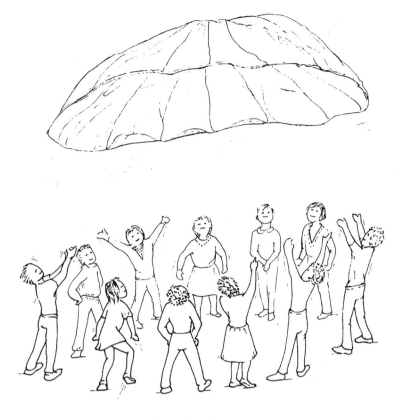

Figure 7.90 Fly-away

The parachute is inflated and, at its highest point, the leader calls a number or numbers. The players who have their number called must attempt to secure the bean bag and get back to their position without being tagged by the opponent. Also, if the chute descends on them while under the canopy no points are awarded. A player who successfully gets back to his team position without being tagged or touched by the descending chute scores one point for his team.

Swamps /crocodiles

Everyone sits on the floor with their legs under the parachute. One person goes under the parachute and becomes the crocodile, who pulls his/her victim under the chute; before doing so, he/she must call out the victim's name; they then change places and the victim becomes the crocodile. With some groups the leader may have to stay under the chute to assist the person who is the crocodile.

Jaws

Everyone sits on the floor with their legs under the parachute. One person becomes the shark who lives underneath the chute (the sea) and is very hungry. By shaking and billowing the chute, a realistic wave effect is produced, which also hides the shark. The shark chooses his/her victim and grasps him by the feet pulling him under the chute, the victim shouting as if in pain from being eaten. He/she then becomes a shark. Eventually the whole group will be sharks.

This game can also be played standing up under a fairly taut canopy. The shark can move quite swiftly under the canopy indicating the path of movement as he maintains contact with the canopy.

Ball Games

Stand or sit holding the edge of the parachute. Place 8 to 12 small foam balls on the chute. Everyone helps to count them. Then all shake the canopy to bounce the balls up and down. Then all stop shaking the canopy and recount the balls.

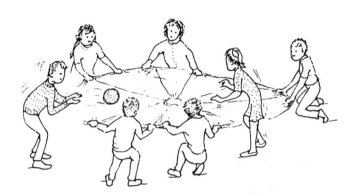

Figure 7.91 Rolling a ball in the parachute

Waves

Everyone stands/sits around the edge of the parachute and holds it taut. Place a large ball, such as a beach ball, near the edge of the chute. The ball is rolled around by everyone raising and lowering their arms alternately, creating a wave effect (Fig 7.91).

Scatterball/Popcorn

Everyone stands/sits around the edge of the parachute which is stretched taut. Place as many balls as possible on the chute and see how quickly they can be billowed off. This can develop into a team game: one team can try to throw off the balls while the other tries to keep them on the chute.

Parachutes can also be used for people with a severe or profound mental handicap (see Chapter 14, p 140).

Skittles (Plastic ten pins)

(See Special Events p 93).

Snooker

The following is a method of introducing snooker (practised at the Newry Special Care Day Centre, Northern Ireland).

To introduce the game of snooker, first encourage the players to practise with a few balls. Always use the white ball to pocket a red ball.

After a period of practice introduce all the red balls in their proper place, ie the triangle. Each in turn uses the white ball to pocket a red ball. If successful, red scores one point and another turn.

The player with the highest score is the winner.

If the players are capable of counting, the other balls can be introduced in their places with their score values printed on them with chalk or felt pen. The aim is to pocket a red ball which scores one point and the 'free' shot can be taken at a coloured ball with a higher score value. At the Newry Centre no points penalty was imposed for pocketing a white ball as this often resulted in a minus score. However, when the players become skilled at the game the full rules can be implemented.

CONTACT SPORTS

Judo

One interesting and successful method of introducing judo has been observed in the Hague, Holland. Students play in a small group with a blanket. They share the blanket, rolling in it, playing under it and feel its tension when all are pulling it against the resistance of those on the opposite side of their small circle. These activities and other variations help them to accept body contact and to respond sensitively to each other. When this sensitivity has been well maintained over a period of time, the first stages of judo are taught. This method might have a wider application when introducing contact sports.

About 30 young men and women with a mental handicap from Ifield Hall (Crawley), Crawley College (Special Needs Group) and Stranford Centre (Horsham), have been taught judo once a week for the past five years.

It is a mixed ability group containing people with, for example, brain damage and Down's Syndrome. They are not taught arm locks or neck locks, and the only Japanese words used by the teacher are the seven in the refereeing vocabulary; the teacher is fairly flexible about language, particularly as one of the group is a deaf mute Down's Syndrome and almost blind without his glasses.

The group, whose hygiene and etiquette is of a high standard, takes part in free practice and contests and also plays some judo games. They all practise the rolling and the impact breakfall. About three or four members of the group could take gradings at an ordinary club, and an internal grading system of badges — 1 badge, 2, 3, 4 and 5 — has been devised. The badges are all black on white so that there is no parallel with the grading

system in the British Judo Association. When the group first started, there was a great deal of talk about black belts, but the teacher pointed out the advantage of having a separate and flexible (and free!) system.

Four students have reached 3 badge level. The original intention was to make 5 badge unattainable, but the system can be changed at any time if it would be beneficial to the students progress.

Several black belts have participated in the teaching.

Kung Foo and Karate Exercises

These exercises are included since they are successfully practised in a few Centres (Fig 7.92). Strong, active young men seem to derive benefit from the vigorous exercise entailed and the discipline involved. At first the men work individually copying the teacher's movement. Most respond well as they have seen the movements on television and in films. The kicks and spin involve movements requiring balance and control, the deep knee bends and jumps with feet apart develop a feeling of sustaining a movement. The strong, sharp blows and positions with the arms, use up a great deal of energy. These movements are equally successful when the men work in twos, the only rule being that they are not allowed to actually touch each other. The men in fact put so much effort into the movements that they are happy to rest at the end of the exercise, and, contrary to general opinion, do not become over-excited.

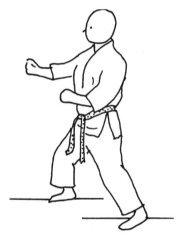

Figure 7.92 Kung Foo and Karate

The movements include: jumps with feet apart, into a strong knee bend; free kicks, to the front and the side, and the back; short run, kick and spin; strong slicing movements with the arms, with the fingers stretched, and palms facing the floor which can be taken in different directions; forward and backward rolls happen naturally and spontaneously.

TRAMPOLINING

The trampoline can be used in two quite different contexts:

1. for people with a mental handicap with minimal physical handicap where the aim is to develop a wide range of trampoling skills;

2. for multiply handicapped people where the aim is usually to provide stimulus and to create a feeling of movement where they are unable to initiate it themselves.

In the first case trampolining is being undertaken as a sport which means all normal safety precautions must be observed, eg four spotters in position, one on each side of the trampoline. In the second case the fact that there is a one-to-one relationship and the activity should always be taken under the supervision of an experienced member of staff ensures safety.

Trampolining as a sport — fundamental skills

1. Mounting and dismounting.
2. Feet bouncing.
3. Seat drop.
4. Knee drop.
5. Hand and knees bounce.
6. Front drop.
7. Back drop.
8. Swivel hips.

Teaching points

1. To kill the bounce (stop bouncing) land with the feet flat, slightly apart, and with knees bent.

2. The fingers should point forward in a seat drop since this bends the arms and prevents any possible jar to locked elbows.

3. Never arch the back in a knee drop.

4. The legs are carried backward in a front drop.

5. The hips are carried forward in a back drop.

6. In swivel hips the arms swing up and the legs swing under the body.

Safety precautions

1. Check the trampoline before use to see that it has been put up correctly and is safe.

2. Make sure there is sufficient headroom from floor to lowest overhanging obstacle.

3. Never jump from the trampoline direct to the ground.

4. See that the four spotters are in position and never jump alone.

5. Jump for a short period only — 45 seconds is enough. This ensures maximum control because fatigue is avoided. It is also more fun for those taking part because there is a quick rotation of turns.

6. Make sure that the trampoline is checked and serviced regularly by the manufacturers.

The use of trampettes

Under supervision, a trampette is a valuable piece of gymnastic apparatus. The landing area must be both spacious and resilient.

Elementary skills

1. Bouncing and making a controlled stop while remaining on the trampette.

2. Bouncing and jumping off with a soft landing. It is essential to train those being taught to hold their heads in an erect position at this stage.

3. Bouncing and jumping off making a specific leg movement pattern in flight, eg legs straight and together, legs astride.

4. Bouncing and jumping off facing in another direction.

These skills develop the enjoyment of flight. They all start on the trampette and therefore avoid the problem of the trampette shifting.

Longer sequences which might include a running start should only be considered when trainees are thoroughly proficient in the above skills.

GYMNASTICS

Dave Rozzell, Hononary National Coach for People with Special Needs, British Amateur Gymnastic Association (BAGA) (Wingate House Sports Holiday Complex) writes: 'There are many definitions of "gymnastics", and to some degree terminology can be misleading. Since the era of Olga Corbutt, gymnastics has tended to be equated with vault, beam and floor. When I started as a volunteer coach for Special Olympics UK, nearly five years ago, many establishments regarded gymnastics as being a sport unsuitable for people with a mental handicap. This was mainly due to the way the word was interpreted. Since then we have managed to change people's concepts and introduce a much broader term for the word gymnastics — "muscular exercise". If this meaning is adopted, the benefits for people with special needs become immediately apparent.

'Undoubtedly, gymnastics is one of the fastest growing sports for special needs in the UK and this is reflected in the greater involvement of local education authorities. Many establishments have of course been providing gymnastics opportunties for several years, but what I have tried to do is to co-ordinate these efforts. In fact, the Wingate House programme has become so successful that governing bodies of other sports are now copying it.

'In general, charitable organisations, such as Special Olympics, Mini Olympics and UKSAPMH, have provided sports opportunities for people with special needs. Wingate House is finding, in relation to the sport of gymnastics, that it cannot just provide opportunities. Someone cannot just be taken in 'off the street' and expected to perform high standard gymnastics skills unless he or she is first subjected to many months or years of training. Skill technique training is what is required, and it is proving to be of great benefit to people with special needs. In October 1986 the first gymnastics coaching awards aimed at people specialising in special needs were launched — the culmination of 18 months' work with BAGA and other organisations representing people with a mental handicap. Since then I have travelled extensively training and examining coaches. And although this have been primarily with people with a mental handicap, the programme is now being expanded to include physically handicapped people as well.

'Being the National Gymnastics Coach for Special Olympics UK and the BAGA, has enabled me to promote gymnastics through the correct channels, thus encouraging education authorities to adopt the programme. In areas such as Liverpool and Leicester it is proving to be extremely beneficial to both teacher and student, and the social implications are very exciting. A team of special gymnasts from Wingate House travels around the country putting on displays, which, apart from promoting gymnastics, educates people about the capabilities of people with a mental handicap. Those who disbelieved cannot help but change their opinion once they have seen for themselves the standards being attained.

'But the adults with special needs must not be forgotten. The training programme can apply to them equally. In the last National Gymnastics Championships for Special Olympics some 30-years-olds were having as much fun and excitement as the youngsters. The message is clear : there is a long way to go and a lot to learn, but with the benefit of the expertise now being applied, gymnastics can be enjoyed by thousands of people once denied the chance. It is hoped that one day the Wingate House programme will be used in every establishment that caters for special needs.

'In late 1987 the new National Sports Holiday Complex for gymnastics was opened. Wingate House, Cheshire, will run training programmes to teach teachers and managers of people with special needs the art of skill technique training in gymnastics. Holiday activities will also be provided.'

For further information about the training programme or Sports Holiday Complex write to: Dave Rozzell, National Coach for People with Special Needs, Wingate House, Wrenbury Hall Drive, Wrenbury, Nantwich, Cheshire CW5 8ES (tel: 0270 780456).

FURTHER READING

Frith, JR and Lobley, R. *Playground games and skills*. London, A & C Black, 1971.

Fluegalman, P. *The new games book*. New Games UK (see Appendix 2).

Know the Game Series. A series of seventy titles covering every major sport and pastime. London, A & C Black.
(Books printed in collaboration with governing bodies of sport which give rules and basic skills.)

Lenel, RM. *Games in the primary school*. London, Hodder and Stoughton, 1974.

New Games Newsletter. 17 Lakeside, Oxford, OX2 8JF.

Physical recreation and sport on the leisure of the adult mentally handicapped — three-tier activity categories to facilitate both participation and competition. *Teaching and Training*. Winter, Vol XX, Nos 4 and 5, 1982.

Project (Adapted Equipment), Physical Education Dept, Clifton Site, Nottingham, NG11 8NS.
(A number of adapted games equipment leaflets are being compiled into booklet form. It is hoped that these will be available in 1989.)

Ruhe, B. *Boomerang book*. London, Angus and Robertson, 1987.

Sports Council. *Handbook of sport and recreation building design* (see sections on dimensions and specifications for sports and on swimming pools). Architectural Press and Sports Council, 1980.
(A condensed version — data sheets — on dimensions is available from the Technical Unit for Sport, Sports Council.)

NOTE: Coaching manuals, rules, wall charts and posters, films and videotape of the major games and sports are available from the governing bodies of sport (see Apppendix 3) and sports shops and large booksellers. The latter will order books not in stock.

Chapter 8

Athletics

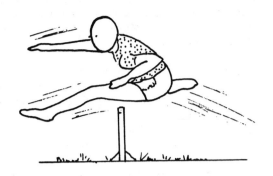

Considerations prior to training — Track events — Sprinting and Staggered middle distance — Relays including baton changing — Field events — Throws (soft ball, medicine ball, small ball, bean bag) — Jumps — Standing long (broad) jump — Long jump — High jump — Safety — Awards for athletics.

Athletics, both track and field events, are part of many hospital, adult training centre and gateway club programmes.

1. The emphasis in one type of programme can be geared to the more able who may in time work alongside athletes in the wider community.

2. An alternative programme may be geared to maximum participation regardless of ability, emphasising the value of social relationships and fun through shared activity.

   In the first programme the rules and methods of training recommended by the national governing bodies of athletics — the Amateur Athletic Association (AAA) and the Women's Amateur Athletic Association (WAAA) — should be observed. In the second programme there should be flexibility.

   The following programme is predominantly based on the methods of training athletics for a sports day by the instructor at the Stonebridge Adult Training Centre in Brent, but takes into account the experience of other hospitals, adult training centres and clubs.

CONSIDERATIONS PRIOR TO TRAINING

1. Know the people you are working with:
   (i) their medical history
   (ii) their handicap (s)
   (iii) their personal interest in particular events
   (iv) their initial standard of performance.

2. Regular fitness training is desirable. If this cannot be arranged, then it is important to gradually build up physical fitness as early as possible before the sports day itself. If possible, practise the events throughout the year.

3. Discuss each event, procedure and visit the sports centre.

4. Interest and incentives are very important and must be offered to the group to get the best out of them. This will help the instructor to discover which trainee is most suitable for which events, and to develop their individual interests.

5. Personal involvement is very important, always in a non-competitive way, by pacing, etc. If trainees see the instructor involved in the sport they themselves derive more satisfaction and consequently are encouraged to work harder.

6. Bearing in mind that a field day or athletics meeting usually takes place only once a year, the concept of athletics will take a longer period of time to develop. Older trainees who have known several sports days get more pleasure from the work involved and the waiting for the big event, in fact the waiting and this 'build up' have possibly been learnt and accepted as part of the event. This is not always true of the younger competitors whose acceptance of the sports may only last for a short time and what they have previously learnt can be forgotten on the day.

7. Develop a certain competitiveness among the group but make sure that this is done in a constructive way, ie only relating to one particular event. Like most athletes, trainees may often develop their own particular event and this becomes their special part of the day.

8. Correct dress and shoes should be worn both on and off the track and a track suit (Fig 8.1) should be put on after and while waiting for an event.

TRACK EVENTS

Sprinting

1. In the early stages the use of blocks is not advised. If the handicapped person feels that it is difficult to learn to use blocks or if it is too involved he can be very awkward, delay the progress of others, or may be put off altogether. Introduce blocks at a later stage.

2. While practising, use a short run to restore energy, say 50m (165').

3. Discuss the starting orders, keep as far as possible to the right sequence.

   Take your marks — on this command the competitors walk forward to the starting line and take up the position behind

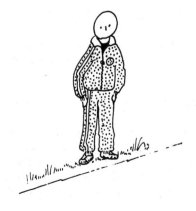

Figure 8.1 Track suit

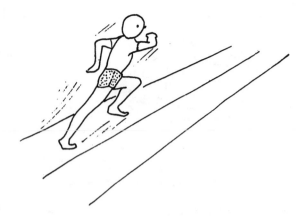

Figure 8.2 Sprinting (keeping in lane)

the nearer edge. All should be motionless — then the starter will command 'SET'.

Set — competitors get into their final position and when all are still:

Go or gun — run.

4. Discuss and practise keeping in lanes (Fig 8.2). Get the group to walk up the track within the lines if necessary.

5. If there is time, use the pre-draw system — this can add to the excitement and avoid any argument as to lane advantage.

6. During and after each run, go across and discuss with the trainees what took place :
    (i)   breathing
    (ii) use of legs, arms, hands, head.

7. Make contact with the respective Athletic Associations.

In the first instance, run with the trainees to encourage them.

Staggered middle distance

Always make sure that, on the day of the meeting, starting procedure has been agreed upon. Use 'Take your Marks — Set — Gun'.

Take your marks. On this command the competitors will walk forward and assume their starting position behind the line and when all are still — Set — Gun or go.

False starts. Competitors must not move a foot or arm over the line.

At first allow three false starts per competitor.
Watch for dangerous jostling crossing lanes.

The finish. The one who crosses the finishing line first is the winner.

In training, discuss and show how to maintain a steady pace and restore energy for the final sprint. This concept is often difficult to convey to people with a mental handicap, who tend always to want to set one pace and try to maintain this for the full distance.

Relays including baton changing

Baton changing is difficult to teach and will take much practice to perfect (Fig 8.3).

1. Discuss the race with the group. Explain it with the use of a blackboard and diagram.

2. Let them handle the baton.

3   Teach how to hold it, support the baton between the thumb and first two fingers and hold with the third and fourth

4. Practise with two, then with the four, placing it in the hand of the person in front. The person in front will probably need to look back at first, in order to get the feel of it being placed in the hand and to grasp it fully. Gradually speed and accuracy will improve.

5. Later take the group on to the track and explain the marking on the field, the start and finishing, and the 20m (66') box.

6. Use a short run at first then gradually build up to a longer, faster run. Check times with a stop watch.

Rules:

1. The first man holding the baton must not hold the baton or any part of it over the starting line.

2. Starting procedure will take the form of the middle distance races.

3. The baton must change hands within the 20m (66') area.

4. No pushing. No throwing of the baton.

5. If dropped, the runner who dropped it must pick it up.

6. After the change-over, the runners should remain within their own lanes.

There is no easy way of gaining this efficiency apart from repeated practice. If the stages are taught correctly and slowly enough, there will be a gradual build up of experience.

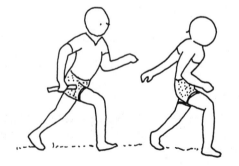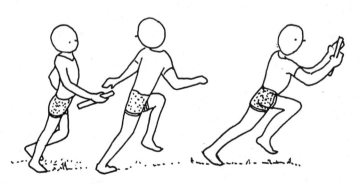

Figure 8.3 Baton changing

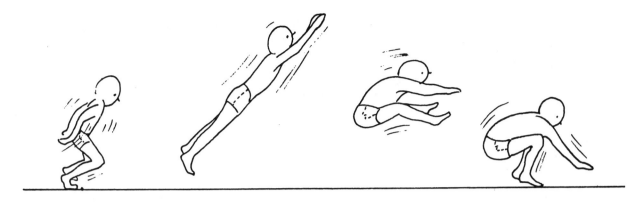

Figure 8.4 Standing long (broad) jump

FIELD EVENTS

Throws

Throws can play a significant part in the physical development of the chest and should always be included in the programme — non-ambulant people can also take part. If the discus, javelin or shot are considered to be appropriate the rules, techniques and safety precautions recommended by the AAA and WAAA (see p. 68) should be followed. Coaches with experience in these events should be invited to assist.

For many people with a mental handicap, easier equipment requiring simpler rules will encourage a greater number of competitors to train and thereby improve their technique, eg soft ball, medicine ball, small ball, beanbag.

Training techniques:

1. Overarm throw (see Chapter 7).

2. Double handed overhead throw as in football or any other adaptation which assists participation.

   Rule: Both feet must be behind the throwing line throughout the throwing action.

   Scoring: Three attempts and record the furthest throw for each competitor.

Jumps

Jumps requiring a running start can give rise to difficulties of co-ordination and overstepping the starting line, therefore standing long (broad) jump is a good starting point (Fig 8.4).

Standing long (broad) jump

Training techniques

1. Place feet a little way apart with toes pointing forwards behind the take off line.

2. Bend and stretch knees several times with relaxed arm swinging forward and back.

3. Push off vigorously from the take off with strong arm swing forwards and upwards to provide lift.

4. Look forward.

5. Land with feet parallel carrying body weight forward.

Rules:

1. Toes must be behind the take-off line.

2. A two-footed take off must be used.

3. Jumps are measured from the take-off line to the nearest contact point on the ground. Ideally this should be the heels but faulty techniques may mean it is the seat or hands.

   Scoring: Three attempts and record the furthest jump.

Long jump

Make sure that the take-off board is stationary and in the correct position — placed at least 1m (3¹/4') from the nearest edge of the landing pit. The runway should be in good condition, the sand moistened and clean to allow for accurate measuring. A long run up is needed.

Training techniques

1. Begin the jump with a steady run building up to the maximum speed towards the latter part of the runway.

2. Practise the timing of the run so that the landing is correctly on the right foot on the take off board. This will only be achieved by constant practice and patient instruction.

3. Remind the jumpers to take a vigorous jump into the air and encourage them to be aware of the use of the arms for balance and extra distance.

4. Help the jumper to throw both legs forward for added distance before landing.

High jump

Experience has shown that very few people with a mental handicap have the ability to do this jump competitively. Where the ability is present then the rules and guidance of the AAA or WAAA should be followed.

Fun and confidence can be experienced by a less competitive approach to this event providing there is a good resilient landing area. In the early stages a rope may be preferred to a bar.

Training techniques

1. Establish confidence by letting each individual run jump and arrive in the landing area with or without a very low bar in position.

2. *Centre jump.* Indicate the starting point, continue as in (1) and jump taking off with one foot. Note which foot each

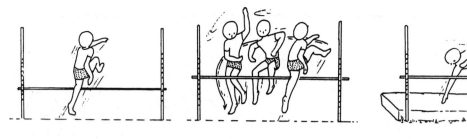

Figure 8.5a Centre jump   Figure 8.5b Side jump   Figure 8.5c Jump and twist

individual uses for take-off. Repeat several times to make sure that same take off foot is used consistently (Fig 8.5a).

3. *Side jump*. Divide jumpers so that those who take off from the right foot go to the right side of the take-off area and those who take off from the left foot go to the left side (Fig 8.5b).

4. *Jump and twist*. Perform the same jumping movements as in a side jump — while in mid air twist or turn to land facing the original starting point.

The twisting of the body after take off is the most difficult part to learn. The landing takes place almost naturally holding the head forward with the arms offering further support. Arms should always be in a supporting position for landing (Fig 8.5c).

Develop a seven step approach, one long enough to generate sufficient speed, yet not so long as to adversely affect speed and timing. Increase speed of approach gradually as confidence and skill improve.

SAFETY

1. Make sure the runway is clear and the landing area measures 5 x 4m (16 x 13'). The material most commonly used is a type of foam rubber covered by a strong protective cover. Ensure that the foam is thick enough to prevent injury. Loose or bagged foam can be potentially dangerous.

2. Gymnastic mats on a hard surface are not adequate.

3. The take-off area should be free from pitting and level.

4. The runway approach should be 8m (26') long.

5. The uprights should be rigid and placed at least 3.55m (12') apart.

6. The supporting peg should have a flat upper surface 40mm (1³/4 ") wide.

7. The crossbars are usually triangular — 30mm (1") diameter and approximately 4m (13') long.

AWARDS FOR ATHLETICS

There are two awards, one for active athletes and the other a coaching award for those wishing to coach them.

Proficiency awards

Through the Amateur Athletic Association there is the Ten Step and the Five Star Award.

Ten Step Award

This is a basic skills award to be taken in ten stages; it covers running jumping and throwing: starting from standing, long jump, a seated throw and shuffle relay. It is appropriate for beginners and can be judged by anyone training athletics at this level.

There is also an excellent scheme for longer distance/cross country running which provides an incentive. Badges and/or certificates can be provided for the number of times the runners go out running rather than length of time or distance.

Five Star Award

This is an award for effort not geared to competition. The scheme caters for a whole range of skills at all levels of ability. It provides an opportunity to learn techniques so as to improve performance. The skills include those of running, jumping, throwing at different levels from One Star to Five Star Awards.

Coaching awards

Those who are interested in teaching athletics could qualify for an Assistant Club Coach Award. Courses for this award are run throughout the country by the British Amateur Athletic Board (BAAB). On request the BAAB might consider organising a course in a local area providing enough people are interested in taking part.

For further information about the above awards apply to: The British Amateur Athletic Board, Coaching Office, Frances House, Frances Street, London SW1 PID.

Athletics meetings

Anyone who is organising a local athletics meeting should seek the help of the nearest athletics club or county association whose members are often willing to help and to give advice leading up to the event and on the day itself.

FURTHER READING

Diagram Group. *Enjoying track and field sports*. London, Paddington Press, 1979.

Know The Game Series. *Athletics*. London, A & C Black. 1986.

Edmundson J and Burnup CRE. *Basic athletics*, (4th ed). London, Bell & Hyman, 1979.

For booklets and wall charts on individual events apply to the Amateur Athletic Association and Women's Amateur Athletic Association, Francis House, Francis Street, London SWIP 1DL.

Chapter 9

Swimming

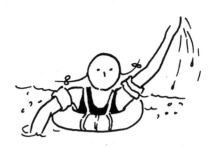

Introduction—ASA coach's method—The Halliwick Method— General hints on the organisation of swimming sessions — Personal hygiene — Tips before going into the pool — Water confidence — Water games — Discipline and safety — Compe- tition — Hints on the organisation of swimming galas — A swimming club for 'any swimmer': the formation of an ATC swimming club and the advantages of affiliation to the Amateur Swimming Association — Swimming at Craig Phadrig Hospital, Inverness — ASA awards scheme and certificates.

Swimming is very high on the list of popular activities available to people with a mental handicap. It offers everything — training in discipline, hygiene, stamina, perseverance. It develops cour- age and self reliance and is in fact a total social exercise.

The ability to swim and be water safe enables people with a mental handicap to enjoy water sports such as canoeing, sailing and angling where local facilities exist or at outdoor pursuits centres, holiday camps, field study centres and youth hostels which are often situated near sea or inland waters.

Practically all hospitals and training centres make every effort to provide an opportunity for some residents and trainees to swim. Rarely are facilities available on the spot, but good use is made of those in sports leisure centres, schools, universities and public and private pools.

Sadly, because of transport problems, high maintenance costs of hospital and private pools, shortage of staff qualified to teach swimming, and of helpers, only a relatively small percent- age have the opportunity to swim regularly. Yet the general feeling is that it is one of, if not *the* most beneficial physical activity for people with a mental handicap and has perhaps the greatest spin-off — educationally and socially.

It is important that any coach in charge of swimming, whether a nurse teacher or instructor, should have *a recognised swimming teacher's life-saving qualification*. The minimum qualifi- cation is the Royal Life Saving Society Bronze Medallion.

Naturally many coaches evolve their own methods of teach- ing swimming in the light of experience. The two methods of teaching swimming to people with a mental handicap described in this chapter are included as examples of good practice. In one swimming aids are used, eg arm bands, rings and floats, and in the other swimmers are taught on a one-to-one ratio of instructor to swimmer. A good teacher teaches pupils *not* the subject — observation and a knowledge of mental handicap accompany normal teaching methods.

AN ASA COACH'S METHOD

A swimming coach holding the Amateur Swimming Association's (ASA) Advanced Teachers' Certificate and the ASA Club Coaches' Award, who is the Senior Swimming Coach at the Gloucester Leisure Centre, uses this method. He is closely involved with the selection and coaching of swimmers who take part in Special Olympics.

In his experience young children with a mental handicap learn to swim much more quickly than the adult with a mental handicap.

A swimming lesson should be structured according to the needs of each individual. Ideally, it is a time when play is a way of learning; when people speak of work in a swimming lesson they should mean putting away the equipment after it is over!

The aim is to encourage the swimmer with many activities involving physical and mental effort.

Remember that people differ, both in their physical and mental capabilities; they therefore require the freedom to explore for themselves and to discover their own natural abilities.

Artificial aids enable the swimmer to feel the sensation of moving in water in a horizontal position as soon as possible. Early success will stimulate enthusiasm to come again.

Stages in teaching the adult with a mental handicap to swim

Stage One

Aids: Each individual is equipped with:
1. inflatable arm bands (the double or single chambered type can be used and should have safety valves);
2. inflatable rubber rings (Figure 9.1) Check that aids are sound and worn correctly.

Entry: Down steps if available. For people with a mental handicap it is best to avoid traditional swivel entry because some have problems of balance.

Allow swimmers to discover:
1. balance and orientation;
2. walking — heel, toe, fairly big steps, with the shoulders under water to avoid slipping — if the head and shoulders are out of the water they move faster than the hips because there is no water resistance.

Bring in direction
    (i)   forwards   (ii)   sideways
    (iii) backwards   (iv) turning.

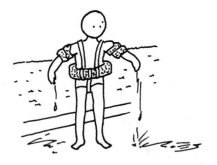

Figure 9.1 Buoyancy aids

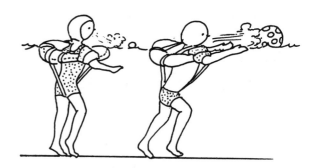

Figure 9.2 Walking – blowing ball

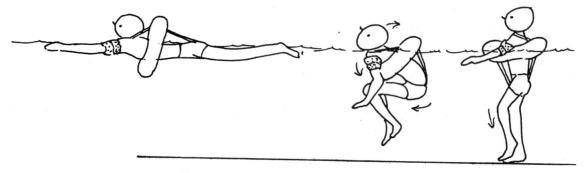

Figure 9.3 Regaining feet from prone floating

Bring in space

  (i) circles

  (ii) squares

  (iii) triangles.

Sometimes guess what pattern the swimmer is making and also point in the direction for the individual to walk. This can be great fun when you change directions.

Walk, blowing a ball (eg table tennis ball). (Figure 9.2)

Stage Two

Buoyancy and propulsion prone

Prone position. Shoulders down, tuck up your knees and spin like a ball, using your hands to pull you around (teacher spins a ball on the water).

Prone floating. Spread arms like an aeroplane and lie down on the water and pretend you are an aeroplane in the sky.

Teaching points:

1. stretch arms and legs;

2. chin down on water.

Regaining feet from prone float. Just ask the swimmer to stand up on the ground (Figure 9.3)

Teaching points:

1. tuck up knees and make body into a ball;

2. bring head back;

3. place feet on ground

Propulsion prone. Lie down on the water again, arms like an aeroplane, legs out straight. Now make a big splash with your feet. Now you are moving like a motor boat.

Ask swimmers to use all of pool, then move from **A** to **B**.

Next bring in the arms. Pull the water with your hands. Show how a dog swims.

Stage Three

Buoyancy and propulsion supine

Supine floating. Lie down on the water on your back, spread your arms and legs and make your body like a star in the sky. (Figure 9.4)

Teaching points:

1. look at the sky;

2. tummy up;

3. toes pointed.

Regaining feet from the supine position. Ask the swimmer to try and stand first. For those who can't:

Teaching points:

1. tuck up knees and make body into a ball;

2. bring head forward;

3. place feet on the ground.

Propulsion supine. Lie on your back, body like a star then put your arms by your sides. Make a splash with your feet and move along like a motor boat.

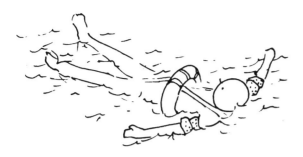

Figure 9.4 Supine floating

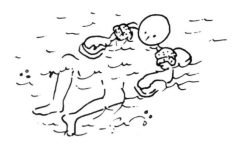

Figure 9.5 Approach to breast stroke

Teaching points:

1.   toes pointed;

2.   hips, tummy up;

3.   look at sky.

Some may find this difficult; sometimes a pair of flippers may be of help in gaining propulsion. If the swimmer is frightened to go on his back then let him stay on his front.

Stage Four

Approach to the breast stroke. Simply ask the swimmer to pull with the hands under the water. If the swimmer pulls with a symmetrical action, his legs will often automatically follow the same pattern. (Figure 9.5).

The swimmer can try the kick on his back or the teacher can sit on a chair and demonstrate the leg action, or even give manual guidance. Kick like a frog!

Teaching points:

1.   feet brought up together,

2.   feet turned out;

3.   feet apart draw a circle;

4.   feet then stretch back.

Those swimmers who are best suited to this type of stroke can be seen at once. Usually it is the ones with very good dorsal flexion, and poor plantar flexion of the feet.

An excellent way to learn the leg action is to lie on the back and kick while watching the feet. A polystyrene float can be used

under each arm to help balance and so promote a symmetrical leg action.

Stage Five

Combination of strokes

Swimmers should be encouraged to try a combination of leg and arm action, eg breast stroke arms, crawl legs; Dolphin legs, breast stroke arms.

Remember the aim at first is to get them swimming any stroke, and any way, then learn the basic strokes

The use of flippers. A swimmer who cannot manage either of these kicks is given a pair of flippers to aid propulsion. Usually the swimmer is taught to make use of them on his back.

Teaching points:

1.   keep flippers under water;

2.   kick from hips. Sometimes manual guidance is needed.

The flippers can be used to teach all strokes

Flippers must be the shoe type and flexible.

When to get rid of the aids. It is surprising the number of people who ask to swim without aids. This is sometimes an indication that they are ready.

Gradually let the air out of the aids until the person is swimming.

Always tell them the air is being let out of the aids.

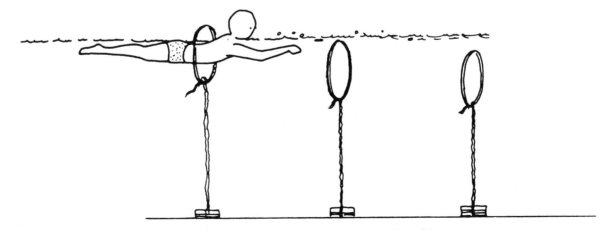

Figure 9.6 Swimming through hoops (tunnels)

When the swimmer first tries without aids always swim towards the rail of the pool. The distance from where he stands to the rail is 'the river'; ask the swimmers to name 'the river', they then swim across it — progress by 'widening the river'.

Water play. Use incentives like 'Who can swim from A to B without putting their feet on the bottom?'

Coloured hoops, partly submerged, represent tunnels. The swimmers are the trains going through the tunnel (Figure 9.6). They are encouraged to make train noises as they swim. This helps breath control. It is fun when each swimmer gets through the tunnel (hoop) and the rest clap.

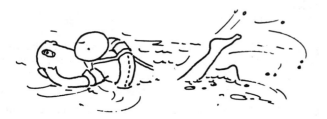

Figure 9.7 Water play

Swimmers hold inflatable toys and kick— eg Dolphins, Donald Duck (Fig 9.7).

There is a special toy to encourage swimmers to go under water, called 'Sammy Magic Star Fish' — a coloured plastic star fish which floats partly submerged. The swimmer goes under water and retrieves it.

With small children, puppets are used successfully: a puppet called 'Swim Tim' can be made to do a kind of breast stroke and can illustrate various ways of floating.

Puppets have not been tried with the handicapped adults but an inflatable Dolphin held by a teacher was the means of attracting a reluctant adult into the pool.

Praise and encouragement. Give lots of praise for effort as well as for progress.

Incentives

Phase 1 — With aids

1. Walk across the pool
2. Blow a ping pong ball across pool
3. Face in water blow bubbles
4. Swim 10 m on front
5. Swim 10 m ON back.

Phase 2 — Without aids

As Phase 1 (1-5).

Phase 3 — Without aids

1. Push and glide — face in water
2. Push and glide — kick on front

3. Push and glide — kick on back
4. Swim 10m recognised front stroke
5. Swim 10m on recognised back stroke.

Phase 4 — Without aids

1. Swim 25m deep to shallow water
2. Tread water for 30 seconds in deep water
3. Jump into deep water
4. When swimmer jumps confidently diving from the side can be taught.

Notes

1. When swimming the 25 m deep to shallow end, keep the swimmer close to the side and carry a pole for swimmer to grasp if he tires — until he is confident.
2. Jump into deep water near to the side (have a pole handy)
3. Diving should always be taught in deep water.

THE HALLIWICK METHOD

The Halliwick Method of teaching swimming was devised by James McMillan who began the work in 1949 at the Halliwick School for Girls in Southgate, London. It is from this school that the method takes its name. It is based on known scientific principles of hydrodynamics and body mechanics. It has proved to be safely applicable to all varieties of handicapped and non-handicapped people of all ages.

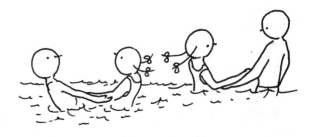

Figure 9.8 Halliwick method – one-to-one – no aids

Swimmers are taught on a one-to-one ratio of instructor to swimmer until the time when complete independence is achieved (Figure 9.8). The swimmer-instructor pair becomes a unit within a group activity so that the swimmer gains the advantages of social interaction with his peers whilst at the same time enjoying unobtrusive but constant attention of an individual instructor. Through the medium of games appropriate to age and ability, groups are made aware of properties and behaviour of water and how to control their own particular imbalance problems.

Handling

Correct handling on the part of the instructor enables the swimmer to experience a mobility unknown on land. After the initial mental adjustments to water are made and balance control principles are learned the swimmers reach a stage where they are prepared to do without instructor contact. Now, often for the first time in their lives, they experience complete independence of movement.

The method teaches swimming as a developmental programme, teaching the mental adjustment to the water, balance and control in the water, and later facilitates controlled activity by the swimmer, and produces a functional swimming stroke. In addition, a carefully thought out system of checks or tests enables the teacher to assess the reliability of the swimmers reactions and the degree of learning achieved.

Swimmers are taught how to maintain a safe breathing position with the face clear of the surface; how to regain such a position from any other given position; and how to control exhalation whenever the face is immersed in water.

They are made familiar with all conceivable body rotation and learn how to initiate, control and arrest such rotations at will.

Water's powers of upthrust, turbulence and, independence to movement are studied, together with metacentric effects. The end product is a secure swimmer whose confidence is based upon sound knowledge of water and his own movement controls.

Halliwick Method used by a physiotherapist

A retired senior tutor/physiotheropist who is member of the National Education Committee of the Association of Swimming Therapy, has used the Halliwick Method for more than twenty years with children and adults with a mental handicap. She says 'I have found that it is applicable to all degrees of incapacity, and believe that it is beneficial to their development. It stimulates the most inactive to some degree of response which appears to be ongoing, and enables the over-active or hyperkinetic swimmer to gain considerable control.

'A further great advantage of the method is that it is able to take account of, and accommodate, any physical disability that may be present concurrently with the mental disability.

'The degree of safety that is achieved by the method is remarkable, almost entirely, I believe, due to the lack of apparatus used: it allows for no swimming aids such as floats, rings, arm bands etc, so there is no danger teaching a swimmer dependence on this kind of support, which in the unreliable person may be inadvertently discarded. Equally, the supervision of the swimmer prevents problems arising from fits etc in that they are coped with in a safe manner if they arise.

'The process of learning whilst seriously and objectively being controlled is essentially recreational. The swimmers do have fun; they are taught to enjoy themselves and most skills are acquired through participation in group games and activities in the water'.

Anyone who is thinking of undertaking this type of tuition should consider care and safety on the bath side. In addition to the team of instructors, a back up team is required to care for people with a mental handicap on the bath side, to:

1. help with dressing and undressing

2. provide refreshments

3. supervise activity and bath side behaviour

4. organise transport if necessary.

Those interested in learning about this method of teaching swimming should contact the General Secretary of the Associa-tion of Swimming Therapy Mr. Ted Cowen, (40 Oak Street, Shrewsbury, Salop. SY3 7RH; tel: 0743 4393) who can put them in touch with clubs in their area which would teach the Halliwick Method and be able to give information of further courses that are organised in all parts of the country from time to time.

GENERAL HINTS ON THE ORGANISATION OF SWIMMING SESSIONS

When organising swimming sessions consider the following points .

Water temperature

It is generally recognised that the temperature of the water should be 82-84° Farhenheit (28-29°C) when teaching people with a mental handicap. For physically active people 80°F (27C°) is adequate — this is the average temperature of most public swimming pools.

Size of group

Ideally each swimmer with a mental handicap should be partnered by a non-handicapped helper (see Halliwick Method above). When this is impossible, a ratio of two instructors to six swimmers is generally accepted.

Frequency of session

Obviously, the more frequent the sessions, the quicker the trainees or residents will be able to swim. A swimming period every day or even three times a week is better than once each week.

Ability in group

In classes of mixed ability some form of grouping is advisable.

Equipment (miscellaneous swimming aids)

Check that aids, floats, armbands when used are suitable, serviceable and available at the start of the session. Inflatable rubber rings can be used: a safety tape over the shoulders should be used to prevent the rings slipping downwards. A tape between the legs would prevent the tape riding upwards.

1. Balls, hoops, ducks, buoys, coffee-jar tops; any intriguing object to challenge the swimmer both above and under water should be used. Colour, texture and shape can be important.

2. Flippers help those who can already swim to achieve a more effective leg kick.

3. Rubber bricks or coffee jar tops can be used for retrieval from the bottom of the pool.

4. Courlene rope. Rope can be used to divide the pool lengthways and widthways — it can also be used to set targets for swimmers to go underneath.

5. Drum. A clear basic rhythm can be set — it is valuable for sculling and change of direction exercises.

6. Rubber mattresses and towels — these are useful for entry and exit from the pool and protection of the skin for multiply handicapped people.

Facilities

Be familiar with the layout and procedures.

Staff and helpers

Make sure that everyone knows exactly what is expected of them.

Swimmers

Be sure to get any medical and parental permission required, well in advance. Be aware of any special disabilities, eg epilepsy.

PERSONAL HYGIENE

1. Where it is required for technical reasons, eg filter plant, swimmers should always co-operate by wearing bathing caps.

2. Men should wash gel from hair and keep it short.

3. The use of tissues, the toilet, showers and footbath are an essential part of preparation.

4. Swimmers suffering from catarrh, sore throat, skin or foot infection, or open sores should not be taken swimming.

5. Wash costumes out after use. Do not wring out costumes into the pool after use.

6. On completion of swim, have a brisk rub down. Dry hair, ears and feet thoroughly.

7. Get changed quickly or there is a risk of catching a cold.

TIPS BEFORE GOING INTO THE POOL

1. Let prospective swimmers come along to watch for just as long as they like, leaving the individual to make the first step into the water.

2. Practise getting the face wet in a bowl of tepid water with a mirror at the bottom to encourage them to open their eyes.

3. Blow bubbles under water.

WATER CONFIDENCE

First and foremost it is essential for swimmers to gain confidence in the water and in the teacher by doing what they want to do with the teacher; sometimes walking, sitting or just talking in the water.

It may take some time to establish this relationship and for the swimmers to be able to move around with or without aids in shallow water without fear.

Encourage jumping up and down — 'washing face', blowing bubbles and holding hands to walk across the pool.

Pull and push the water with the hands.

Touch head, shoulders, knees, feet etc; make shapes with hands, arms, knees and legs.

WATER GAMES

The learner's pool is an ideal place for water games as the depth is 1 m (3' 3") — as an alternative use the shallow end of a large pool roped off. An occasional game introduced into a swimming session often maintains enthusiasm and interest. The following are examples of water games.

1. **Fishing Net**

Trainees standing in 1 metre area of the pool. Two trainees join hands and the others spread out anywhere in the area. On hearing a given signal the two holding hands begin to chase the others. Anyone whom they touch joins them and the game continues until all the trainees are in the chain with their hands joined.

2. **Team passing**

Equipment: Floats and plastic ball.

Trainees are divided into two equal teams. One team stands on one side of the pool and the other team opposite. Floats can be used for goal posts and left on each side of the pool about four metres apart. A light plastic ball is thrown up between two centre swimmers to start the game and team passing begins until a score of ten is reached by either side. Team scores a point when ball is hit or thrown between the two floats.

3. **The retrievers**

Equipment: Two rubber rings

Trainees are divided into two teams. Two rubber rings are placed in the centre of the roped off area of the pool. The teams line up on opposite sides. On a signal a member from each team retrieves the ring either by walking, swimming or running, and hands it to the next swimmer who replaces it in the centre again. This is continued until the first team with the ring over the first swimmer and in a straight line, shouts 'stop'.

4. **Relay race**

Equipment: Floats

Swimmers are divided into two teams. Half of each team on one side and the other half on the other side of the pool. First swimmer of each team, with float, jumps or climbs into the pool and swims or walks to the other side, gets out and hands the float to his team mate who repeats this until one team wins by finishing the relay and all team members are gathered together on one side in the pool in a straight line.

5. **Push partner**

Equipment: Floats.

Swimmers are paired off with a float between them at arms length in a prone position. They hold tightly to the float and do a leg kick and try to push each other to the side of the pool. A good game for balance and equilibrium.

DISCIPLINE AND SAFETY

A swimming bath is an obvious source of potential danger and therefore a teacher or instructor must take all the necessary safety measures. Discipline is essential. Certain rules which must be obeyed, together with an acceptable code of behaviour will ensure a happy, relaxed atmosphere and minimum risk.

1. No trainee may enter the water until instructed to do so.

2. Do not chew gum or other sweets.

3. No running along the bathside or pushing each other into the water.

4. Signals by hand or whistle should be promptly obeyed, especially those indicating stopping and getting out of the pool.

5. Diving only permitted under supervision.

6. Long poles should be placed at the side of the pool to be used in case of emergency.

7. If not in the 1 m (3' 3") pool, a rope should show the limit of shallow water appropriate for the class lesson.

8. All must leave the water immediately when instructed to do so.

9. Supervision is important in the changing room. Make sure an enthusiastic swimmer does not wander back into the pool. If aids are put on in the changing room, safety on the pool side is ensured.

10. Never swim without a qualified life saver with a whistle on the pool side whose sole job is to watch every individual and to blow the whistle in the case of an emergency to stop all activity — use of the whistle should be practised from time to time.

11. The teacher or instructor with the swimmers should be aware of all the safety apparatus available and be acquainted with the necessary and normal emergency arrangements provided at the pool.

12. The teacher should be qualified in methods of resuscitation and first aid.

13. When bathing or swimming in inland waters or in the sea, special attention should be paid to all safety precautions, especially those laid down locally. The teacher/parent should know about the local tides, dangerous currents, depth of water — weirs, rocks and any other hazards.

If you have any doubt — don't!

COMPETITION

Many people with a mental handicap once they have learned to swim like to test their ability in competition. This is arranged in clubs and at regional, national and international level by many organisations. There are various methods of competition. Some Inter-Adult Training Centre annual swimming sports and galas are run under the Amateur Swimming Association rules and with the help of ASA officials.

Awards

These can be devised locally or by a national organisation, eg Scottish Amateur Swimming Association. These awards provide an incentive to both swimmer and teacher.

HINTS ON THE ORGANISATION OF SWIMMING GALAS

The following officials should be appointed:

Gala Co-ordinator; Referee; Chief Whip; Pool Supervisor; Life Saver; Starter; one Time-keeper for each lane in use;

Recorder; one or more Placing Judges; Chief Judge; Chief Time-keeper; Announcer.

The responsibilities of the officials shall be:

Gala Co-ordinator — shall be responsible for the overall efficient conduct of the Gala and shall appoint such further assistants as required. He shall have overriding authority in all matters.

Referee — shall give a decision where the opinion of the Chief Judge and Chief Time-keeper differ. If in the opinion of the Referee a competitor has been fouled to a degree that endangers his or her chance of success, he shall have the power to re-run that race or enable that competitor to compete in the next round or final. He may disqualify any competitor he considers guilty of wilfully obstructing another competitor.

Chief Whip — shall ensure that all competitors are at the starting point at a reasonable time prior to the commencement of their race.

Starter — shall satisfy himself that timekeepers and judges are at their appropriate stations and are aware that the race is about to start. He shall start the race by giving a preliminary command 'take your mark' followed by a starting signal.

Time-keepers — shall start their watches at the starting signal and shall stop their watches when the swimmer in the allocated lane completes the appropriate distance. The time recorded shall be made known to the Chief Time-keeper.

Place Judge — shall note the order of finish and advise the Chief Judge accordingly.

Chief Time-keeper — shall resolve any timing dispute and enter each swimmer's time on appropriate form for submission to the Recorder.

Chief Judge — shall resolve any dispute between Placing Judges and shall enter the placings on the appropriate form for the submission to the Recorder.

Pool Supervisor — shall ensure that suitable arrangements are made for competitors to enter and leave the water and that helpers in the water are properly instructed in their duties in that they neither impede, physically assist, or swim directly in front of any competitor. He shall ensure that free passage is maintained at the bathside.

Recorder — shall have a record of all times and placings as submitted by the Chief Judge and Chief Timekeeper. He shall prepare a list of award winners for use at the time of presentation.

Note — The presence of at least two life savers, usually four, on the pool side and lane ropes are desirable at all times.

A SWIMMING CLUB FOR 'ANY SWIMMER'

'Sport for all', the Sports Council's slogan triggered off a member of the staff of the Birkbeck Adult Training Centre in Leytonstone, Essex, to form a swimming club for 'any swimmer'. Club members include people with a mental handicap physically handicapped people as well as other swimmers — a good example of integration.

Affiliation

Affiliation to the Amateur Swimming Association was accepted and consequently opportunities to take part in competitions — water polo — diving and swimming awards have been provided. Some members are now training for their ASA Bronze personal survival awards.

Club grades

For those members who are less able swimmers an easier set of swimming grades has been compiled. These are proving to be an invaluable asset to members in achieving some form of self confidence not only in themselves as swimmers but as people.

The conditions of each of the five grades are:

Elementary: Swim 23 m

Intermediate: Jump (or dive) in and swim 32 m

Grade I

1. Jump in and swim 23m of a recognised stroke.

2. Tread water for 3 minutes

3. Swim 46m of a recognised stroke without touching the sides or bottom.

4. Get out of the baths unaided without using the steps.

Grade II

1. Jump (or dive) in and swim 46m of a recognised stroke.

2. Tread water for 5 minutes.

3. Swim 69 m of **ONE** of the following strokes without touching the sides or bottom of the bath:
   (i)   Front crawl
   (ii) Back stroke
   (iii) Breast stroke.

4. Do one surface dive during the 69m swimming.

5. Get out of the baths unaided, without using the steps.

Grade III

1. Dive in with a pair of pyjamas (top and bottom) over swim suit.

2. Swim 91.5 m within a set time of 10 minutes.

3. Tread water for 5 minutes, whilst discarding pyjamas.

4. Swim for 275 m of **ONE** of the following strokes without touching the sides or bottom of the baths:
   (i)   Front crawl
   (ii) Back stroke
   (iii) Breast stroke.

5. Do 2 surface dives in the 91.5 m swimming.

6. Get out of the baths unaided without using the steps.

   Safety. When undressing in water, all discarded clothing must be removed from the pool immediately.

SWIMMING AT CRAIG PHADRIG HOSPITAL, INVERNESS

This hospital is fortunate in having an excellent pool, purpose-built, opened in 1970. Three full-time qualified instructors with the Royal Life Saving Society's Teachers' Award are employed, two men and one woman.

All residents swim unless they are excused on medical grounds. There is an excellent standard of personal hygiene with special care for incontinent patients who wear rubber pants. Everyone showers both before and after swimming. People with epilepsy swim but wear red costumes for quick identification.

Small groups

Residents swim in small groups with a one-to-one helper-swimmer ratio when paraplegics are in the water and with others when possible. The helpers are nursing staff who are encouraged to attend the instructors' class and to go into the water with the residents. Voluntary help is given from boys from the Inverness Academy as part of their community service training.

New residents

New residents start in a very warm paddling pool and progress to the big pool as confidence increases and they feel they want to.

Programme

The daytime programme has an educational bias and groups are graded where possible. Recreational groups swim during the evenings and at weekends. Anyone can join in whatever age or ability, but must have nursing staff with them.

Competitive swimming events

These are run within the hospital. The size of the teaching group varies. Paraplegics have two lessons a week and other residents who can swim using the pool during recreational hours provided there are instructors present. Some other active patients are able to swim every day and this is of great benefit to them.

The pool is not open to the public, but children from a nearby school for physically handicapped people use it.

The pool is used a great deal for teaching purposes and residents who can swim are given the opportunity to do so at any time during recreational hours.

ASA AWARDS SCHEME AND CERTIFICATES

Details of: (i) teachers/coaches qualifications and training; (ii) award schemes for personal performers can be obtained from: The Amateur Swimming Association, Harold Fern House, Derby Square, Loughborough, Leics LE11 0AL, and the Association of Swimming Therapy, Dr J Martin, 66 Church Street, Kensington, London W8.

WELSH INTEGRATED SPORTS PROGRAMME: WALES AQUATICS

The scheme sets out to integrate disabled and able-bodied people; increase participation in swimming; reward effort in improvement of personal performance; contribute to the safety of young people in water environments; and emphasise the social and enjoyment aspects of the sport.

The emphasis in this scheme is on the integration of able and disabled people. Therefore, awards will be made to pairs and not individuals. Each disabled person wishing to take an awards must recruit an able-bodied partner of either sex to accompany him/her in the scheme.

Who can join? Any 2 people, one of whom must be disabled in some way. For further details contact: Aquatics, Sports Council for Wales (Sophia Gardens, Cardiff, CF1 9SW).

NOTE: Some Gateway Clubs include swimming as part of their programme (see Chapter 18 p. 173)

HEALTH RELATED FITNESS SCHEME

Following the success of the Aquatics Awards which the Welsh Amateur Swimming Association has agreed to incorporate into its award scheme, the Sports Council for Wales has launched a new element in the Welsh Integrated Sports Plan.

Marilyn Godfrey, of the Sports Council for Wales, reports that: 'Sponsored by ASW the scheme consists of one session of low impact aerobics per week for 10 weeks. Originally intended to run for 10 weeks only, such has been the demand that we now have the original 20 participants on a maintenance session and 20 newcomers on the next 10 weeks.

'The tutor is a young American who has had considerable experience of working with fitness and health for all abilities, although her previous experience of mental handicap is minimal. However, people with a mental handicap are joining the sessions and since care staff are also encouraged to attend, a caring, social atmosphere has resulted.

'Reports indicate that the personal benefits of participation have been manifold, ranging from a blind couple finding recreation together, to a lady with a severe mental handicap learning to plan ahead and have her kit ready each week.

'The scheme will continue and is planned to extend into other areas of Wales.

'Initially piloted in south Glamorgan at the National Sports Centre for Wales, the sessions will move into Rhondda Valleys in February 1989.

'All participants receive a free T-shirt and take part at no cost to themselves.'

For further details contact: Marilyn Godfrey, the Sports Council for Wales (see Appendix 3).

FURTHER READING

Amateur Swimming Association *The teaching of swimming*. ASA, Loughborough, 1987.

Amateur Swimming Association. *The teaching of swimming for those with special needs*. ASA, Loughborough, 1985.

Association of Swimming Therapy. *Swimming for the disabled*. London, A & C Black, 1981.

Association of Swimming Therapy. Leaflets: *Forming a club; Lifting and handling; Swimming and epilepsy; Facilities; Medical considerations; Classification systems in competitive swimming*. AST 4 Oak Street, Shrewsbury, Shropshire SY3 7RH.

Diagram Group. *Enjoying swimming and diving*. London, Paddington Press, 1979.

Elkington, Helen. *Swimming*. Cambridge University Press, 1978
Lovesey, J. *Swimming a lifelong activity*. Tadworth, World's Work, 1980.

Royal Life Saving Society. *Life saving*. Royal Life Saving Society, London.

Williamson, DC. The transition swimming approach in instructing people with disabilities. *British Journal of Physical Education*, Vol. 19, July/Oct. 1988.

Wilson, C. *Swimming*. London, Barrie & Jenkins, 1977.

Chapter 10

Special Events in Sport and Physical Activities

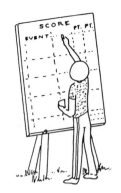

Displays - Tournaments: American or League; Knockout tournament; Progressive games tournament - Ladder and 'house' competitions - Matches - Athletic sports - Tabloid or potted sports - 'Mob sports' - Swimming sports or galas - It's a Knockout - Superstars - Miscellaneous events - Displays and festivals - Indoor or outdoor 'Have a Go' sports meeting - League finals day - Inter-hospital skittles competition.

Several types of events are suitable for single players, couples, teams or a number of teams from one establishment—some competitive some not. Providing the players have practised the necessary skills to an adequate standard, competition can be challenging and fun for participants and spectators alike. Some events such as displays, sports days and swimming galas, give parents and friends the opportunity to see for themselves just how high the standard of performance can be. It is possible to organise many types of events, and the rest of this section contains suggestions as to how such events can be organised.

DISPLAYS

Displays promote enthusiasm and a better standard of performance; they inspire confidence and help the social training of those taking part.

Displays can be of one or a series of items according to the purpose of the display.

The venue. This can be indoors or outdoors, on a stage or at ground level with the audience seated round or in rows. Entrances, exits and dressing room accommodation should be taken into consideration.

Music. If music is required check the availability of piano or other instruments and sound equipment.

Lighting. Check what lights can be used if required and what additional lights are necessary.

Programme

1. Decide on the length of the programme including intervals.

2. Select items which ensure variety and in which as many as possible can take part. The inclusion of a guest item such as a gymnastic or dance group can add interest, introduce a new activity and bring in more spectators. This special item can be professional or amateur.

Commentary

A good compère can 'make' a display. The audience should be given some information about the performers and the purpose of the display both verbally and in writing (programme) to ensure maximum and accurate publicity.

Organisation

Detailed organisation will, of course, vary but helpers will be required:

>   to look after performers, costumes,
>
>   equipment, audience, programmes,
>
>   first aid etc, press and radio coverage (if applicable).

Sources of help. Other members of staff, students, sixth formers, members of voluntary organisations, local sports council, regional officers of the BSAD (see Appendix 2), parents and friends.

Invitations. Written invitations should be sent to civic dignitaries, local and hospital authorities, sports councils press, UKSAPMH and any notable sports personality in the area.

Rehearsals. Performers should be rehearsed sufficiently to give them confidence and a feeling of achievement, but not to such an extent that they lose interest and spontaneity.

The compère

The compère is the key person at the performance itself. Select someone with a good voice and sense of humour who will ensure the continuity of the performance and keep the audience informed; someone who will talk enough, but not too much.

TOURNAMENTS

American Tournament - League System

This league system is suitable for soccer, cricket, hockey, basketball, netball etc (Fig 10.1).

Points: Win = 2 points. Draw = 1 point. Lose = 0 points.

Tie: In the case of a tie, the position is decided on goal average.

Knockout tournament (How to conduct the draw)

The number of entries in the competition, if not already a power of 2, ie 4-8-16-32 etc, must be made so by means of 'byes' — if there are 5 entries in a competition, the number must be brought to 8 by giving byes to three competitors. All byes are decided in the first round. The best means of drawing is to put the names of all entries in a box.

The following is an example: 12 entries — there must be 4

	Team 1	Team 2	Team 3	Team 4	Won	Lost	Draw	Points	Place
Team No. 1		Won 3–1	Lost 1–3	Draw 1–1	1	1	1	3	2nd
Team No. 2	Lost 1–2		Lost 2–4	Draw 2–2	0	2	1	1	4th
Team No. 3	Won 2–1	Won 1–0		Won 3–1	3	0	0	6	1st
Team No. 4	Draw 0–0	Draw 3–3	Lost 1–3		0	1	2	2	3rd

Figure 10.1 American tournament – league system

byes to bring the total to 16. The first 4 names drawn will be byes while the remaining 8 play (Fig 10.2).

Further examples:

Number of entries	No of byes	No of matches in 1st round
9 7 short of 16	7	1
15 1 short of 16	1	7
24 8 short of 32	8	8
29 3 short of 32	3	13

Progressive Games Tournament

A well organised tournament of this type can provide vigorous exercise for many at the same time. As with all mass events, success depends of thoughtful preparation and good organisation.

Layout of ground: Draw a plan of the ground — the positioning of the various games is important. Make sure that there is plenty of space between pitches so that there is no danger of competitors from one game getting in the way of those in another, of colliding or of being hit with a ball. Pitches should be numbered (see Fig 10.3). Mark out pitches before players arrive and see that all fixed equipment, goal posts, wickets, etc. are readily available and safe.

Choice of games: Choose games suitable for those taking part, this particular example is a tournament for men and women (mixed play) — and ones which do not require lengthy explanation and involve specialised techniques.

Alternate very energetic games with less vigorous ones. As each team plays all the others, the number of games should be **uneven.**

Course officials: Appoint a competent leader/referee to be in charge of each game. When the teams move on to the next game, these referees should stay on their own pitches and be responsible for teaching, umpiring and scoring. Also appoint a controller whose job it is to ring a bell or blow a whistle at the start, half-time and at the end of each round of matches.

Each team should have a leader/helper to see that players progress quickly to the next game.

Competitors: Divide players into an even number of teams with the two sexes in the same ratio in each, not more than twelve players in all, then arrange for the election or appointment of a team captain. Number each team A1, A2; B1, B2 and so on. By the end of the tournament all the 'one' teams will have played against all the 'two' teams. When the teams are ready, explain the organisation of the tournament, how the teams change, the time allowed for each match and the method of scoring.

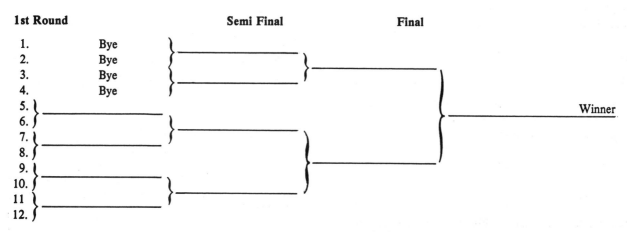

Figure 10.2 Knockout tournament: the draw

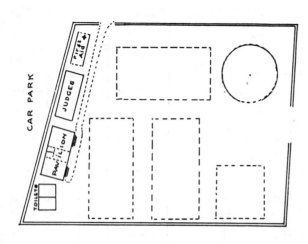

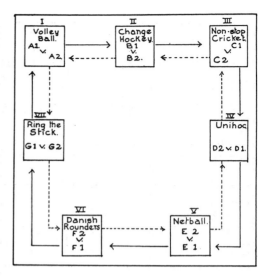

Figure 10.3 Layout for progressive games tournament

Order and time of play: In the first period of play, A1 will compete against A2 at game No 1, B1 will compete against B2 at game No 2 and so on.

At the end of the first round, all the 'one' teams move clockwise and the 'two' teams counter-clockwise on to the next game.

At the start of the next round, allow five to ten minutes for the leader/referee in charge of each game to check that the players understand the rules before the match begins. The time allowed for each match will vary according to the time available for the whole tournament; 5 to 7 minutes each way is suggested.

Scoring: At the end of each round the captain or leader of each team takes the result to the controller (helper) who enters the score on the scoreboard:

a win scores 2 points

a draw scores 1 point.

At the end of the tournament, gather teams together at the scoreboard (Fig 10.4), total the points and announce the winner. If two or more teams tie, arrange a simple relay to decide the winner.

LADDER AND 'HOUSE' COMPETITIONS

Ladder

Ladder competitions are a useful means of maintaining interest over a period of weeks. Individual couples or teams can compete in such games as: badminton, table tennis, short tennis, quoit tennis, team hand tennis, volley ball and many other minor and major games.

Each competitor (individual couple or team) is given a number. The draw is then made and the competitors are listed in the order in which they are drawn (Fig 10.5).

Any competition may challenge the one immediately above on the list (ladder). If the challenger wins, he moves one step up the ladder; if he loses, there is no change in the order. All matches must be played according to agreed rules. It is often necessary to encourage players to challenge the player above. The ladder should be made so that the name tabs can be pulled out and slotted in the new order.

House

The principle of this type of competition is the same as for the ladder competition, but it allows more scope for challenging. Starting at the chimney of the 'house', position all the competitors according to the order of the draw (Fig 10.6).

A competitor may challenge any other in the same row of bricks. If he wins, he may then challenge anyone in the row above; if he wins again, he then takes the place of the competitor he has beaten.

MATCHES

Matches can be arranged in almost every game between groups from hospitals, adult training centres, Gateway clubs, hostels, wards etc., and against school and youth clubs. Matches against schools and youth clubs provide an opportunity for integration and the subsequent social training.

ATHLETIC SPORTS DAYS

These should be run as near to the Amateur Athletic Association rules as possible (see p. 68 for address).

TABLOID OR POTTED SPORTS (For men, women or mixed teams)

Tabloid or Potted Sports, played indoors or out-of-doors, can provide a considerable number of people with varied, objective and enjoyable exercise. Events can be of different types involving the skills of throwing, aiming, running, dexterity and balance.

Each competitor is competing against a high or a low standard and scores points towards a team total at each event.

The events selected should vary according to the standard and interests of those taking part, the space and equipment available, and the occasion—for instance, at a social function, the aim is not so much to test physical ability as to provide the maximum amount of fun. No miniature sports meeting will be enjoyed unless it is well organised.

	1	2	3	4	5	6	7	Total Points			1	2	3	4	5	6	7	Total Points
A1										A2								
B1										B2								
C1										C2								
D1										D2								
E1										E2								
F1										F2								
G1										G2								
Section Total										Section Total								

Figure 10.4 Scoreboard for progressive games tournament

Preparation

Know the exact position of each event in relation to the surroundings. Take any hazards into consideration. Make a plan of the space available. Be sure that all the apparatus is to hand before the start of the meeting. If possible, find a few reliable volunteers to make the ground markings, to set up the events before the rest of the competitors arrive, and to help with judging, scoring, assisting competitors.

Selection of events

In selecting events, remember that they must be suitable for the competitors and that they should call for different forms of skill and effort, eg speed, accuracy in aiming at target, balance, endurance, skill in handling, spring. Arrange the course so that the less vigorous events alternate with the strenuous ones.

Competitors

Divide the competitors into teams of not more than ten players in each; no one should be left out. If a team is one short, player No 1 can have two turns at the first event, player No 2 at the second, etc.

Collect the competitors together to explain the general organisation of the meeting. When all are in their places at the first event, the judges explain the events and make the scoring clear.

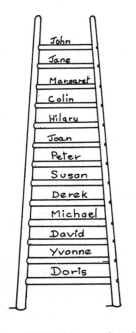

Figure 10.5 Ladder scoreboard

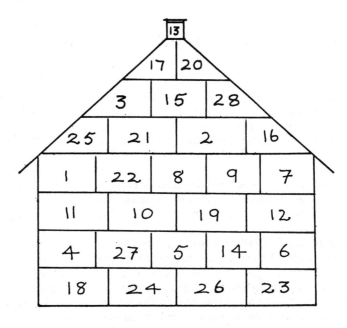

Figure 10.6 'House' scoreboard

Organisation

Start team A at the first event, team B at the second and so on. When all the members in every team have completed their turns at their first event, the signal for the teams to move on to their next event will be given.

Try to choose events which will take approximately the same time; otherwise some teams may get restless while waiting. If there are more than 8 teams, duplicate the events, and run two parallel meetings. Thus, teams A-E and F-J will be working round different courses, but in the end all will have a turn at the same events.

Officials

Provide a judge for each event, and a recorder to summarise the scores. Get each team to appoint its own leader, and make him responsible for moving it from one event to the next.

The recorder gives the signal for the team to move from one event to the other.

Scoring

There are various methods of scoring, but perhaps the best known is the double standard system (sometimes referred to as the A and B standard system). In this, high and low standards are set for each event; those attaining the higher standard win 2 points for their team, and those gaining the lower standard, 1 point. In order to decide the standards, ask a few players of average ability to try out the various events before the start of the meeting.

At the same meeting double and single standard systems can be used for different events. To remind all competitors of the standards, display them on small cards, or chalk them on the floor at each event. As each event is finished, the judge fills in a score card, signs it, and gets one of the team members to take it to the recorder. A specimen card might read:

TEAM:	A	
EVENT:	Throwing a ball for distance	
Points scored:	High standard — 6 players 2 points	12
	Low standard — 4 players 1 point	4
		16

Judge's signature ....

The recorder places the teams in their correct order of merit and enters on his summary (Fig 10.7) the number of the place gained. In each event the winners score 1 point, the second team 2, and so on. If two or more teams tie for a place they are awarded the average of the places tied for, eg two teams tying for a second place score 2^1/2 points each. At the end of the meeting the 'place points' for each event are totalled, including those awarded for the relay, and the team with the lowest number of points wins. It is a good idea for the recorder to use a blackboard, so that the teams may see their progress.

An alternative method of scoring — which can be used when all the events are being judged on the single standard system — is to count the actual points gained. This is a simpler method for inexperienced leaders, and competitors sometimes find it less confusing and more stimulating: when looking at the scoreboard they can easily see how their team stands. It may not give, however, a completely true result, particularly if there is a wide range between the number of points which can be scored for the various events. The actual points won at each event are entered on the scoreboard and at the end of the meeting the team with the **greatest** number of points is the winner.

Final relay

If, when the points are finally added, two or more teams have tied, arrange a simple relay to decide the winners of the whole meeting. Such a relay can be run, in any case, as a grand finale. Award points to each team according to its place in the race, the winners gaining 1, the second team 2 and so on. (If the alternative method of scoring mentioned above is used, the winning team will score the highest number of points and the last 1.)

An ingenious leader will be able to think out a great variety of events, and competitors will enjoy making them up for themselves. Those suggested below are merely samples. Although standards vary considerably, according not only to the ability of the competitors but also to the conditions, eg outdoors, indoors, grass or asphalt, the leader should set a high and low standard bearing in mind the most able and least able in the group.

Examples of events

Aiming

1. 12 throws of a tennis ball into an inclined bucket, from a distance of 2-3m (6-10'). the ball must remain in the bucket. Score 1 point for each successful throw.

2. 12 throws of a rubber or rope quoit to ring a peg 450mm (18") high, from a distance of 2-3m (6-10'). Score 1 point for each successful throw.

3. 6 single-handed overarm throws of a football at a netball ring, from a distance of 4.9m (16') i.e. edge of circle. Score 1 point for each successful throw. Throwing points within the circle area can be selected.

4. 10 underarm bowls with a cricket ball towards two skittles 300mm (12') apart, from a distance of 7-8m (23-26'). Score 1 point when the ball passes between the skittles without touching them.

5. 4 throws of a football to knock down a skittle, from a distance of 6m (20'). Score 1 point for each successful throw.

Speed

1. Dribbling with a unihoc stick and ball over a course of 20m (66'), with three obstacles (poles or chairs) separated by 5m (16.5'), the first being 5m (16.5') from the start.

2. Circular potato race. A circle of 6m (20') diameter is drawn and 8 potatoes are placed at regular intervals round its circumference. A bucket is placed in the centre of the circle and a starting line is drawn 1.8m (6') from the circumference of the circle. Starting from the line, run and pick up each potato separately and put it into the bucket: then run with the bucket to the starting line.

TEAM	Speed		Spring		Balance		Aiming		Skills		Relay	TOTAL PLACE POINTS	FINAL PLACE
	POINTS	PLACE	POINTS	PLACE	POINTS	PLACE	POINTS	PLACE	POINTS	PLACE	PLACE		
A	8	2	6	1	4	5	10	1	6	$1\frac{1}{2}$	2	$12\frac{1}{2}$	1st
B	2	5	1	5	10	1	7	4	6	$1\frac{1}{2}$	4	$20\frac{1}{2}$	5th
C	4	3	5	2	6	4	9	2	4	4	5	20	4th
D	10	1	4	3	7	3	6	5	2	5	1	18	2nd
E	3	4	3	4	9	2	8	3	5	3	3	19	3rd

Figure 10.7 Potted sports scoreboard

Spring

1. Hop, step and a jump, from a stationary start.

2. Three consecutive forward jumps with feet together. No hesitation allowed between jumps.

3. 'Haphazard hops'. 8 circles (300mm (1') in diameter) are drawn in zigzag formation and numbered 1-8. Stand on one foot in circle 1 and hop to circle 2, then to circle 3 and so on to circle 8. Hopping must be continuous, the feet must not be changed and the ground between the circles must not be touched. Two turns, one with either foot. Score 1 point for each successful round.

Balance

1. Balance walk along a bench (narrow side up) or a plank supported at both ends, balancing a book or beanbag on the head without touching it with the hand.

2. Mount and dismount three chairs in a line, balancing a book or beanbag on the head without touching it with the hand. Score 2 points if successful with three chairs and 1 point if successful with two.

3. Flower-pot walking. Stand on two strong flower-pots (or bricks), balance on one and move the other forward with the hand. Walk forward in this way for 6m (20'), turn and walk back to the starting point. Dismounting is not allowed. Score 2 points for the double journey and 1 point for a single journey.

Miscellaneous

1. 'Juggling' with two small balls
   (a) both hands
   (b) one hand.

2. Balance a pole on the fingers of one hand and change it to the other without the hands touching.

3. Blow a table tennis ball along the ground between parallel lines 200mm (9") apart with one breath. (Only suitable for indoors).

4. Reaction. Two judges (or competitors) hold a stick, 600-900mm (2'-3') long, at hip height. When the competitor is ready he says 'Go!' At any time after this signal, those holding the stick release it and the competitor tries to catch it before it touches the ground. When waiting for the stick to be released, the competitor may hold his hand over it but must not touch it. Six attempts. Score 1 point for each success.

'MOB SPORTS' (A variation of Potted Sports)

Arena

30 - 40 - 50m (100' - 132' - 165') long according to ability.

Formation

2 competing teams A and B divided into two streams each (Fig 10.8). Two against two in each head. (3 teams A, B, C can compete.)

Heats
8 7 6 5 4 3 2 1

A race is a complete series of heats in one event.

1st race (Each heat). Players run and remain at the far end in heat places — points awarded 1 - 2 - 3 - 4.

2nd race (Each heat). Players race back but with some variation in the race. Continue *ad infinitum*.

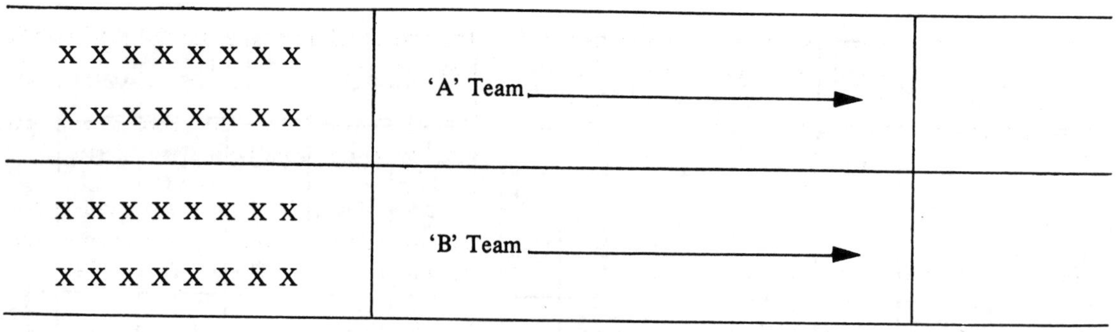

Figure 10.8 'Mob sports' – formation

Note: 1. The 2nd heat can be started before the 1st heat has passed the winning line and so on.

2. It is possible to run 120 heats in 45-50 minutes.

Variations

1. Straight sprint

2. Jump over balance bench at halfway stage

3. Run to a hoop. Pass it over head, step out and run on.

4. 2 hoops on the ground, throw 'objects', eg bean bag, from 1 hoop to the other and run on.

5. Erect a deck chair

6. Crawl under a net

7. As (3), but with 2 hoops instead of one.

Scoring

1. Points are totalled at the end of each race or at the end of the meeting.

2. Have separate score cards for each race, 'A race' 'B race' etc.

3. The team with the lowest total is the winning team.

4. Scorers only use Team Initials 'A' and 'B'. No names should be taken.

Team 'A' has the **lowest** number of points and is the winner (Fig 10.9)

Indoor events

1. Bouncing a ball into a bucket — box — bin (5 times).

2. Quoits (5) throw quoit over post — turn.

3. Deck Quoits (5) use a soft broom to push them into circles, each circle a different number of points in value.

4. Tossing shuttlecocks (5 old ones), into a hoop or circle on the ground from a given distance.

5. Standing broad jump.

The principle in all these sports is to have maximum participation. In the 'Mob Sports', nobody should be barred — a team could consist of 40 players.

SWIMMING SPORTS OR GALAS

For details of the organisation see swimming, Chapter 9, page 75.

IT'S A KNOCKOUT

Pat Brudenell, who has worked as a Further Education Lecturer specialising in mental handicap, and who is a qualified swimming teacher, describes how the project developed.

When 1981 was designated the Year of the Disabled, the Lions Club of Harrow felt it important to identify a group in the community who were not only disabled, but who were often forgotten. A group of adults with a mental handicap was chosen.

The club then suggested to eight Adult Training Centres in North West London that they should stage a day of fun and games on a sponsored basis — a suggestion received with great enthusiasm!

It envisaged that the day would be run along similar lines to the popular TV programme It's a Knockout, but on a sponsored basis to enable each centre to raise funds as well as have fun.

Races	1	2	3	4	Points 'A'	Points 'B'
	A	B	B	A	5	5
	B	A	A	B	5	5
	A	A	B	B	3	7
Total Points					13	17

Figure 10.9 'Mob sports' – scoring

RAF Stanmore kindly offered its sports arenas for the day. The Commanding Officer arranged for the Station charity fund to pay for the rental of the premises, and also mustered manpower, facilities and equipment.

Working together

Five months before the proposed date, a comprehensive planning meeting was held with all interested parties. In that first year it was important that each stage of the proceedings was carefully documented and discussed. At the time everyone thought that this was to be a one-off event — no-one dreamt it would become a major annual occasion.

Share and share alike

Each Centre was delegated certain responsibilities. Initially this involved selecting and organising two games — simple enough to be played by all participants. Once this had been decided, copies and instructions for the games were made available to the other Centres. This gave the eight Centres time to practise the 16 games. Each Centre nominated a Team Manager, responsible for 'training' the team of eight competitors. Two staff from each Centre were nominated as Games Referees — specific responsibilities being to run their two games and ensure that they were played correctly.

Making it accessible

As with many athletic events, inevitably the 'best' are those that take part. It was felt important that It's a Knockout should be made as accessible as possible to people with a mental handicap of all abilities. Obviously, there was a strong element of competition involved, but each team was allowed to have up to four substitutes — thereby giving some of the lower ability members the opportunity to take part in one or two events.

Each team was allowed to field a 'joker' card for one event, so that each Centre had an opportunity to run its own competitions at home for the best card.

Poster competitions were also organised; and, on the day, each Centre displayed its entries around the hangars in the Station — bringing a lot of colour and creativity to the event. Prizes were awarded to both individual and group entries — thereby enabling a great many people to be involved in the day's activities.

Scoring

As the competition was being sponsored it was vital that the scoring system could accommodate close, yet high scoring:

the winning team scored 7 points, 15 if it played its 'joker';

the losing team scored 6 points, 10 if it played its 'joker'.

Therefore, a team losing every single game would score 100 points, and the team winning every game would score 120 points.

Trophies

All competitors were individually presented with certificates, and each captain proudly accepted a trophy on behalf of his team.

The overall winners received the challenge Trophy which they held for a year.

All entries for the poster competition were also acknowledged by individual certificates.

The spirit of It's a Knockout places the emphasis on taking part — and not the winning — and this aspect of the competition was emphasised as strongly as possible.

The day dawns. . .

The timing of each event had been carefully worked out in advance, but it was crucial that the schedule was closely adhered to so that all the games could be played. Each Centre brought bus loads of banner-bearing supporters who took their places in designated areas.

RAF volunteers were attached to each team for the day, and dozens of Harrow Lions took up their places as stewards and scoring marshalls.

Each game had been designed to run for no more than 10 minutes — and much to everyone's surprise, this actually worked! team managers were supplied with a detailed guide to the day which outlined where each team should be at any one time — and most importantly, what they should be doing and against whom.

Although complex at first glance, the formula was really quite a simple one, as follows.

Each arena was divided into 2 sections, with a game set up in each. The 16 games were lettered ABCDEFGH and abcdefgh.

Each team was given a starting point, and progressed according to the plan from one game to the next. When all 8 teams had completed the first 4 games these games were dismantled and 4 more set up during a break of 10 minutes.

The process was then repeated — each team playing in both arenas.

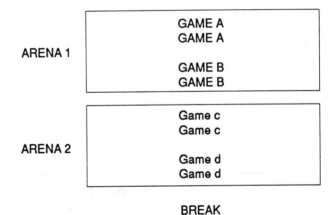

Team 1 start in Arena 1 and play Game A against Team 2. Both teams progress to Game b. Both teams move to Arena 2 and competing against different teams, play Games c and d.

At all times 2 teams are playing each of the 4 games.

After a 10 minute break, the 4 games are dismantled and 4 new games set up. Each team continues to move around both arenas, thereby completing 8 games in total by lunch time.

ARENA 1	GAME E
	GAME E
	GAME F
	GAME F

ARENA 2	Game g
	Game g
	Game h
	Game h

LUNCH

The remaining 8 games are played using the same format in the afternoon.

Team 1 programme

Time	Arena	Game	Opponent
11.00	1	A	Team 2
11.10	1	B	Team 2
11.20	2	c	Team 3
11.30	2	d	Team 3

Break for 10 minutes

Time	Arena	Game	Opponent
11.50	2	h	Team 5
12.00	2	g	Team 5
12.10	1	F	Team 6
12.20	1	E	Team 6

Lunch break

Time	Arena	Game	Opponent
13.00	2	a	Team 7
13.10	2	b	Team 7
13.20	1	C	Team 4
13.30	1	D	Team 4

Break for 10 minutes

Time	Arena	Game	Opponent
13.50	1	G	Team 8
14.00	1	H	Team 8
14.10	2	f	Team 6
14.20	2	e	Team 6

Games referee chart

Team 1 – Games A and a

Game A ARENA 1

11.00	Team 1 v Team 2 .... Winner ....
11.10	Team 3 v Team 4 .... Winner ....
11.20	Team 5 v Team 6 .... Winner ....
11.30	Team 7 v Team 8 .... Winner ....

Game a ARENA 2

13.00	Team 1 v Team 7 .... Winner ....
13.10	Team 6 v Team 2 .... Winner ....
13.20	Team 3 v Team 5 .... Winner ....
13.30	Team 4 v Team 8 .... Winner ....

Favourite games

The games varied enormously. In subsequent years some were dropped and new ones introduced. But the following were the definite favourites.

Jaws (Team 4 Game D)

Equipment: Polystyrene fish (metal/magnet in centre); tray; fishing rod with magnet; 1 whale; sou'wester.

Team lines up and, when the whistle blows, first team member takes fishing rod to tray of fish half way along course. Hooks fish (no hands — must use magnet) and runs to end of course — throwing fish into the jaws of the whale. Returns to next team member and hands over the rod. Last person, on return, puts on sou'wester.

Balloons (Team 5 Game E)

Equipment: 8 chairs; 1 cone; 8 balloons.

Chairs have a balloon attached to each and are placed equidistant in a straight line. First team member runs to furthest chair — and sits on the balloon. When it bursts, the next team member runs to next chair and so on. The first team to burst all the balloons is the winner (Fig10.10).

Hanging out the washing (Team 2 Game B)

Equipment: 1 washing line; 16 pegs; 8 tea towels; bowl.

Team lines up at start, and when the whistle blows, first team member runs to bowl of pegs and washing — collecting 2 pegs and 1 tea towel. Runs to washing line and pegs washing out. Runs back to team and tags next team member. First team to peg out all the washing is the winner.

Crackers (Team 1 Game A)

Equipment: 1 hurdle, Christmas crackers.

Team line up at start, and when the whistle blows, first team member runs to collect cracker furthest away, under the hurdle and back to team, to pull the cracker with next person. The first team to pull all the crackers in sequence is the winner (Fig 10.11).

Welly bash (Team 8 Games H)

Equipment: 8 pairs large wellies — each pair tied together; hundreds of balloons!

On the whistle, all team members put on their tied wellies and hop to end of course where balloons are on the floor. By jumping on them — all balloons must be burst. First team to return to start — winners.

Slalem (Team 3 Game C)

Equipment: 1 broom handle; 1 tray; 6 cones.

On the whistle, first team member pushes the tray with the broom handle round the outside of the cones — handing over to next team member on completion of the circuit. When all team members have completed the circuit, the first team back in place is the winner (Fig 10.12).

(NB. On the day — the teams ran in opposite directions to each other.) This was voted the favourite game of all. The staff game used this principle — but with only 1'6" broom handles!

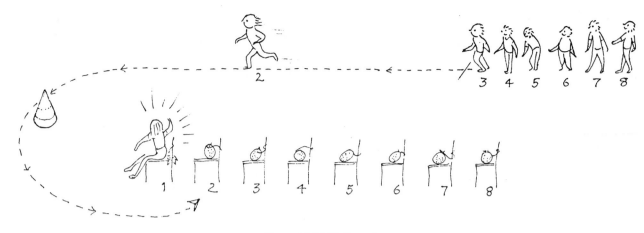

Figure 10.10 'Balloons'

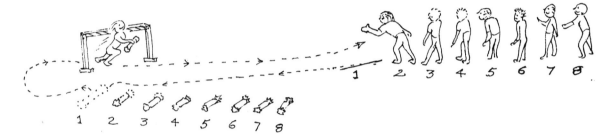

Figure 10.11 'Crackers'

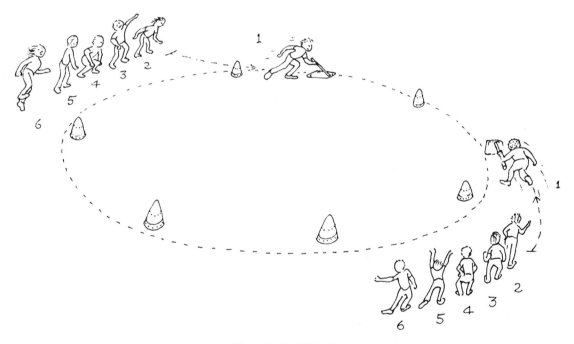

Figure 10.12 'Slalem'

Halfway through the day, a half an hour lunch break gave everyone a chance to prepare for the afternoon session. Score boards in each arena gave up-to-date information on who was winning what — and the excitement grew as each game progressed.

Staff game

At the end of the afternoon, to allow time for official score marshalls to make the final calculations, team managers and games referees took part in a staff game — which gave teams and supporters tremendous delight.

At 3pm the results were announced! And everyone knew that they were a winner! Exhausted, everyone rushed home to add up the sponsorship totals!

In 1981, the total sponsorship collected was £3450; in 1984, this figure rose to over £4000, and is still rising.

It's a Knockout now features as the major sporting and fun event on the calendar of the eight Centres.

What has happened since 1981?

A reunion was held three months after the event to discuss the 'repercussions' and share the photos and videos which recorded the event so vividly.

The RAF volunteers who had worked hard on the day, were so attracted to the people they were 'helping' that they soon became involved in other Centre activities, and eventually requests to join the club were received from Adult Training Centres outside the North West Thames region! In 1987 another It's a Knockout competition was organised by the Lions to accommodate this obvious need. Harrow Lions, through their very thorough documentation, have been able to provide other Lions clubs with the formula for success.

It is almost impossible to outline just how beneficial the event has been for all the people with a mental handicap who participated. The most obvious benefit — that of being able to have fun competitively — is just a small part of what has been gained.

The competition has given a great many people the opportunity to be responsible for the day, to look smart as representatives of their respective Centres and to work hard and do their best.

Team members themselves were involved from the outset— designing the games and preparing equipment and props created a democratic competition. It also provided opportunities for people with a mental handicap to have some say in just what types of games would be played. Built into all this, of course, was the chance for them to be able to decide if games were too complex or too simple for some of their peers.

For the staff, this venture was a new experience. In contrast to other major sporting events, the staff were not simply the people in charge of their teams; everyone was responsible. The teams knew where they had to be — often when the staff did not — and it was a refreshing change for them to share all the responsibilities. At lunch time one member of staff was told by the team captain to go away and have a drink — he said she looked as if she needed one! "Don't worry about us," he said reassuringly, "after what we've just done, we can cope with anything!"

The games that made up the competition became useful tools for the team to use in other training sessions. They could see the relevance of the skills involved and were able themselves to make the adaptations appropriate to other situations.

Choosing a team of eight with four substitutes seemed a formidable task at first. But after the first year, the members all had a good grasp of what was needed and selected the team themselves. They took into account every variable, and made sure that their choices accommodated people's needs and capabilities. They were always quick to point out that to spectate was far more fun than to participate! At least as a spectator you could see what was going on!

The competitive creative element allowed everyone to be involved. A great many handicapped people have no burning desire to do something 'sporty', but are delighted to have the opportunity to paint a picture or make a banner — or simply be there. At summer athletics meetings, everyone is aware of how boring some of the proceedings can be for spectators — but at It's a Knockout there is so much to see all the time — and all of it highly entertaining — being bored is impossible!

Raising money for much-needed extra pieces of equipment is a tireless and thankless task. It's a Knockout made fund raising a new experience.

Those who work in the field of mental handicap are constantly having to 'work hard' at something. If more establishments involved themselves in activities such the one described here then before long an international It's a Knockout might be a possibility.

SUPERSTARS

Superstars, another popular TV programme, inspired Pat Brundenell to use this idea with her students.

Superstars is an adventure! It generates pleasure and enjoyment for those participating, and can be used as a central focus for teaching a great many subject areas. It is very adaptable and can be geared towards any client group, but careful planning is essential. Superstars is certainly not something that can just happen spontaneously.

What is Superstars?

It is a group activity: each group member competes in a series of games — working against the clock or working against other competitors. The highest scoring competitor at the end of the series is the winner.

Who can play?

It is unrealistic to make the claim that anyone can play. Superstars has been used as an activity for a wide cross section of people with a mental handicap. It has been particularly beneficial for hyperactive youngsters and some individuals who tend to withdraw from group interaction and play.

How many can play?

After four consecutive years of running superstars, Pat Brudenall has a group of 32 mixed ability 20 to 47 year olds. But it is advisable to start with a small group of 8 to 12 people. This allows time and space for people to familiarise themselves with this way of working, the group being sufficiently small and manageable to sort out any teething problems as they may arise.

Who wants to play?

It is very important that those who **do** play actually **want** to!

Democracy is the best policy

The best results are always achieved when the entire group has had some say in what goes on. Although the leader will be directing proceedings, try to ensure that decisions are made democratically. People with a mental handicap spend their lives having decisions made for them — this is one occasion when we can help to redress the balance.

Before you begin

Planning is essential. The leader should carefully prepare for this activity before taking it to the group. This may appear to be time consuming — but not time wasted; once the master copy is prepared, it can provide a successful format for future use.

Getting started

Try to organise a Superstars at a time when there is not a lot going on, and then check with the administrators that what is being proposed is a viable proposition. If at all possible, try to cajole other members of staff to share the load.

Timetable the activity. Depending on the size of the group, the leader will need to plan ahead for at least eight weeks. Whenever possible, try to ensure that the session runs at the same time each week, in the same place. At some point, it would be ideal to take some of the activities outside — but this is not imperative. The most important factor is that the activity has a recognised slot—which other staff are aware of so that it does not overlap with other programmes of the individuals concerned.

Set the scene for the group carefully. It is one thing to explain something, but quite another for the concept to be fully understood. Superstars needs a numeracy base. Eventually, group members will be responsible for their own files and scoring. Many will be unable to do this unless first of all they are taught the necessary skills. This can be achieved quite easily within the sporting context.

A great many handicapped people can count from, 1 to 10/20/100 and so on, but many have no concept of what numbers actually mean. To understand how numbers can work, they have to be experienced. The following games are taken from Pat Brudenell's Superstars experiences.

Oxford and Cambridge

Two teams sit opposite each other on the floor, with legs outstretched and straight, feet touching. Each pair is given a number.

The leader shouts out a number, and corresponding people have to run round the back of their respective teams, carefully jumping over the remainder of the outstretched legs, back to their place. The first person to sit down in their place scores a point for their team.

Two teams standing in straight lines. Starting with the person at the front, each team member has a number — corresponding to their place in the line.

The leader asks Team A to call out its numbers — 1, 2, 3, 4, 5, 6, and so on.

Team B then does the same.

When each team is familiar with its numbers, the leader then asks each team to call out its numbers again, but, on reaching the final number, the team has to repeat but in reverse — 6, 5, 4, 3, 2, 1.

If team members are then asked to change places, the leader can ask each team to find out what their new numbers are. This can be repeated until both teams are familiar with what the numbers mean.

Combining the teams, the numbers become greater, and the game becomes more demanding. There may be people who simply cannot, at first, grasp what is going on, but leaders will find that many of them will be actively encouraged and helped by the more able group members. Leaders should give encouragement and support, but allow the group to find its own level.

Scoring

This can be difficult! Although not the solution to all problems, the following can be tried.

Using rolls of unwanted wallpaper, make a chart as follows:

Position	Points
1st	10
2nd	9
3rd	8
4th	7
5th	6
6th	5
7th	4
8th	3
9th	2
10th	1

If most of the group have little concept of what Positions are, cover up the Points side of the chart initially and spend time discussing what Positions are, and how they can be recognised.

Split the group into two teams. The first team member runs round an obstacle course, to a bucket placed at the end, whereupon he picks out a card. He then identifies the position on the card and indicates it on the chart. When this is successful, he then tags the next number in his team. The first team to complete the circuit correctly is the winner.

As soon as the group are confident with Positions, uncover the rest of the chart and bring the Points into play. This again is best achieved through more games.

The leader can use any type of equipment, and, if sporting equipment is not available, alternatives can be buttons, money, shoes.

Depending on the ability levels of the group, split them up into either pairs, threes, fours, teams. Give each group a card with a Position written on it. Ask them to refer to the chart to establish just how many points relate to the prescribed position. When this has been established, ask them to collect the same number of pieces of equipment. Encourage people to follow the dotted lines across from the Position to the Points side, so that mistakes can be kept to a minimum. Again this can be run as a team tag game. Whilst the leader may have to spend some time working on numeracy, he or she will still be incorporating sporting elements.

During the numeracy games, the leader must remind the group of the importance of scoring in relation to being able to play Superstars. Concentration spans may be short, and the leader should ensure that the group stays alert and well motivated. If the leader's energy levels are high enough, this will be easily transferred to the group. Whilst involved in numeracy games, leaders will become aware of how group members function on a more academic level.

What activities and games?

Ten activities are needed. All activities are attempted, and each competitor takes his best eight scores for his final total.

The following list of activities have all been selected by students. Over the years, adaptations have been made — some activities became quite complex, whilst others were made simpler. There are no hard and fast rules — save that they must be within reach of the group for whom they are intended.

Unless indicated otherwise, all activities are timed against the clock.

1. *Obstacle race*
   Course designed by the group.

2. *Football*
   Dribbling around a short obstacle course and shooting at goal.

3. *Hockey*
   Dribbling a hockey ball around an obstacle course and shooting at goal.

4. *Hoops*
   i   Two hoops placed next to each other. Participant jumps into first hoop, then second hoop, picks up the first hoop and places it in front of hoop on the floor — and so on. Starting line to finishing line = 2.1 m (7').
   ii Line of 10 hoops placed. One foot only in each hoop, participant runs along the line and back.
   iii 'S' shape made with hoops. As above.

5. *Basketball*
   i   Starting 3 m (10') away from net, participant approaches the net, bouncing the ball. Three tries are allowed for a basket. On the third try, participant returns to start, bouncing ball.
   ii $1/2$, $1^1/2$, 2 minutes to go from start to net. Maximum number of nets counted.
   iii Participants starts at net. Fastest time to score 3 baskets.
       (Impose time limit otherwise you could be there all week!)

6. *Sit-ups*
   Number achieved in set time — ie. $^1/2/1$ minute. This has to be tailor made to suit each group and each member's individual ability level.

   Cheating is easy! Ask participants to start off by lying down with arms outstretched behind their heads, back of hands on the floor. On sitting up, elbows cannot be used to lever the person up, and one sit-up is counted when hands reach the toes.

   Alternatives: lying with knees bent, feet flat on floor, hands behind head, when elbows touch knees on sit-up — this counts. This can be very difficult for many people; if necessary, use a bench to anchor the feet. The sit-up is counted when (a) the elbows touch the bench, or (b) when hands touch feet.

7. *Bench jumps*
   Participant stands feet astride bench. One jump is allowed and both feet must land on the bench simultaneously. Time for $^1/2$ minute as this is very strenuous. One jump is recorded for correct completion of both parts of exercise.

   This is very difficult. Using floor markers, ask participants to complete the exercise on the floor.

8. *Squat thrusts*
   Place markers on the floor. With hands and feet placed in the prescribed positions, participants have to 'jump' both feet forward of the marked line, and then 'jump' both feet back of the prescribed line. This is another strenuous activity and should not be timed for too long.

9. *Flying aircraft overhead*
   This is an elimination game, not played against the clock, and there are lots of variations.

   The instructions are called out by the leader, and the last person to reach the prescribed position is out. The winner is the last person to remain in the game. The instructions are as follows:

   'Port, Starbord, Bow and Stern' — if the group finds this confusing, use something from the room instead, eg 'wall side', 'kitchen side', 'door side'.

   'Scrub the decks' — group members kneel on the floor 'scrubbing'.

   'Salute the captain'. Standing to attention, saluting.

   'Man the rigging' — pretend to climb.

   'Flying aircraft overhead' — participants throw themselves on the floor, lying very flat and still on their stomachs.

10. *Swimming*
    In any mixed group, there will inevitably be some members who cannot swim. Alternatively, the work setting may be such that swimming is not an activity undertaken with any regularity. But for practitioners with access to a pool, the following can be used: (i) 25 m (83') any stroke; (ii) 25 m with the help of a float board; (iii) 25 m walking.

    Once again this activity will be determined by the ability levels of the group. When working with a high ability group, it may be necessary to employ a more complex structure. The distance can be increased, and a wider selection of strokes can be used. When working with a lower ability group, then more water games may have to be introduced, eg blowing table tennis balls across 5-10m ($16^1/2$-33') or walking 5 m with the help of float boards and so on.

    Having a grading system enables each person to find his own level. If the task is too difficult, then this will be off-putting.

11. *50m (165') sprint*
    This can be changed to any distance.
    A fun alternative is to create a 10/15/25 m walk backwards.

12. *Egg and spoon race*
    Glueing table tennis balls onto wooden spoons is sometimes easier than the more traditional interpretation of this game.

13. *Darts*
    Lots of variations for this one.
    i   Against the clock — the highest score with a never ending supply of darts!
    ii Highest score with 6/10/15/20 darts.

14. *Rolling a ball a certain distance along the floor.*

15. *Hurdles*
    i   Used in the normal way over a set distance.
    ii Set out over a prescribed distance, but instead of jumping over them, participants crawl under them.

The activities outlined are by no means exhaustive. Leaders can use their knowledge and experience of the groups they work with to devise other appropriate activities.

Whatever activities are selected it is important that the

	Obstacle Race	Sprint	Basket Ball	Sit ups	Hockey	Squat Thrusts	Hoops	Bench Jumps	Swimming	FAO	TOTAL
Robin B	1st 10										
Susan B	3rd 8										
Tom C	4th 7										
Karen E	5th 6										
Margaret H	6th 5										
Lisa H	2nd 9										
Peter L	11th 1										
Philip M	7th 4										
Sally P	10th 1										
Valerie S	8th 3										
David S	9th 2										
Michael T	12th 1										

Figure 10.13 Master Score Chart

team have some say in the selection process. Sometimes leaders will need to curb some of the more over-adventurous suggestions. One group became very irritated when the leader refused to include canoeing and a 12' high wall!

Plan of action

The next step is to work out a plan of action.

If the activities are numbered 1 to 10, it is important that a good cross section of them are played each session. Some are more strenuous than others, and this needs to be kept in mind.

Depending on how the leader organises the 'scoring', it may be advisable to play fewer games each session so that time can be spent working out charts and scores and enable discussion to take place on all sorts of related subjects. One of the main aims of Superstars is to broaden the context of sport, and leaders must make time to cover all eventualities.

If leaders decide, on the first occasion, to do the scoring themselves, this will leave more time for activities. But it is most important that those taking part understand what they are doing.

Leaders must be seen to be keeping to the rules! If games are played over a set distance, then it is important that the distance is clearly marked out. Should repeats occur the following week, markers should be placed in the same positions.

Allowances should be made for absences, and leaders must

ensure that when group members do not attend, they have the opportunity to catch up the following week. Since personal and inner discipline is very much a part of sport, two ground rules are useful:

1. unless a group member refuses to come to the session, arrangements can be made for him to catch up with activities when he returns. This makes allowances for dental visits, sickness, and other centre activities;

2. it should be understood that all games will be attempted. If someone does not complete an exercise — eg through lack of confidence — then one point should be awarded for trying. There is no incentive for anyone if points are not awarded for effort made. Leaders should encourage, never actively discourage.

When the leader has organised ten activities/games, a master score chart will be needed. This can be set out as in Figure 10.13

It is also useful to have a wall chart that can stay *in situ* in a prominent place. This will help to reinforce the work completed, and give people a focal point. As the leader completes his master chart, the wall chart can be updated; this acts as an incentive for team members and helps to create added interest from other staff and clients.

It is important to acknowledge that there are times when the boys do better than the girls, and although experience has shown that the girls outshine the boys in some respects, the boys nearly always win. To be fair, the master chart should always be drawn up alphabetically, and although the current chart leader should be prominently displayed, the organiser should always make a point of ensuring that the girls can see at a glance who is leading the 'ladies table'.

Each team member needs to have their own personal file, and be responsible for bringing this to each session. It is important that families and other practitioners involved are aware of what is going on, and the file can be a useful public relations tool. When files are started, send a note home explaining what the file is for, and stressing the importance of it arriving at the session each week. If leaders do their homework properly, the lost file should be a rare occurrence.

The leader may want to run a side competition for the best decorated file. Giving people a free reign to decorate their files can produce some wonderful results. The more involved people can become about their files, the more responsible they will feel for their safe keeping and update.

Once the ten activities/games have been selected, draw match stick diagrams to explain some of the more obscure ones. It is important that people can see at a glance what is meant by 'Squat thrusts' or 'Bench jumps'. Print in bold letters and explain the games simply.

Score sheets also need to be clear and simple as in Figure 10.14

Off and running

A stop watch, master chart and pencil are all the leader needs.

As with all sporting activities, make sure that groups are warmed up. If the group is a small one, the waiting period between each activity will be minimal, but leaders of large groups must be mindful of working cold muscles. Track suit trousers can help to keep the legs warm. Explaining the importance of warming up can save a lot of trouble later on, and remember that the aim is that the client groups should be independent and responsible.

As each participant completes an exercise, leaders should immediately give a result. The group will have their files open, and will want to record their achievements straight away. If they are unable to write the correct entry, try to find another group member to help.

Never rush people. They will all get there eventually.

Calculators

Ask group members to bring calculators to help with the sums. There are a large number on the market which have digits large enough to cope with poor co-ordination and dexterity skills. It is easier to ask someone to copy something visible, than it is to ask them to add up a column of figures.

In a few short weeks, the majority of the author's group were becoming efficient at using calculators, and parents were delighted that their sons, and daughters had at last managed to master these pocket machines. Through Superstars they were beginning to **use** them, whereas before they were simply **playing** with them.

The value of winning

When people respond with enthusiasm and energy, especially

Name . . Tom C . . . .
Day of session . . Tuesday . . . . . Time . . 2–3 . . . .

Event	Date	Position	Points	Totals
1. Obstacle race				
2. Sprint				
3. Basket ball				
4. Sit-ups				
5. Hockey				
6. Squat thrusts				
7. Hoops				
8. Bench jumps				
9. Swimming				
10. Flying aircraft overhead				

Overall total =

2 lowest scores = event . . . .

. . . .

Final total =

Position in Superstars =

Figure 10.14 Score Sheet

where competitions are involved, leaders should recognise this.

One way of acknowledging this response is to invest in two trophies — one for girls, and one for boys. Trophies represent effort made, and they are very much the outside confirmation of being 'the best' there is. If a competition is called 'Superstars' then there ought to be some visible and tangible evidence that whoever wins such a competition is a Superstar.

Certificates

All participants need some acknowledgement from staff and their peers that their hard work has been recognised. It is an inexpensive and easy task to design certificates. By running competitions for various events, staff can select the motifs most suitable for each occasion; by careful photocopying they can be transferred onto A5 size certificates.

Continuity

There is no reason why Superstars should be a 'one-off' activity. The whole event will be much more relaxed and enjoyable the second time round. By keeping a careful note of the previous year's records, the leader will be able to monitor progress. Inevitably, some games will be repeated and this will offer an ideal opportunity to establish if group members are improving upon their Personal Bests (PBs).

After the first year, the leader might consider introducing a new ground rule — that those who have been Superstars should not be allowed to compete the following year. They can participate in any event but their scores, while noted in their personal files, will not appear on the master chart. Superstars have a responsibility towards the rest of the group; their ability has been acknowledged, but they should now be encouraged to take on the added responsibility of assisting in the smooth running of the competition. They may wish to set up the activities/games, be responsible for the care and placing of equipment, or they may prefer to take on an administrative role. This has worked successfully, and it is very rewarding to see people with a mental handicap being encouraged by their peers, as opposed to being helped by staff. Very often, the peer group can explain in much clearer terms how the calculator works or which line to enter the numbers on and why.

Having extra help also eases the leader's load and creates a greater sense of sharing among the group.

Widening horizons

Having established the ground rules during the first year, it is important that the leader begins to introduce new group members. If some members of the original group are willing to help with the administration and are available to help the new members, the latter can feel their way gradually without holding up the rest.

It is crucial that leaders try to ensure that each person taking part feels that their contribution is of value.

Superstars helps to boost people's confidence in themselves and generates a sense of sportsmanship and team work, while respecting the capability levels of each individual. It offers an incentive to try out and experiment with the unknown, and in addition, is something to talk about, look at and be involved in. And last, but not least, it is fun!

MISCELLANEOUS EVENTS

Displays and festivals

Many movements and dance organisations arrange displays and are now including items for groups of people with a mental handicap, eg the Gainsborough Morris Dancers, Manor House Hospital Keep Fit Team, a fitness training group in Tower Hamlets, London, a Gateway Club dance group in Ealing, London, and the National Gateway Festival held bi-annually at the Festival Hall in London.

Indoor or outdoor 'Have a Go' sports meeting

The purpose of an indoor or outdoor sports evening is to give people with a mental handicap and opportunity to 'have a go' at various games and activities. If some young people who already take part in these activities, together with trained coaches, teachers, instructors, nurses, leaders etc, offer to coach the games, referee and take part, people with a mental handicap will have a chance to see and join in a selection of activities from which they can make a choice. Also those planning a continuing programme

of sports and physical activities will have an opportunity to discover which activities are most enjoyed by the clients.

The organisation of a 'Have a go' meeting is similar to a Progressive games tournament (see p. 79) but without the competitive element. Refreshments at half time will, of course, add to the enjoyment and give people a chance to get to know one another.

League finals day (indoors or out-of-doors)

Out-of-doors. In some counties the season is ended with a League finals day to which parents and friends are invited, together with mayors, councillors and officers of the various authorities, voluntary and sports organisations. These usually take place on a football ground, hospital or industrial sports ground or park.

During the day the final matches between the sections of the various games such as football, netball, volleyball and unihoc etc, are played off. Usually a buffet lunch is provided and there is a prize-giving ceremony at the end of the day. Such a day encourages healthy competition and enables parents and all others present to realise the standard of play which can be reached with patient coaching and practice.

Indoors. A similar event held in a sports leisure centre differs only in the games played — for example: basketball, unihoc, trampolining, badminton, volleyball, archery quoits, short tennis and table tennis. Games such as netball and archery can be played as part of an outdoor or indoor finals day.

Inter-hospitals skittles (plastic ten pins) competition

(As played in the Inter-hospital Sports Association South of the Thames.)

Twenty three hospitals play to these rules.

Apparatus: A set of plastic ten pins (skittles). 2 balls

Formation: Arrange 10 pins in a shallow triangle, sufficiently far apart to allow a ball to pass through without touching any skittle.

Two teams of 5 players

Game: No 1 bowls 1 ball — any skittles knocked down are removed. No 1 then bowls a second ball. The total number of skittles knocked down are scored.

Note: If all the skittles are knocked down by the first ball, they are replaced before the second ball is bowled.

Scoring: Each team plays 3 rounds to complete a game. The total number of skittles knocked down in the 3 rounds are scored, the highest number wins the game. Games points are awarded: 2 points for a win; 1 point for a draw.

A match consists of 3 games (15 players from each side). At the end of a match, all games points are totaled and compared:

	A team	B Team
1st game	1	1
2nd game	1	1
3rd game	2	0
	5	1

The A team win by 5 points to 1

FURTHER READING

Ministry of Defence Army Sport Control Board. *Small side team games and potted sports.* Ministry of Defence: Army Sport Control Board, Clayton Barracks, Aldershot, Hants.

Chapter 11

Movement and Fitness Training

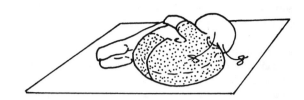

1.   *Movement training — Laban's principles — An example of a basic movement lesson — Examples of movements with emphasis on different body parts — Musical accompaniment and selection of music for movement — Two lessons based on Medau Rhythmic Movement — Sequences of movements using balls, hoops, scarves or ribbons — A Keep Fit lesson including hand apparatus — Two examples of Keep Fit in hospital; (i) Keep Fit at Manor House Hospital, Aylesbury (demonstration team) (ii) Keep Fit at Harperbury Hospital*

2.   *Fitness training — Fitness training exercises — Fitness training schemes — (circuit training; obstacle course; ropes course; Trim tracking; weight training and weight lifting; yoga; regular daily fitness training sessions; examples of two daily dozens (with and without chairs) — Weight watching — Assessment*

Movement and fitness training is a general term used to cover the many different systems of training which aim, to a greater or lesser degree, to:

> improve general health and maintain a high degree of fitness:
>
> teach management of the body;
>
> preserve normal movement in all the joints;
>
> maintain all muscles and organs in a healthy condition;
>
> improve stamina by increasing the power of the heart and the capacity of the lungs (circulation and respiration);
>
> increase mobility and strength;
>
> facilitate the learning of specific skills;
>
> give each individual an opportunity for creative physical activity;
>
> encourage communication of feelings and ideas;
>
> increase the span of concentration.

(See also Chapter 1.)

Some form of movement training is important for both men and women and can be enjoyed by and be beneficial to all. Although movement training, particularly when it is accompanied by music, could be said to be more suitable for and popular with women, there is evidence that groups of men and women working together benefit, providing the movements are selected carefully.

All different systems of movement training can be successfully adapted to meet the needs of people with a mental handicap. There is no 'one way' but the choice depends on a number of factors — on the knowledge and experience of the nurse, instructor, club leader and teacher, the availability of experi-enced teachers of movement in the area, what facilities exist within the hospital, centre or club and in the community, and on how much time can be allocated to movement training within the framework of the daily or weekly programme. This section includes information about the different types of movement training and good practice being carried out in hospitals, adult training centres and clubs. A number of adult education estab-lishments run fitness training classes which people with a mental handicap can attend. Movement and Dance Liaison Groups exist in each Sports Council Region. Membership is open to any movement or dance organisation. For further details contact: Regional Sports Councils (see Appendix 3).

For the sake of clarity, the activities involved in movement and fitness training are divided into two sections.

MOVEMENT TRAINING

Most of the movement training lessons are based on either Laban's principles of movement training, Educational Rhyth-mics, Keep Fit or Medau Rhythmic Movement.

On whatever system the lesson is based, all parts of the body need to be thoroughly exercised. There should be a balance between movements which emphasise stretching to counteract the all too common 'slouch' posture and relaxing movements to relieve tension.

The content of the lesson and the method of teaching, which should be lively, interesting and enjoyable, may have to be adapted not only to the ability of the group members, but to far from ideal conditions. The teacher may have to use her ingenu-ity. Versatility will ensure that interest is maintained and that the training effect is comprehensive. There must be a sound purpose behind all that is selected and taught.

LABAN'S PRINCIPLES

One method which is being taught increasingly in special schools is that based on Laban's principles.

Veronica Sherborne, former Senior Lecturer in Special Education at Bristol Polytechnic, who has for thirty years been training teachers of children with a mental handicap, has devel-oped ways of using these principles for such children and is now, as a free-lance teacher of movement in special education, intro-ducing them in hospitals, adult training centres and schools in many parts of the world. Briefly, her aims, which are equally valid for adults with a mental handicap, are to help develop children to experience ways of moving which they have missed and which are necessary if they are to acquire sensory awareness of their bodies and the ability to be aware of other people and form relationships.

'Feeding in' body awareness

The parts of the body which it is most important that the person should become aware of are those which bear weight, particularly the knees, and the centre of the body, the trunk. Initially, much of the work involves using the floor, or mats, as a surface against which someone can experience the body in such activities as rolling and sliding. Many ways of 'feeding in' bodily experiences, both parts of the body and the body as a whole, are described in *Physical and creative activities for mentally handicapped children* (see Further Reading p.112.).

Development of relationships

The different kinds of relationship play include ways of giving support and of being supported; the use of free flow experiences such as sliding, rocking and swinging; containing and being contained; and a variety of ways of experiencing the control of strength through pulling against or pushing a partner.

Relationship can be adjusted to the individual, ranging from work with the severely retarded — who appear to make no response to activities — to those who can take responsibility for the care of a partner. Finally, many adults and children can collaborate in groups of three or more. This aspect of movement teaching is described in detail in *Physical education for children with special needs* (see Further Reading p.112.).

The movement activities are presented in an enjoyable way, and the movement teacher, and any helpers, should join in the sessions. Veronica Sherborne's methods can be adapted to the needs of hyperactive people, to those with autistic tendencies, and to those who are multiply handicapped.

It is essential for the teacher using these methods to have had personal experience of developing his or her own bodily awareness and of building relationships. Although Veronica Sherborne's approach is essentially very simple, it requires intelligence, intuition and considerable powers of observation as well as experience in working with children or adults with a mental handicap.

New developments

In hospitals for people with a mental handicap Veronica Sherborne frequently works with a multi-disciplinary group of nurses, physiotherapists, occupational therapists, speech therapists, aides and teachers . Movement plays an important part in the school programmes, and nurses and therapists, working together, are experimenting in using movement with some of their patients.

In the Adult Training Centre it is the deputy manager, trained under her, who is responsible for the movement training, and the results are already most encouraging. These developments under Veronica Sherborne's guidance are proving valuable in linking the work in special schools with the adult training centre and the hospital programme (Groves and Upton see p.112).

Although the plan of a lesson will vary with the principles of the particular system of movement and fitness training followed, the following outline of a lesson and examples of movement may be helpful to those with little specialist knowledge and experience.

AN EXAMPLE OF A BASIC MOVEMENT LESSON

Since the length of lessons, the ability of class members and other factors will vary (whether they take place in hospitals, adult training centres and clubs) the content must be flexible, but should include:

Movements

1. *A warming up activity* to prepare the group members for the lesson.

2. *General body movement* ie movement of the whole body with emphasis on one or more body parts.

3. *Movements* designed to strengthen the muscle groups (a) extending the joints (particularly those of the spine); (b) of the abdominal wall.

4. *Group activities.*

NOTE: (2) and (3) can be performed in standing, sitting or lying positions. Foot and hand movements can be included in any part of the lesson. More times should be spent on (3) and (4) than on (1) and (2).

A lesson can be varied by including: apparatus — hoops, balls, clubs, scarves, ribbons; the use of fixed or portable gymnastic apparatus — benches, ladders, beams, box, climbing apparatus and agility activities using mats; a national or other form of dance at the end; training ending with a game or relaxation.

EXAMPLES OF MOVEMENTS WITH EMPHASIS ON DIFFERENT BODY PARTS

Warming up activities

1. Run a little way and stop still.
   Run further, stop and curl up small near the floor.
   Run again, stop. Arms stretched high — V-shape — wide stretch.

2. Stand with feet a little way apart knees easy.
   See how many parts of the body you can slap lightly — knees, thighs, back, chest, shoulders, head, toes, ankles, backs of legs, neck.
   Variation: use a light springy touch instead of a slap.

3. Stand or sit, rub the arms, hand, thighs, shoulders, legs, feet.

4. Shrug shoulders up and hold, down and hold, up down, up down. Circle shoulders singly and together vigorously.

Movements with emphasis on the shoulder girdle

1. In any starting position, trace various patterns with the hand in front of the body, eg '0', 2,3, and to the side.
   Variation: lead with the elbow instead of the hand.

2. In any starting position, clap the hands lightly in any direction round the body, concentrating on the outward movement after the clap and varying the levels above the shoulder.

3. Sitting or sitting on heels: beat a strong rhythm with the fists on the floor in a wide circle, then stretch both arms slowly in any direction. Gradually change the level of movement by reaching higher during each stretch.

Movements with emphasis on hip girdle

1. Standing, with one knee leading, circle it towards the supporting leg and outward — draw a circle with the knee.

2. Step with wide steps in different directions across, behind, sideways, cross behind, diagonally forward and back; each leg in turn and then alternately. Trace a variety of shapes on the floor.

3. In various kneeling, sitting and lying positions, draw one knee up to the chin then stretch it away from the body in various directions. Vary the speed of the movement, changing legs and starting positions.

4. Standing in lines or pairs (hold hands lightly for support) swing left leg forward and back — keep the body upright and the supporting knee straight. Change legs — change to swing back and forward.

   Variation: Swing right leg forward and back — repeat (1-4). Step right, left, right, lift left leg behind ready to swing (5-8). Repeat, swing left leg — repeat 1-8 continuously. This can be performed moving up the room.

5. 'Walking': sit upright, legs stretched in front, hands relaxed on knees. 'Walk' forwards and backwards from the hip joint, bouncing off the seat. Lift and push right leg forward past the right. Repeat these 'walking' steps rhythmically with the music.
   16 forward and 16 backwards, then cut down to shorter phases of 8 or even 4.
   Note: The effort of sitting upright is often difficult; give a short rest in between turns.

6. Rocking: sit upright, the palms of the hands resting on the floor at the sides. Rock rhythmically from side to side, taking weight alternately on each side.

Movements with emphasis on the whole spine and abdominal muscles

1. Sitting with legs apart, knees slightly bent, turn to the right, left arm reaching forward and downward to touch the floor as far outside the right foot as possible (1), return to sitting position (2). 'Stretch up tall', repeat 3 times (3-8), repeat turning to the opposite side (9-16).

   Variations: (i) 2 turns to each side; (ii) alternately right and left.

2. Lying, draw one knee up and stretch it out. Repeat with alternate legs, with both legs together. Vary direction and level.

3. Sitting with one leg straight and one leg bent up, change the position of legs at different speeds — lift the legs as they change. Use hands as support; later repeat exercise without support of hands.

4. In any starting position, draw circles with the arms in all directions round the body; small quick circles, large slow circles, circular floor patterns, arms singly and arms together. Facing a partner, shadow the other's movement with variations of speed, strength and levels. Other shapes can be invented.

5. Lying on the back, with the arms stretched out in a low V, palms upwards, slowly stretch arms up to a high V, keeping backs of hands on the floor, stretch the legs, and point the toes. Hold this position for 8 counts. Slowly curl up onto one side into as small and round a shape as possible for 8 counts.

Foot movements

Foot movements can be introduced at any stage in the lesson except immediately before or after movements involving strong use of the feet.

1. Move each joint in the feet separately: (i) lift heel and lower — keep toes on the floor, (ii) lift heel, then the whole foot to stretch the toes, but keep contact with the floor; (iii) lift the whole foot off the floor through stages (i) and (ii) 'peeling off'. Repeat each stage several times; develop into running on the spot.

2. (i) Sitting, bend and stretch the ankles alternately and together — pull the toes up — stretch them down; (ii) cross one leg over the other at the ankle, ankle circling outwards; repeat with other foot — repeat circling inwards — encourage the drawing of a large 'O' with the big toe.

3. Sitting — open and close the toes.
   Different combinations of the last three movements can be made into short sequences.

4. Suggest simple movements involving changing the weight from one foot to the other in various directions, forwards — backwards, diagonally forwards and backwards — sideways — across in front and behind.

5. Walk on toes.

6. Walk quickly, slowly, quietly, loudly, with short and long steps, stamp. Combine any two, eg: (i) 4 long steps followed by 8 short steps; (ii) stamp (1-4) walk quietly (1-4); (iii) walk on toes (1-4), walk with short steps (5-8); (iv) walk quietly (1-4). Stamp on the spot (5-8).

7. Practise dance steps, eg skip, polka, slip.

Hand movements

1. Clench fingers tightly. Open hands sharply and fully. Repeat, slowly clenching the fingers and slowly stretching them apart.

2. Shake the hands freely in different directions and levels, encourage relaxation in the wrist.

3. Sit on the floor — play on imaginary instrument, encouraging individual use of the fingers.

4. Kneel or sit — pretend to 'glue'; the palms of the hands onto the floor. Slowly peel the hands off and away, lifting the wrist and palms first then the fingers, Chant: 'Stick, lift, stick lift.'
   Repeat this movement but 'glue' the hands together or to parts of the body, eg to the legs, sides. Chant: 'Push it away'.

5. Sit or stand, stretch hands: (i) move first finger to thumb, repeat with the other three fingers; (ii) play a five finger exercise in the air or on the floor. Repeat (i) but when each finger in turn is touching the thumb, press together gently. Chant: 'Touch and press', 'touch and press'. Can the thumb touch all the fingers together?

6. Circle the wrist outwards and inwards, keeping the elbows to the sides. Stretch arms forwards, palms turned to face the floor. Turn palms up and down continuously.

7. Sit or stand, pretend there is a door in front, push it open. Encourage the palms and fingers to be stretched before pushing.

Composite lesson

A short warming up period of general exercise selected for example from the above movements — one or two from each section — can be followed by a dances, games, movements using balls, hoops or scarves or simple gymnastic agilities.

MUSICAL ACCOMPANIMENT AND SELECTION OF MUSIC FOR MOVEMENT TRAINING

Accompaniment

Accompaniment can either be provided by the teacher's voice, piano, recorded music (record and tapes) or by a percussion instrument. A steady pulsating rhythmic beat will help the trainee develop more feeling for movement. In creative work, it can enhance movement, quality and expression. The music so 'reinforces' the movement that, as soon as a particular tune is played, the trainee may well perform a specific movement automatically. Include where possible music selected by class members; perhaps some members could produce their favourite tune to which a special movement sequence could be devised for all to perform. Music should help the class to improve their performance as well as providing enjoyment. It should help them to move more lightly on their feet, swing their limbs more freely and give them a feeling of stretch or poise where necessary. To achieve this, suitable tunes must be chosen to fit the movement: ie for their rhythm — smooth, dotted or swinging, pattern — rise and fall of melody, number of phrases — and for their character — heavy or light, sharp, flowing.

Voice

The teacher's voice is all-important: by giving clear explanations and indicating the rhythm, speed and quality of the movement, both to the class members and to a pianist (when one is available) the teacher can create the right atmosphere in the class. The teacher can use words to encourage, prompt and coach by chanting them in time with music.

Piano

Played by a good pianist who can improvise for different movements, the piano accompaniment is perhaps the ideal. The advantages of using a pianist are:

(i)   the continuity of the lesson is more easily maintained since the teacher is not involved with records and tapes;

(ii) the speed of the music can be varied, the quality of movement enhanced;

(iii) a greater variety of tunes can be used;

(iv) adaptations can be made on the spot.

Percussion

The most useful percussion instruments include clappers, cymbals, tambourines, drums, triangles and a tunable tambour with a round-headed beater. Simple percussion instruments can be improvised and made quite cheaply. A beat can be indicated by tapping two sticks together.

Recorded music — Tapes and records

Recorded music is less suitable because the speed cannot be varied and the phrasing is often not consistent throughout the record. Non-vocal records are generally more suitable since the rhythm is clearer. It is also difficult to teach the component parts of the movement using the music as the teacher cannot be continually putting the record on and off in order to correct and coach details. With the help of a good pianist, tapes can be made of a selection of suitable music for simple movement sequences including pauses during which the teacher can prompt and coach. After a pause, the music can be repeated at a slower or quicker speed as necessary; in fact, a tape can be 'tailor-made'.

If a pianist or musician who can improvise is not available, well known tunes can be used but only if they are simple and their tempo is suitable to the movement; complicated music will tend to dominate the movement.

Music for movements of different types

Skipping — 6/8: for skipping, galloping, pas-de-bas steps and jumps, eg '100 Pipers', 'The Lancashire Poacher'.

Walking — 4/4: many familiar marches, provided they are played without too marked an accent, eg 'Waltzing Matilda'.

Running — 2/4: 2 runs to a bar, eg 'Bobby Shaftoe'.

Swinging — 6/8: continuous rhythm, eg 'Skye Boat Song'

Swinging — 6/8: with accent, eg 'My Bonnie Lies Over the Ocean'.

Swinging — 3/4: triple runs — lilts, eg Many Chopin waltzes.

Sharp, light — 2/4: eg 'This Old Man' — 6/8 eg 'Bonnie Dundee' 'Little Brown Jug'.

Smooth, flowing — 4/4: eg 'All Through the Night', 3/4 'The Ash Grove'.

Strong sustained — 4/4: eg 'The Volga Boat Song', 'Old Man River'.

Beaten, accented — 4/4: eg 'John Brown's Body'.

Combined swinging and stretching — 6/8: eg 'Blow the Man Down', 'Rio Grande'.

Combined beating and lifting — 6/8: eg 'Girls and Boys Come Out to Play'.

Polka — 'See me Dance the Polka'.

Waltz — Strauss waltzes.

Mazurka — Mazurka from Coppelia.

Rope skipping — syncopated 4/4: eg 'Scatterbrain'.

TWO LESSONS BASED ON MEDAU RHYTHMIC MOVEMENT

Two lessons based on Medau Rhythmic Movement are included for the following reasons:

> to show how movements are built up in simple stages over a period of time;

> to show how hand apparatus, balls, hoops and scarves can be used to aid the movement and to add variety and interest.

Sequences using a ball, hoop or scarf can be memorised and used for a display or be introduced into the ordinary lesson. (Figures 11.1, 11.2, 11.3)

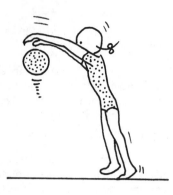

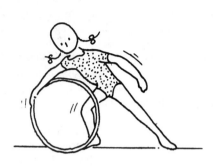

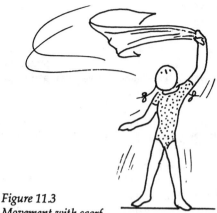

Figure 11.1 *Bouncing a ball*

Figure 11.2 *Using a hoop*

Figure 11.3
Movement with scarf

Lesson 1

Opening activities

1.   Clapping and stamping.
     Stand in a space. Clap hands in any direction, eg towards the ceiling, the windows, the floor. Clap hands 4 times moving arms to full stretch followed by 4 claps on the knees. Repeat No 2. 4 claps in any direction and 4 claps touching either knees, calves, ankles. Repeat clapping upwards with 3 claps and stretch higher on the 4th beat, bend to clap over the knees 3 times. Stamp feet 8 times lifting the knees up high. Repeat clapping as in No 4, then 4 stamps facing front, 4 stamps to turn around on the spot.

2.   Transfer of weight with body swings and partner work. Stand with feet apart, weight on the right foot, swing body and arms to the left, right and left, and clap out to the left side. Repeat to the right.

     Partners face each other, with one hand joined and weight to the same side, swing arms to transfer the weight from side to side with a swinging action in the legs and hips. Repeat all with the other hand joined. Partners face each other as in 7, swing across and out, swing across and run forward with partner side by side. At the end of the phrase change hands and repeat.

3.   Walking and running.
     Following a leader, walk and run according to the changes in the rhythm of the music.

Main section

(with a ball, 17.8 cm (7") diameter, 0.5 kg (1 lb) weight)

Aim: To exercise the whole body rhythmically, encouraging a stretch through it.

1.   Sit on the floor in a circle, with legs wide apart and the ball between them. Hit the top of the ball with the palm of the hand using alternate hands to a given rhythm.

     Repeat making a fist with the hand on the slow beats and using fingers on the quick beats.

     Repeat making a fist with the hand on the slow beats and rolling ball away from the body and back on the quick beats.

     Repeat above movement with the ball by the side of one hip keeping a hand on the ball; roll it as far sideways as possible and back again. Repeat to the other side.

     Sit with the legs apart, the ball by the right hip. Roll the ball down outside of right leg Then roll down the inside of the left leg around the foot and up the outside of the left leg to finish by the left hip.

Repeat in reverse.

Repeat No 4 but as ball reaches the left hip, continue to roll it behind the back and change hands behind the back, finish with the ball by right hip.

2.   Sit with legs wide apart, bounce the ball — a continuous movement keeping hands on top of the ball.

     Repeat, bouncing the ball with both hands, also one hand at a time.

     Bounce ball 4 times, followed by one strong bounce, stretch up towards the ball and catch.

     Bounce, the ball, gradually changing to standing whilst bouncing. If this is too difficult, stand up and then start to bounce.

3.   Bounce, roll and catch with partner.

     Stand with a ball facing a partner, bounce the ball for the partner to catch. Encourage a good stretch through body. Face partner. Strong bounce across to partner, who catches the ball, and bounces it back to partner. Bend down and roll the ball across to partner to pick it up.

     Face partner — a little distance away. One partner rolls the ball across to the other who bends the knees to pick it up and throw it upwards and across to partner. Repeat the movement with the other partner starting the roll.

     One ball each, start from the end of the hall. Bend and roll ball forward, run by the side of the ball as it rolls, overtake it to come in front of the ball, bend and pick it up into a throw, stretch and catch. Repeat movement to continue rolling ball down the hall.

4.   Walking.— bouncing a ball continuously.

     Collect the balls by throwing them into a large bag held open by 2 class members.

Final Section

Aim: To encourage mobility in hip joints and a feeling of spring.

1.   Stand in a circle with hands joined. Stand on left leg, swing right leg forward and back, 3 times, stamp right, left, right.
     Repeat leg swinging on right leg.

2.   Step forward on right leg, swing left knee up high, and step back on left leg, back on right leg. Repeat on left leg. Repeat 2, swinging the knee out to the side.

3.   In a circle, a wide step to the right, close left foot to right; repeat to the right 3 times; repeat all to the left.

4.   Gallop to the right for 8, repeat to the left.

5.   Facing a partner, hands joined, repeat gallop step sideways, adding a variety of claps or stamps.

Teaching

When *bouncing the ball*, follow the bounce with the body to give a feeling of resilience or elasticity. Keep the hands on top of the ball to give a feeling of drawing the ball up like a yo-yo.

When *throwing the ball*, stretch towards it with arms and body before catching.

When *rolling the ball*, bend the knees, keep the seat down, with a long back.

Lesson 2

(using a hoop. 61 cm-76.2 cm (24-30") diameter)

Opening activity (warm-up).

Stand with hands joined in a circle.

1.   12 walking steps to the right. 4 stamps with alternate feet, and on the spot turning to face the opposite direction.

12 walking steps to the left. 4 stamps on the spot. Repeat taking longer steps to the right, 12 steps. Stamp alternate feet 3 times — rhythm: quick, quick, slow.

Repeat walking to the right.

Repeat this phrase walking and stamping to the left.

Practise the rhythm with hand clapping and stamping separately — quick, quick, slow.

Repeat to the left: finish facing the centre of the circle.

6 walks forward to the centre of the circle, clap hands — quick, quick, slow.

6 walks backwards, clap — quick, quick, slow.

2.   Combine the two movements as follows:

In a circle hands joined.

6 walks to the right and 3 stamps — quick, quick, slow. Repeat to the left.

6 walks into the centre, 3 claps — quick, quick, slow.

6 walks away from the centre, 3 claps — quick, quick, slow.

3.   Repeat 2 with running steps.

Main section

(with a hoop)

Aim: Work with a hoop to increase the mobility of the spine, to twist, stretch and curl it.

Stand inside the hoop holding it with one hand on each side, with straight arms.

1.   Turn the hoop so that one hand comes forward and the other back, the body twisting at the same time, twist back to the starting position. Repeat in the opposite direction.

Repeat so that it is a continuous twisting first to one side then the other — twist and a twist and a twist.

2.   Repeat twist 4 times

Lift hoop vertically up to stretch to the ceiling. Lower hoop over the body to the starting position. Repeat.

3.   Repeat twist 4 times.

Lower hoop to put it onto the floor, slowly. Stand up without hoop and stretch both arms to the ceiling.

Bending knees and keeping back long, pick up the hoop and return to original starting position.

4.   Repeat twist 4 times

Lift hoop down over the body and bend to lower the hoop to within a few inches of the floor. Return to original starting position.

5.   Partners standing side by side with one hoop: one partner holding the top of the hoop in a vertical position with the lower edge of it on the floor. The partner without the hoop bends down to crawl through it, returning to standing position to take the hoop for the other partner to crawl through. The movement could be done to a set rhythm, add rhythmical clapping after crawling through the hoop and before holding it for the partner to repeat the movement.

6.   One partner holds the hoop as in 5, with feet apart and weight to one side, with a swaying action through the legs and hips, gently roll the hoop from side to side 4 times.

Hold the hoop still whilst the partner bends to crawl through it and to take the hoop for the other partner to repeat the rolling from side to side.

7.   Each person with a hoop. Start from one end of the hall. Roll the hoop from side to side with a swinging action in the legs, as in 6, 4 times, followed by rolling the hoop forward. Run with it to catch it — 'roll — roll — roll — roll run — run — run and catch'. Repeat continuously.

8.   Roll hoop running with it, clap a short rhythm before catching it and repeating the movement.

Floor section

Aim: to encourage mobility of the spine.

1.   Hoop flat on floor. Sit in it with feet outside, with alternate hands, reach out to touch the hoop in different places, so twisting the body, eg touch in front, at the side, behind, sitting as before. With right hand, touch in front, twist and touch on left side, twist further and touch towards the back and come back to original position.

Tap the floor with a simple rhythm.

Repeat with the other hand.

2.   Sit behind the hoop — flat on floor — reach to touch different parts of the hoop. With alternate hands, stretch 4 times and tap a simple rhythm on the floor, with hands in the middle of the hoop to end of phrase. Repeat, stretching alternate legs so that the foot touches different parts of the hoop, then tap a simple rhythm with the feet.

3.   Sit slightly sideways to the hoop with legs to one side. Trace the shape of the hoop using one foot, repeat with the other foot.

Continue to trace the shape of the hoop, using the hand and arm or foot and leg as if painting the hoop.

Final section

Standing in a circle.

1.   Stand on the right leg in a circle with hands joined, tap the floor in front with the left heel, then left toe twice, feet

99

together and pause. Repeat with the right heel and toe.

2. Heel and toe with right foot stamp right, stamp left, stamp right — quick, quick, slow. Repeat left.

3. Stand on right leg with left leg stretched forward. Make a large 'pawing' movement with left leg twice and stamp, stamp, stamp, — quick, quick, slow. Repeat with the other leg.

4. Partners side by side travel up the hall. Repeat 3 once with right leg and walk forward for 8 steps. Repeat movement with the left leg.

5. Walking, either following a leader or with a partner, change to a phrase of running and return to a phrase of walking change to a phrase of skipping and return to a phrase of walking.

SEQUENCES OF MOVEMENTS USING BALLS, HOOPS, SCARVES OR RIBBONS

Movement sequences are only suitable for more able trainees/residents. Teach each movement separately and then combine them in any order, gradually working towards a sequence of all the movements.

1. Music of 'Eye Level' or a similar rhythm. Bounce ball 8 times, followed by strong bounce, stretch catch, strong bounce, stretch catch.

   Repeat 3 times.

2. Hold the ball in both hands, feet apart and weight to one side.

   Swing changing weight from one side to the other 4 times; swing the ball into a large circle and swing.

   Swing the ball into a large circle and swing.

   Repeat the 1st movement again.

A sequence of movements with a hoop
Music: 3/4, eg 'Edelweiss'.

1. In two's face partner of equal height, partners hold hoop horizontally between them, with hands under the hoop and at the sides. Weight to one side, swing, changing the weight from side to side, 6 times then slowly swing and lift the hoop up high, turning under it as if to turn the hoop right over — pancake turn.

   Repeat. Finish holding the hoop horizontally with right hand.

2. Waltz steps (1, 2, 3) round each other in a clockwise direction, slightly pulling away from the hoop, then change hands.

   Repeat waltz steps in an anti-clockwise direction. Repeat.

   Finish with one of the partners holding the hoop in a vertical position with the edge of the hoop on the floor.

3. Twist and spin the hoop in a vertical position, both partners run round the spinning hoop — finish in original places. While one catches the hoop, replaces it on the floor and spins it again, the other partner claps hands to the rhythm of the music.

   Repeat, the other partner catching the hoop.

   Finish holding the hoop flat between partners as in 1, ready to repeat the sequence.

Movements with scarves or ribbons

These movements are suitable for and enjoyed by people with a mental handicap. Scarves — one metre square. **Big** scarf movements can increase the range of movement. Holding the scarf by the corner, make the following movements:

1. swing it from side to side or back and forward;

2. make circles in front, at the side and around the body, also above the head;

3. run, trailing the scarf;

4. for dexterity: fold the scarf with both hands, or one hand only;

   screw it up in one hand and throw it high;

   watch it as it floats down;

5. use it as an obstacle for stepping over;

6. dance with the scarf (own interpretation) while a piano plays various styles of music, eg Spanish, Ballet, Can-Can, gypsy.

A KEEP FIT LESSON INCLUDING HAND APPARATUS

The Keep Fit lesson at the Chelmsford Adult Training Centre is taken by a member of the centre staff who is also a keep fit teacher. Through the experience of working in two centres, she has found that the following type of lesson is both educationally and socially beneficial.

Part 1

General warming up and intermingling using lively music to stimulate and setting the mood for the lesson.

1. Walking in any direction using the whole space. 16 walking steps, finish with feet apart, sway right, left — feet apart.

   Four slip steps to right, sway left, sway right. Four slip steps to the left, sway right, sway left.

   Repeat.

2. Walk 16 steps to meet a partner, finish with feet apart, side by side holding inside hand.

   Sway right, left — feet apart (1-4). Repeat 6 times (5-16).

   Repeat to meet another partner.

   Variation: (a) Sway facing partner with both hands joined. (b) Substitute slipping steps sideways for swaying.

Part 2

Using small apparatus.

Hoops

1. Standing with feet together, hoop held undergrasp in right hand and out to the side.

   Swing hoop in front to the left and to right continuously, repeat with left hand.

   Variation: (i) Repeat swing with right hand (1-6), pass hoop into left hand and out to the left side (7-8). (ii) Repeat exchanging the hoop overhead (7-8). (iii) Repeat with feet apart and swaying from foot to foot.

2. Standing with feet apart, holding hoop in front and parallel to the ground with both hands.

   Swing hoop across body to left, swaying from right to left foot, repeat to right repeat continuously left and right — increase the width of the swing.

3. Sitting on floor with feet on right hand side. Holding hoop on floor in front — palms facing upwards. Lift hoop in front and high towards ceiling. Lower hoop over head to touch floor behind. Return slowly, pausing overhead, with a high stretch and lowering hoop to floor in front.

Balls

1   Stand with feet apart holding ball in right hand. Throw ball from right hand into left hand and back, continuously.

2.   With feet together, throw ball up and catch four times (1-8).

   Pass ball at waist level around body, twice (9-16).

   Repeat throw and catch (1-8).

   Repeat passing ball round body in the opposite direction (9-16) 4 times. Suggested tune 'Eye Level'.

Streamers

(Made from short dowelling rods 250 mm (10") long with streamers of ribbon or crepe paper 50 mm (2") and 1.5 m (60") long. This part of the lesson encourages class members to make up their own movement patterns, the only instruction being a verbal reminder that there are different 'levels' to move in, i.e. low, medium and high, and that one can balance on different parts of the body, eg left or right side, left or right knee, both knees, sitting, lying, using both hands in turn to manipulate the streamer. Each member should decide on their own starting and finishing positions.

   Suggested music: Slow waltz-time.

Part 3

Calming down, relaxing period.

   Suggested music: waltz-time.

   8 waltz steps anywhere in the room — 8 bars (1 step to 1 bar).

   Raise both arms to shoulder level — 2 bars.

   Lower to sides — 2 bars.

   Relax head and shoulders forwards — 2 bars.

   Stretch to standing position — 2 bars.

   Repeat several times.

   Variation: Single or double arm raising sideways, forwards or upwards, downwards in any combination of directions.

TWO EXAMPLES OF KEEP FIT IN HOSPITALS

Keep Fit at Manor Hospital, Aylesbury (demonstration team)

In 1971 the Manor House Hospital in Aylesbury approached the Buckinghamshire Keep Fit Association for a teacher to take a keep fit class with a group of young women resident in the hostel attached to the hospital. Two teachers volunteered. They started with a group of 8 young women with moderate and severe mental handicap, their ages ranging from 22 to 37 years. From the beginning all wore white shorts, yellow cotton shirts and white plimsoles. Keep fit classes, including other age groups, continue at the hospital under the same leaders.

Progress

At first only very simple movements were taught in a circle formation and singing action games. After some weeks, 6 young men joined the group and the lesson was adapted to include not only keep fit exercises but country dancing which provided opportunity for social training. Gradually hand apparatus was introduced — hoops, clubs, scarves and ropes. Later, special attention was given to freedom of expression at one stage in the lesson. The teachers were surprised to see how the class remembered what had been taught, and how well they were able to make up movements of their own. Later the boys were involved in outside rehabilitation training, and were too late back to join in. More young women joined the class bringing the numbers up to 12. They responded well to the music and greatly enjoyed moving. After a visit to one of the Keep Fit Association functions, they asked to wear leotards. The hospital fitted them out with black ones, which they wore with their ordinary tights and plimsoles. They were not yet prepared to work with bare feet.

Demonstrations

The group have given demonstrations at various functions with great enjoyment. Their latest demonstration is performed with scarves 1 metre square in all shades of blue green. Not only does this group demonstrate the pathway or pattern of the movements but also strength and lightness and other qualities of movement. (For details of this sequence see end of section.) Each member of the group was a member of the Buckinghamshire Keep Fit Association.

Integration

Members of the teachers' other keep fit classes have shown interest by helping to teach the young women health care and the art of make-up and grooming. Each summer the teacher invites the group to a country party in her cottage, and at Christmas the other teacher arranges a party for them in Aylesbury.

Co-operation

Much can be achieved when there is co-operation between the hospital and hostel staff and the outside world; a second class has now started for a group of overweight young women. This is being taken by 2 members of a keep fit class (one a teacher) under guidance. Being more severely handicapped they need greater persuasion to join in, but progress is being made.

   The teachers say: 'After 7 years we are delighted with the results, and really enjoy the work. If others could help in the same way elsewhere, they would find it most rewarding and interesting'.

Spin-offs

These women have acquired poise, walk well, become more sociable, outgoing and friendly, and have made friends in the community. They have been stretched to demonstration standard, enabling them to show their enthusiasm and achievement to others. There has been improvement in their health and fitness and in their appearance — considerable loss of weight was a must for most of them if they were to wear leotards and tights.

   A number of people in the community understand more about mental handicap and that people with a mental handicap **can** keep fit and, given time and patient teaching, **can** achieve a good standard.

Demonstration Using Scarves

Music: 'Love can make you happy' or a tune like 'Somewhere over the Rainbow' (Record MER 313 - 'Cocktail Piano'). Once through was found to be insufficient, therefore a repetition of this music minus the introduction was added to the tape.

Scarves: 1 yard square nylon material in shades of blue green, from light to dark. The women wear black leotards and tights.

Formation: In a circle all facing anti-clockwise.

Starting position: Hold scarf square on with both hands, left hand to centre waist and right arm extended to right side — weight on the right foot. After 4 bars of introductory music has been played:

1. Swing right arm round and across to left — transferring the weight on to the left foot (bars 1-2). Repeat swing in the opposite direction (bars 3-4). Repeat twice more, 3 times in all (bars 5-12). Turn on the spot to the left and finish facing the centre of the circle (bars 13-16).

2. With right hand hold the scarf by one corner. Run into the centre of circle throwing scarf up high (flames) (bars 1-2). Run out backwards dragging scarf low (bars 3-4). Repeat in and out three times, running to finish (5-16) in a space.

3. Throw scarf overhead from right to left slowly to touch floor 3 times (bars 1-16). Finish sitting or kneeling in various ways on the floor.

4. Each performer improvises with slow scarf movements, eg swing scarf round head. All forms of stretching in various directions, with various scarf holds. At the end of the phrase run into groups, ie lines of 4 or 5 holding scarf by one corner with right hand giving opposite corner to the performer on the right, joining into a line (bars 1-16). The number of bars of music used becomes flexible here, allowing time to get a strong feeling in the stretch.

5. Each line runs in an open circle, stop. The leader threads a little way through an arch made by the last two in the line, all stretch strongly in various directions keeping hold of the scarf. Return to open circle. Repeat starting from the opposite end of the line. Repeat both threading sequences again.

   Having opened out, all join up in one single circle linked one to another by scarves.

6. Walk into the centre of the circle raising arms up high. Turn on the spot to face outwards, lowering arms overhead to end with them crossed low in front. Lift arms and scarves up to face centre again, opening arms up and out.

   Repeat.

   Leader drops right hand hold and runs to lead into a 'maze'. Unwind 'maze' and run off. Music is 'faded out', as last person exits.

   NOTE: Illustrate directions to aid memory, eg 'flames' of a fire, when running in, 'over the moon' for alternate side bends, 'flowers growing in the garden'; when sitting down, go to 'Jennifer's house', 'Sylvia's house'; to indicate to which line to run.

Keep Fit at Harperbury Hospital

In 1960, at the instigation of a parent of one of the long-term patients, a keep fit class came into being at Harperbury Hospital, Hertfordshire. The mother was not only concerned for her own daughter, now too handicapped to move, but for the many others becoming more apathetic and immobile each day. At first she took the class herself, doing everything to encourage and stimulate the patients in her daughter's ward. She realised that someone with 'knowledge of movement' should take the class and she consequently approached a keep fit teacher.

A challenge

The teacher accepted the challenge, although she had never had any previous contact with people with a mental handicap. After the first lesson she knew she wanted to continue and for three years she took the class single-handed with the help of a 78 year-old pianist. She says: 'It was hard going but I won the patients' affection and when I achieved, through coaxing, some movement from them, they were as happy with themselves as I was with them. I knew by then that this could go on throughout the hospital if I could first gain the co-operation of the staff and, secondly, gather in some of my keep fit colleagues. I managed to find a team of 16. We covered all the wards in the female wing and a few of the children's wards. The sisters of the wards did not accept the scheme very easily, but with the Matron's support, most of the sisters soon became our friends'.

Move involvement

For another four years the teachers visited the hospital every Wednesday, the residents eagerly awaiting the visits. The teachers packed and delivered Christmas parcels for all the female patients in the hospital; this has continued each year with the support of hundreds of members of the Middlesex Keep Fit Association and has now been extended to some male wards.

Educational rhythmics

In 1969 the teacher attended a course in Educational Rhythmics for Mentally and Physically Handicapped People, under Ferris and Jennet Robins. She came away with many new ideas but needing equipment and records with which to implement them. The Lions gave £25, and with this the records and small apparatus, such as tambourines, were bought; the teacher made her own coloured flags and a large wooden clock. HMV provided a record player. The patients responded well to this different approach — over a period of time they were able to move and sing a rhythm at the same time — pick out colours and use their arms as the hands of a clock. 'By now our reward was tremendous — I say 'our' as I encouraged my colleagues to take my class and work on the new method'.

She herself then worked in the wards where the patients were more severely handicapped.

Co-ordinator of voluntary services

During the past few years a 'Co-ordinator of voluntary services' has joined the hospital staff and now all voluntary workers are welcomed and directed. The classes continue with as much enthusiasm as ever, as do the Christmas parcels and entertainment by the Middlesex Keep Fit Association each year.

FITNESS TRAINING

FITNESS TRAINING EXERCISES

These exercises generally include training techniques for specific sports. If the training programmes are carefully prepared according to the likes and dislikes and the ability of the group members, they can be enjoyed equally by men, women and men and women together.

A lesson

Limbering and warming up exercises. Before taking part in any exercise, particularly of a strenuous nature, the body should be 'warmed up' to prevent unnecessary strain. Limbering exercises are often seen being practised by athletes, footballers, gymnasts and dancers on television. The trainees or residents like to associate themselves with the 'stars' and as a result more willingly take part in these movements without too much explanation.

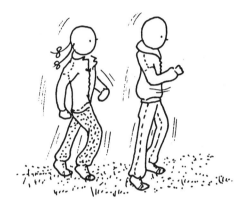

Figure 11.4 Jogging

1. **Jogging.** Run on the spot, lifting the knees high using the arms in a natural way — jog in different directions — once the beat can be maintained, introduce a simple pattern: 8 forwards, 8 backwards, 8 turning or chalk a pattern on the ground, eg letters of their names — diamonds — triangles — squares and circles. This will enable the class to jog for a longer period and add interest. At the end of the jogging, pause for breathing to be restored to normal (Fig 11.4).

    Those who cannot jog can sit or stand and lift alternate knees up and down or, if they are mobile, walk along the patterns and, if necessary, be given help to change direction.

2. **Galloping** (slip steps). Galloping develops spring, speed and quick change of direction, eg

    8 gallops to right — repeat left

    4 gallops to right — repeat left

    2 gallops to right — repeat left

    Gallops combined with jogging or springs;
    (i) 8 jogs forward — 8 jogs backwards
    (ii) 4 gallops right — 4 gallops left, repeat
    (iii) 8 gallops right followed by 8 low springs on the spot with feet together.

3. **Stride jumps.** Stride jumps develop spring, co-ordination and balance, eg
    continuous stride jumping, slowly and quickly.
    Chant: Out rebound — in rebound — slow
            Out in — out in — quick.
    Jumps can alternate with clapping in different directions on the spot.

Body movements

1. **Back rocks.** Sit on a mat with knees bent up, arms round the knees with fingers interlinked. Rock backwards onto the mat, uncurling the spine (head last), push up and rock forward. If the swing is broken and the momentum is lost it is difficult to rock forwards again. Take the movement slowly at first, then gradually quicken it.

2. **Side rocks.** Lie on the mat with knees bent onto the chest and elbows in at the waist with hands clasped on the chest. Rock onto right side maintaining a curled up position. As soon as the right side is in contact with the floor, push off and roll over onto the left side. This movement should be taken smoothly as many people are disorientated when lying down. It is helpful to chant instructions such as: 'to the door, to the clock' or 'right side, left side'. If the arms remain on the chest there is no chance of them being squashed.

    NB. These movements are necessary, particularly if simple vaulting or forward rolls are to be attempted, with a relaxed landing.

3. **Sit ups.** This is an easy introduction a series of movements designed to strengthen the abdominal muscles. Work with partners suitably matched. **A** is the worker, **B** is the helper. **A** lies on his back with hands on the floor at the side. **B**, firmly but without squeezing, holds **A**'s ankles. to prevent him raising his legs whilst he is moving. **A** lifts his head forward and gradually sits up, keeping his legs in contact with the floor. He uncurls gently to lying position, being careful not to bang his head. Repeat with **B** working and **A** helping.

    Note: Those with possible heart or respiratory problems should not attempt this movement!

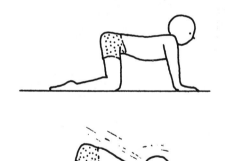

Figure 11.5 Simple press-ups

4. **Simplified press-ups.** Kneel with hands on the floor, right angles at hip and shoulder, keeping the hands still, move the head and body forward by bending the elbows. Return to the original position by straightening the elbows (Fig 11.5)

5. **Press-ups.** Lie on the front on the floor, hands under shoulders, fingers facing forwards, elbows bent and toes curled under. Gently push the body up, by straightening the arms. Return to starting position and repeat continuously. It is important not to repeat this movement for too long (Fig 11.6).

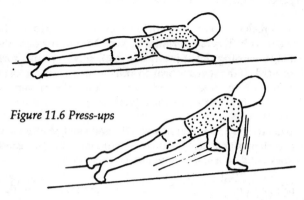

Figure 11.6 Press-ups

Agilities

A great number of agilities, both with and without hand apparatus, movable and fixed equipment, can be included in a movement and fitness training lesson with a gymnastic bias, eg:

Moving through, under or over obstacles, climbing up and along and through wall bars, ladders and climbing frames.
Moving along benches — various methods, eg walking, running, bunny hop, side to side, on and off.
Jumping to touch obstacles at various heights.
Forward and backwards rolls.
Cartwheels.
Jumping off the box at various heights onto a mat into a forward roll.

Movements interpretation

In some instances fitness training can be introduced through movement interpretation of:

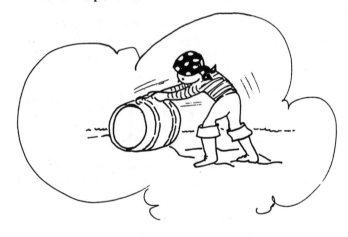

Figure 11.7 Movement interpretation

Indians, stalking, preparing to fight;

cowboys, cracking whips, rounding up the cattle;

pirates, hauling ropes, rowing, fighting, looting;

shipwrecked, waves striking and beating, floating, rescue;

astronauts, walking on the moon, take off;

machine, punching, rolling, swinging, turning movements;

energetic tasks, chopping wood, hammering, digging, pneumatic drilling, painting, hauling a heavy load (Fig 11.7).

Negro spirituals or Afro/Caribbean Musicals provide suitable music for the above.

Simple gymnastic exercises

The following gymnastic activities — successfully taught in Muckamore Abbey Hospital, Northern Ireland—should be kept **very simple** unless the instructor has had some training in teaching gymnastics.

Activities with ropes

Climbing with ropes with
(i) crossed legs
(ii) hands only (warn them not to slide down rope).

Travelling sideways from rope to rope.
Upward circle (using two ropes).
Heave vault (using one rope).
Heave vault (using two ropes).

Activities with beam

Crossing beam with hands
(i) travelling sideways
(ii) travelling sideways with rotation.

Downward circle.
Side vault.
Heave vault between two beams.
Balancing on inverted beam.

Activities with benches

Climb an inclined bench — using feet and hands.
Pull self up inclined bench — using hands only.
Circle round raised bench.

Balancing activities on inverted bench:
(i) walk along
(ii) roll ball along
(iii) walk along avoiding obstacles.

Activities with box

Face vault on vertical box.
Through vault on vertical box.
Overswing vault on horizontal box.

Activities with wall bars

Vertical climb.
Horizontal climb.
Vertical twist (upwards).
Horizontal twist.
Diagonal twist (upwards).
Diagonal twist (downwards).
Hanging
(i) knee lifting; (ii) leg lifting; (iii) reverse hanging.

Floor work

Forward roll.
Backward roll.
Head stand.
Cartwheel.
Handstand.

FITNESS TRAINING SCHEMES

Various fitness training schemes can be introduced into the physical recreation programme.

Aims: (i) to develop strength and stamina;
  (ii) to help participants to realise and develop their own potential in the skills practised;
  (iii) to stimulate interest.

1. Look After Yourself
(Helping you to better health)

This is the title of the Health Education Authority's scheme. Schedules and detailed information obtainable from: The Health Education Authority, 78 New Oxford Street, London WC1 (tel: 01 631 0930).

2. Circuit training — two examples

The first example, practised in a hospital, is a simple circuit for which obtainable equipment is used; the other, practised at an ATC, utilised more sophisticated equipment.

Simple circuit

Muckamore Abbey Hospital, Northern Ireland, has devised this circuit, suitable for active young men (Figure 11.8).

Equipment: benches, skittles, canes and skipping ropes.

(i) Step ups;
(ii) sit ups;
(iii) jump ups;
(iv) press ups;
(v) jumping and running zig-zag;
(vi) skipping.

If fixed apparatus is available, the following could be included in the circuit:

(i) chin ups;
(ii) rope swings;
(iii) bench lifts;
(iv) rope climbs.

Circuit using more sophisticated equipment

Hornbeams Adult Training Centre, Welwyn Garden City, Hertfordshire, has gradually acquired some interesting apparatus and equipment. The instructor says: 'experience has shown that advancement has been made and there is no doubt that it is noticeably demonstrated in the workshops and many other activities'.

Equipment: chair, rowing machine, cycling equipment, punchball stand, medicine balls, footballs, logs — 2$\frac{1}{2}$ m (7') long, sliding strengthening equipment, mats.

This programme starts with ground work and ground exercises, chair work coupled with brain stimulators, followed by standing activities, eg catching and throwing using medium and heavy balls from varying distances — these can be organised as team work and on a competitive basis.

The trainees are first shown how the equipment should be used. A time target is set.

3. Obstacle course

The obstacle course is an activity especially effective for people with a mental handicap as it contains equipment requiring a variety of movement, responses and skills. Different obstacle courses can be set up both indoors and out of doors (Figure 11.9).

Arm and shoulder strength development. Hanging or climbing obstacle — climbing and swinging obstacle — obstacle for developing arm and shoulder strength.

Total body development. Climbing ladder — vertical climbing obstacle — apparatus for climbing over and through — large tractor tyre mounted for crawling and climbing.

Balance and agility. Balancing beams and logs — ladder used for balancing tasks — stepping stones made from tree stumps — balance obstacles made with inclined logs or discarded tyres climbing obstacle made from logs.

Indoor equipment. Balance equipment — balance beam and support constructed from strong timber — balance board — rocking board.

The teacher must be aware of each trainee's disability. Each must develop as an individual aiming to reach his own maximum potential and at the same time work together with others in a team.

Sturdy, imaginative equipment can easily be made as long as it serves the purpose of the programme. A wide variety of

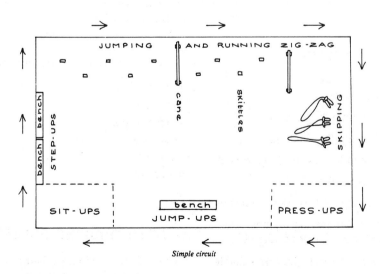

Figure 11.8 Simple circuit

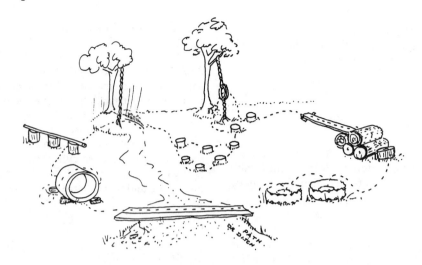

Figure 11.9 Ostacle course

equipment that complements a well development programme will provide adventure, social play and the development of co-ordination and manipulative skills.

Example of a simple obstacle course

Twenty suitable chairs in a line. Trainees crawl under all chairs one following on after the other. Repeat this, pushing a football in front.

Fix square pieces of cardboard together in various shapes. Arrange these shapes in different positions for trainees to climb over and step across.

Logs can be tied together to jump over and to use for balancing.

The programme starts from ground level and finishes in standing.

4. Ropes course

A course consisting of ropes attached to trees or other stable supports which are used for swinging, climbing and hauling.

5. Trim Tracking (Trim trails)

The Trim (meaning 'fitness') concept was first developed on the Continent. It is applied to a specific physical recreation facility known as a Trim Course, built of 'stations' of logs, specially designed to make general exercise as 'easy, enjoyable and beneficial as possible'.

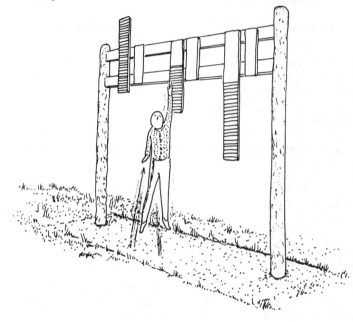

Figure 11.10b Trim tracking - exercise station

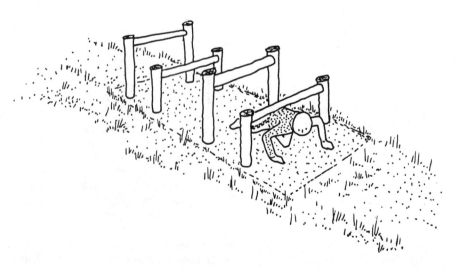

Figure 11.10a Trim tracking - exercise station

Aims

Trim trails have two main aims:

1. to encourage those not normally engaged in active physical recreation to enjoy it at a level which suits them, and
2. to provide additional and more intensive fitness training for those already in regular training for competitive sport.

Trim trails

A Trim trail can vary in length, shape and content and can be individually designed to make the best use of the grounds available and to suit the needs of the potential users. It can be a simple training path requiring simple route marking, a kind of jogging course. Most courses, however, incorporate carefully planned exercise stations at intervals along the pathway.

The pathway design

The length of the pathway varies with the space available, 400-1500 m (437-1640 yds). The start and finish of the route should be at the same place. A figure-of-8 or clover-leaf shaped route is particularly suitable for longer courses as it provides intermediate finishing points, coinciding with the start for those who do not wish to cover the full distance.

Exercise stations

There is no set ratio of number of stations to the length of the course but experience shows that users are comfortable with 1 station to 50 m (165') over shorter courses and 1-75 m (3'3" - 248') over longer courses, ie a 400 m (437 yds) course would have 8 exercise stations and 1500 m (1640') course might have 20. When designing the stations follow a sequence which avoids exercising the same muscle groups at consecutive stations, eg the stations might be designed to exercise the whole body, then the arms, then the trunk, then the legs and so on. Stations, usually constructed of timber and logs embedded in concrete, may be simple in design yet still attractive. Many hospital grounds lend themselves to Trim trails as do some of the smaller spaces nearby or surrounding some adult training centres, particularly those in the country areas. Figures 11.10a and b of exercise stations and their use may inspire those with space available to construct a Trim trail. Before embarking on a project, consult the regional or local Sports Council.

6. Weight Training and Weight Lifting

Weight training can be a valuable method of building up a reasonable degree of strength and energy. It is essential for the teacher to have expertise in this activity in order to set the right target for each individual (Figure 11.11).

It is also necessary to seek expert advice and medical sanction. If the handicapped person has any degree of spacticity, care must be taken to ensure that the extended wrist grip is used.

The well planned programme must be aimed at at a gradual increase over a period, it must not be an unplanned exercise destined to discover who can lift the heaviest weight.

Weight training is being practised in centres and hospitals, often included in a programme of circuit training. Equipment consists of barbells and weights which are fairly inexpensive and practically indestructible.

Carefully selected young men can benefit by weight training as an aid to fitness and weight lifting as a sport. Huw Price, a member of the British Weight Lifters Association, has worked with boys with a mental handicap He says, 'These boys had a record of failure in everything and it was necessary to find something to give them success of a deep, satisfying nature so that they could improve educationally and socially'.

He already had the simple equipment necessary. The exercises taught can be easily learned and, to improve, all that is necessary is repetition. The boys enjoy doing this once the exercise is mastered. As weight lifting is a very individual sport, they are only competing against themselves, and soon see that there is almost daily improvement. As Huw Price says 'They can see that they are getting stronger and are aware that strength is a quality to be admired. In this way they achieve standing in the eyes of their peers'.

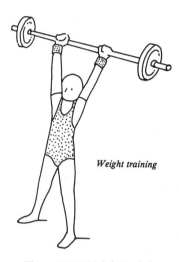

Weight training

Figure 11.11 Weight training

Spin off

Soon these boys wanted to read about weight lifting — in many cases they were non readers; they wanted to write about the sport and even draw themselves performing. At the same time their attitude to their friends and to adults improved dramatically.

'In the same way', Huw Price says, 'weights can be used as successfully with young adults with a mental handicap. In no way do the rules or apparatus have to be altered or adapted to cater for them. Once they have learned the exercises they would be sympathetically welcomed into adult clubs, and this could do much to ameliorate their lives'. He is certain that weight training and weight lifting can be used to enable some to live a more normal live.

7. Yoga

Yoga has been taught to young people with a mental handicap at the Kingsway College of Further Education, London, where adults with a mental handicap joined a Yoga class. The results were enlightening and it was found to be quite practical to integrate people with a mental handicap with ordinary class members who were made aware that the main attention would be given to those who were handicapped. In this way, handicapped people have other people to copy and this makes the class easier to handle.

Each week one of the young people is chosen to stand in front of the class to act as a demonstrator. This works well and there is keen competition to take this role.

It is surprising how quickly people with a mental handicap pick up the different postures — in this respect they differ in no way from the ordinary class members. Some of the postures involve balance, standing on one leg; these are enjoyed so much that it has been easy to progress to the more advanced stages. The work is based on stretching and strengthening the body, at the same time increasing stamina. 'We aim to get the body back to its correct shape'. This system of Yoga is designed to act on the internal organs — each posture tends to have a stimulating effect on one or two parts of the body. Yoga is an activity which gradually refines the body and there is no reason why people with a mental handicap should not reap the benefits.

Stiffness is a major problem. Young people, unlike older people, do not have the same endurance. Progress is, therefore, bound to be slower and the teacher needs to encourage the students more than usual and to devise routines which will keep their interest.

The teacher is trained by BKS Iyengar and he recommends that any hospitals/training centres wishing to introduce Yoga to their residents or trainees should investigate the Iyengar method This system is now widely accepted throughout the world by many educational authorities as the safest and most comprehensive. The teachers are meticulously trained before they can gain a qualification.

8. Regular daily fitness training session

Experience has shown that daily fitness training sessions benefit all those attending hospitals and ATCs. One centre in the London Borough of Havering has successfully introduced such sessions.

Fitness training at Havering ATC

Members of the Havering staff, having decided that most of the students did not get enough physical exercise while attending the centre, devised a programme to involve as many of the students as possible in a fitness programme. Attendance was voluntary but as many students as possible were encouraged to take part, particularly the less able, who tend to miss out on exercise provided by the other organised sporting activities.

The keep fit fitness training session commences shortly after the trainees arrive at the centre, and lasts for about 45 minutes. Initially the Health Education Authority recommended exercises were used, omitting those which were too difficult. Shortly afterwards, music was introduced to vary the programme. This was a great success and added to the students' enjoyment. The Music and Motion LP 'Popmobility' record which involves exercising to pop music was also used, and it was found that the trainees follow the instructions more easily on the record and that this allows the staff more time to spend helping individual trainees.

Special clothing for the Keep Fit Club is optional — most women wear leotards and plimsoles; the majority of men wear shorts or jeans, T-shirts and gym shoes. The objectives in providing the Keep Fit Club are to improve health, mobility, stamina, strength and posture. It has also helped to establish a group relationship with staff from various departments within the centre and, of course, the students benefit from the team work involved in performing the various sequences of exercises.

Examples of two daily dozens

1. Without chairs

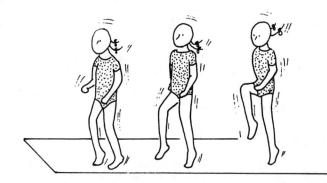

Figure 11.12a Warming up

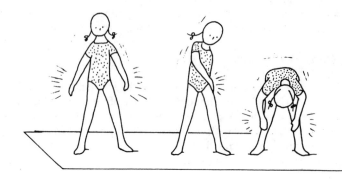

Figure 11.12b Beating

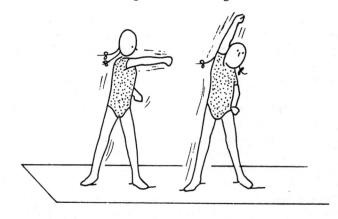

Figure 11.12c Punch and twist

Warming up. Running on the spot. Keeping the feet near to the ground gradually increase the height of the knee lift, decrease the height of the knee lift, repeat continuously higher and lower (Fig 11.12 a)

'Beating'. Stand with feet apart, fists clenched loosely. Beat the thighs, eg front, side, back, continue beating other parts of the body — arms, knees, shoulders, chest, ankles, legs, back. Move the body as much as possible, eg to beat behind, so twisting the body. Combine 1 and 2 until everyone is warm (Fig 11.12b).

Punch and twist. Stand with feet apart, fists clenched. Alternate arm punching forward with a body twist. Repeat punching to one side — across the body — repeat in different directions — upwards, downwards, obliquely (Fig 11.12c).

Hip swing. Standing, shoulder grasp with partner or holding on the back of a chair for balance. Swing the right leg across the left leg to the left. Swing out to the right (1-2),repeat twice more, 'across and out, across and out' (3-6). Stand still (7) lift the left leg low sideways (8), ready to repeat the swing with the left leg. Repeat right and left continuously (Fig11.12d)

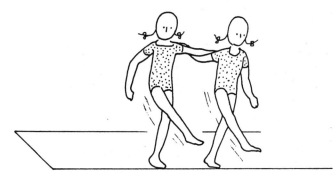

Figure 11.12d Hip swing

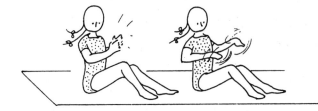

Figure 11.12e Hands

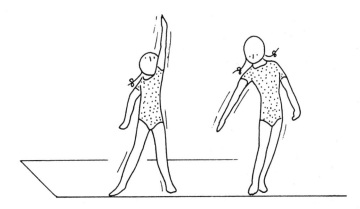

Figure 11.12f Stretching

Hands. Standing or sitting. Various hand movements, eg opening, closing, spread fingers out, circle the wrists in and out, wrist bend up and down, clap hands, shake hands. Take any two or three hand movements and make up sequences, eg 'open and close, open and close', wrist circle outwards and inwards (1-8) Fig 11.12e).

Stretching. Stand with feet a little apart. Slow stretching alternate arms in any direction above shoulder level and out to the side. Stretch through the body to the end of the fingers (Fig 11.12f).

Bend and twist. Standing with feet apart, arms relaxed. (i) Body bending sideways to left and right continuously (Fig 11.12g). (ii) Body turning — twist to look behind — left and right continuously (Fig 11.12 h). Combine (i) and (ii), eg bend right, left, right and up (1-4) followed by body turning right, left, right and forwards (5-8). Repeat starting to left.

Brisk walking. If space allows: (i) walk briskly in different formations, eg round the room — in circles — files — pairs or freely (Fig 11.12i). Using the whole space, walk freely (1-16) find a partner, link arms or join hands and walk round on the spot (1-16).

2. Using chairs

Ordinary chairs with or without arms. Be sure that the chairs are in good repair. Move chairs quietly and in a controlled way. Teach class members to sit with thighs supported on the seat of the chair but with the whole foot firmly on the floor, feet forward. The back should be erect but not stiff — 'lift out of the waist'. 'Sit tall'.

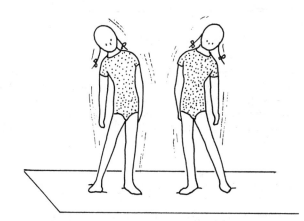

Figure 11.12g Side bend

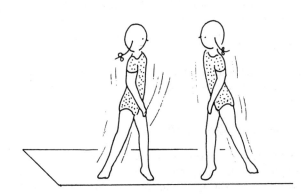

Figure 11.12h Twist

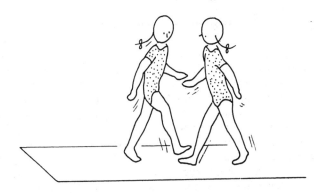

Figure 11.12i Brisk walking

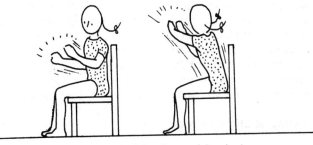

Figure 11.13a Warming up (clapping)

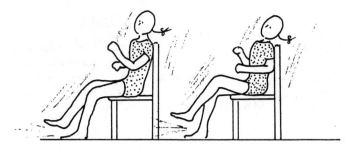

Figure 11.13b Marking time

Warming up. Clap hands with big circular arm movement — in front of the face — out to the side — below knees — towards the back with a body twist. Clap in one direction several times at first — gradually clap in other directions, eg 2 claps forwards 2 claps to one side, repeat to the other side, 2 claps high — 8 claps (Fig 11.13a).

Marking time. Marking time, slow beats followed by quick beats; finish by accelerating the speed (Fig11.13b).

Hip and back. Hold the side edges of the chair seat or chair arms firmly throughout, keep the elbows straight. Lift 'seat' off the chair swaying slightly forward. Lower 'seat' on to the chair swaying back. Increase the range of movement so that the feet are lifted off the floor on the back sway (Fig11.13c).

Variation:
(i) move the 'seat' forward over the feet and back; (ii) lift 'seat' up, keep feet firm — swing knees to right and left alternately in the lifted position.

Hands. See Daily Dozen No 1 above.

Stretching. Raise arms sideways and upwards to put hands lightly on head. Keeping the back erect, lower arms slowly to sides — keep the whole movement slow and sustained (Fig 11.13d).

Variation:
as above but stretch arms to touch hands high above head.

Combine the two movements.

Wriggling. Wriggle the spine, shoulder girdle and head. Slowly at first — gradually increase the movement and the speed (Fig 11.13e)

Knee lifting. Grasp one knee with both hands. Pull it up as near to the chest as possible and put it down. Repeat with the other leg (Fig11.13 f).

Circles or lines. Hold hands lightly round a circle or in lines — sway from side to side with as much body movement as possible — repeat swaying forward and back (Fig 11.13g).

Relax. At any point in the lesson the following movement can be introduced. Bend forward slowly to put forehead on knees slowly uncurl to erect position — let the arms hang easily to the side.

The teacher can devise many variations of the above movements for warming up and giving general exercise. *All movements should be repeated a number of times to be effective.* If music is used the tempo should be slow enough to allow full range of movement. Use 4/4. 6/8, and 3/4 rhythms. See Music p. 97.

Everyone should feel thoroughly warmed up at the end of 15 minutes continuous exercise.

Note: Where there are ambulant and non-ambulant people in the same class — exercises can be selected from 1 and 2 to make a Daily Dozen suitable for both.

WEIGHT WATCHING WITH PEOPLE WITH A MENTAL HANDICAP IN SCOTLAND

Many adults with a mental handicap are overweight — a hindrance in the development of physical activities and sport. The Lothian Regional Council (Social Work Department) decided to investigate this problem through their Diatetic Adviser.

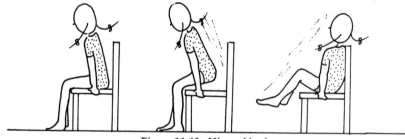

Figure 11.13c Hip and back

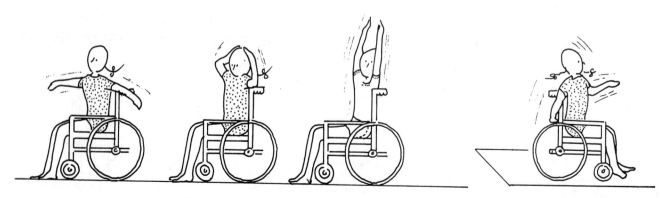

Figure 11.13d Stretching

Figure 11.13e Wriggling

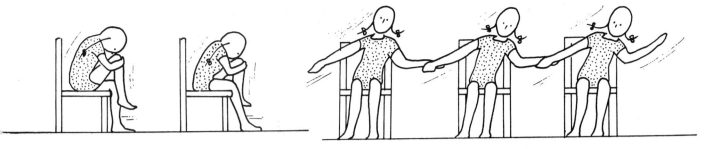

Figure 11.13f Knee lifting

Figure 11.13g Swinging from side to side

Firstly, adults with a mental handicap seem to have difficulty in knowing when to stop eating. Secondly, they usually have a few dislikes and consequently eat anything and everything offered. The consequence of inactive leisure pursuits is both a cause and an effect of overweight. This cycle can be broken if relatives and friends encourage physical and mental activity during leisure time rather than allowing passive pursuits such as watching television.

The risks linked with obesity include heart disease, strokes, diabetes, respiratory disorders, arthritis, piles, flat feet, and also an increased rate of accidents in the home and in the street due to decreased mobility. Apart from these medical reasons for losing weight, weight loss also has social benefits — improved looks and improved choice of clothes. These latter are more immediate advantages and can be used to inspire will-power.

Since many members of the Adult Training Centres in the Lothian Region had weight problems, Weight Watchers Clubs were started in each of the eleven centres by the Social Work Departments' Dietetic Adviser. All the trainees were weighed and measured, and their target weight determined from ideal weight charts. Each trainee was instructed on the dietary alterations necessary and the importance of exercise in the weight loss programme. A simplified diet sheet was designed to reinforce the message, and a copy given to each overweight trainee.

A talk was given to the parents at one of their meetings in each centre, and they were encouraged to participate in the programme themselves if they had a weight problem. They were all advised to check with their general practitioner before embarking on the diet.

As many fatty and starchy foods as possible were removed from the midday meal — potatoes were cut out and vegetables and salads increased. Puddings were replaced by fresh fruit, yoghurt, biscuits and cheese or jelly. During the winter, vegetable soups were allowed instead of sweet. The fact that many of the staff in the centres participated in the weighing and dieting greatly helped the trainees to both understand and comply with the restrictions. Extra physical activities were organised in the centres including keep fit, football and swimming.

During the first year monthly weigh-ins assessed progress. During the summer months results were very encouraging but losses during the winter slowed down. The difference in losses between different centres indicated the level of enthusiasm and interest of parents in helping the trainees to continue their diets at home. The response from parents was, in general, good, but some parents refused to deprive the trainee of anything. Individual consultations were held with parents who refused to co-operate. 42% of the trainees were overweight to some extent and the average weight to be lost was 16 kg ($2^{1}/2$ stone). In the first year the average loss was $^{1}/2$ stone, but there were individual losses of 9.5-12.7 kg ($1^{1}/2$ to 2 stone) in several cases. This average rate of loss is not as good as was hoped, but any loss is encouraging.

When weighing all the trainees and checking their weights against the Ideal Weight Chart, it was found that several trainees were underweight to a worrying degree. Advice has been given and a diet sheet provided, but the success rate has been disappointing. The biggest problem to be overcome if these trainees are to gain weight is the lack of feeding facilities in the Centres and also lack of finance. Regular high protein, high calorie snacks need to be provided in addition to the main lunch-time meal.

ASSESSMENT

There is no right or wrong way to teach movement and fitness training, as long as the teacher is always aware of the needs of the individuals in the group, and plans each lesson with these in mind — the teacher carefully assessing the progress of the group as a whole and of each individual. The method of recording the progress is the teacher's concern, but some record should be kept. Some centres record achievements on charts displayed on their notice boards — trainees and staff alike taking a great interest in the ticks or square-filling.

Assessment activities

Phase 1

(i)   Crawl a distance of 9.5m (30') (Fig 11.14).

(ii) Lying face down, using arms, travel forwards 6m (20').

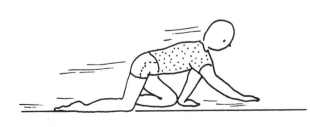

Figure 11.14 Crawling

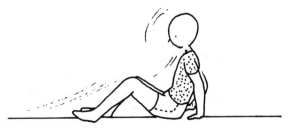

Figure 11.15 Moving backwards

(iii) Sitting, travel backwards 6m (20') (Fig11.15).

(iv) Lying, achieve 6 push ups.

(v) Lying, roll sideways 3.6m (12') to the right.

(vi) Lying, roll sideways 3.6m (12') to left.

Phase 2

(i) Slide under a partner who is kneeling on all fours.

(ii) Slide through a tunnel made by 3 people kneeling on all fours and then help to make the tunnel.

(iii) Roll a partner sideways like a log for 3.6 m (12')

(iv) Sitting on seat only, spin right round using hands only to help.

(v) Roll a large ball to the other end of the room and then collect it (any method accepted).

(vi) Throw a large ball to a partner 3 m (10') away — sitting or standing.

Phase 3

(i) Jump a distance of 1 m (3'3")

(ii) Jump over an obstacle about 305 mm (1') high.

(iii) Slide a partner along the floor for 6 m (20').

(iv) Stand with arms extended to wall, lean against wall, achieve 6 push ups.

(v) Bounce and catch a large ball 3 times.

(vi) Dribble a large ball to the opposite end of the room.

Phase 4

(i) In twos 3 m (10') apart. Throw and catch a large ball 3 times.

(ii) Give a partner a ride round the room for about 6 m (20').

(iii) Sitting back to back with partner, stand up and sit down twice.

(iv) Keep moving round the hall, eg jogging for 30 seconds.

(v) Keep moving round the hall, eg jogging for 1 minute

(vi) Create a mini circuit, eg crawl under a table, over a low obstacle then run round a skittle at the opposite end of the room and return to the starting point — once, twice, three times without any pauses.

This method of encouraging movement is recommended for senior adolescents and adults. It can be used where there is no specialist help or where facilities are very limited. Tasks will constantly need to be revised to meet the particular disabilities of an individual or group. Distances mentioned are only intended to be guidance for the leader and should not be adhered to rigidly. There must always be the *potential for success*.

In this particular set of tasks Phases 1 and 2 provide scope for large body movements and can be attempted by the ambulant and non ambulant. They should often be repeated as warming-up activities for those attempting the more difficult tasks in Phases 3 and 4. These demand increased concentration, co-operation, effort and motor skill. A playful presentation of these activities should always be encouraged.

FURTHER READING

Amateur Gymnastics Association, *Gymnastics*, London, A & C Black, 1986.

Anderson, M E. *Inventive movement*, Edinburgh, Chambers, 1970.

British Judo Association, Working Party for the Disabled. *Judo for the disabled*. BJA, 16 Upper Woborn Place, London, WC1.

Brown, A. *Active games for children with movement problems*. London, Harper and Row, 1986.

Buckland, D G. *Gymnastics*. London, Heinemann Educational, 1969

Cameron, W M and Pleasance P. *Education in movement*. Oxford, Blackwell, 1963.

Colson, J. *Getting into rhythm; music and movement and recreational activities for hospitals*. Yorkshire Regional Health Authority, 1974.

Don, A. *Keeping fit for all ages*, London, A & C Black, 1986.

Fentem, P H, Bassey, E J and Turnbull, N B. *The new case for exercise*. London, Health Education Authority, 1988.

Groves, L. ed. *Physical education for children with special needs*. Cambridge University Press, 1979.

Jennings, S. *Creative therapy*. London, Pitman Publishing, 1975.

Know the Game Series — *Karate and Keeping fit*. London, A & C Black.

Kent County Council, Education Dept. *Physical education for pupils with special educational needs in mainstream schools*. KCC, 1986.

Lancashire County Council, Education Dept. *Lancashire looks at physical education in the special school*. Preston, LCC, 1985.

Oram, Chris. *Every woman: her guide to fitness*. Tadworth, World's Work, 1978.

Playtrac. *Dance and drama activities*, Shenley, Playtrac, c/o Harperbury Hospital, 1988.

Robins, F and Robins J. *Educational rhythmics for mentally handicapped children*. Ra Verlag, 8713 Veriken Schwize, Switzerland, 1963.

Robinson, C M et al. *Physical activity in the education of slow-learning children*. London, Edward Arnold, 1970.

Smith, A B S. *Expressive movement: ideas for lessons*, Jordanhill College of Education, 1984.

Thomas V. *Better physical fitness*. London, Kaye and Ward, 1979.

Upton, G. ed. *Physical and creative activities for mentally handicapped children*. Cambridge University Press, 1978.

Chapter 12

Movement and Dance Therapy

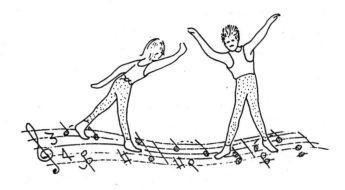

Interest in movement and dance therapy has increased in recent years, particularly for people with a mental handicap, and many individuals are doing interesting pioneer work in co-operation with various organisations. The following are two viewpoints on movement and dance therapy.

AN AMERICAN VIEW

Joanna Harris, a leading dance therapist in California who has visited the UK on several occasions to advise and train therapists, believes that 'Dance therapy is a process by which client and therapist interact using words, movement, music, images and artistic activities of varying kinds. The emphasis, however, is on building a safe environment, both personal and public, in which a safe "sense of self" can be developed. That means, in therapeutic terms, that the client determines the tempo and nature of whatever interaction and activity ensues. The therapist responds by being ready and capable of response when and however is appropriate.

'When teaching in a group, the therapist offers "the art of the possible" presenting ways into competence by re-enforcing whatever skills the group can share and achieve. It is a slow process, one that repeats the "positive mirroring" of optimal parental nurturing — nurturing that allows an accomplished self to grow through a sense of social, physical and personal well-being.

' The dance activity reflects the evolving self. As positive encouragement and authentic movement produce a creative person, the dancing self becomes free to bring security and expanded energy to everyday life.'

AN ENGLISH VIEW

Jasmine Pasch, who trained at the School of Contemporary Dance (Goldsmith College, London), holds the Teachers Certificate in Education. She has wide experience of teaching people with a mental handicap in social education and day centres, and in training teachers through the Association of Movement Therapy, the United Kingdom Sports Association for People with Mental Handicap, and at the Laban Centre. She says that dance therapy addresses itself directly to the presenting problem, disorder, difficulty, disturbance, behaviour, or areas of conflict, and there are a number of approaches and theoretical models (see page 114). It effects change in feelings, cognition, physical functioning and behaviour, confronting and resolving deep needs, fears and conflicts.

'An educational or arts activity on the other hand is more concerned with tapping the creative talents of the students, having fun while learning, enjoying the process and developing pride in achievement and in the final product. This may be a

dance shared with others in class, or the experience of performing in front of an audience, for example the work of Wolfgang Stange which brings together students with various disabilities and able-bodied people. Such pieces as 'Ruckblick' and 'Silence' are judged on their artistic merit, and compete on equal terms with the professional dance and theatre world.

Aesthetic and educational criteria

'Aesthetic and educational criteria (not behavioural) are employed. The outcome of the activity may be therapeutic; students may feel better as a result of enjoying themselves or achieving something. It is possible to employ a therapeutic approach to an educational or arts activity, being mindful of problems and difficulties experienced by the students, but not making them the focus of attention. For example, in my work at the Royal Free Hospital — in the psychiatric wing, acute admissions ward — a number of difficulties need to be taken into account: students may find it very difficult to tolerate a group; their attention span is short and they come and go during the session, or sit out and smoke a cigarette; there may be emotional outbursts, irrelevant comments and interruptions; the energy levels of individuals in the group may range from very lethargic to those who are hyper-active; and attendance is often erratic. It would be foolish to imagine that anyone can prepare and teach a straightforward dance class. A therapeutic approach is required, coupled with clear but flexible learning objectives responsive to the ever changing needs of the group.

'Secondly, the nature of the contract between the parties needs to be stated: What do the students and tutor, clients and therapist agree to come together to do?

' This concerns the *choice* of the individual, which should be defined clearly, articulated and respected. It is arrogant to assume that people with disabilities, or "special educational needs", need therapy any more than anyone else does. This is connected with commonly found able-bodied attitudes towards people with disabilities: that they are in need of some sort of help, even though they may not have asked for it, and that they are thought to be incapable or ineducable ... the "Does he take sugar?" syndrome.

'It also concerns the requirements of the institution or employer, and the expertise of the practitioner: what sort of class do they want? and what am I equipped to do? It is important to define clear boundaries and responsibilities with all parties concerned, and know in your own mind what you are doing.

'Having defined the major differences, there are many similarities between the outcomes of good therapy and good educational practice. They both provide an opportunity for people to reflect, re-learn, re-experience, clarify their understanding, increase their ability to cope effectively with new demands and situations, open up fresh horizons, and effect a change in perspective. They both work on "blocks" or difficulties: one to free the creative process or to facilitate deeper learning; the other to allow the individual to integrate a previously denied opportunity. Things done in a creative dance session may be similar to those done in a dance therapy session, but for different reasons and to achieve different ends.

Creative dance with adults

Preparation for a lesson

'I work creatively with dance and movement at a "functional" level, eg to improve breathing, balance and coordination, increase flexibility and mobility, develop awareness of body parts, and promote relaxation. I also use it as a means of "communication", working with partners in small groups, and as a whole group, encouraging social interaction and relationship building. Thirdly, I try to stimulate the "imagination" using creative improvisation structures as a framework from which to draw out students' own ideas, giving them an opportunity to express themselves, and watch and learn from one another.

'In addition, we play games, based on the non-competitive "New Games" ideas, and explore issues such as taking a leadership role in the group. I also use a whole range of equipment such as beach balls, garden canes, hoops, ribbons, masks, parachutes, balloons, dressing-up box, pictures, drawings, and a varied selection of music.

'Such is the range of ability within each group, and the differences in attention span that, in order to get the most out of each student, I have to work in a "flexible" way, providing as stimulating an environment as possible to motivate and capture their interest.

'I use some repetition to give security, and to create safe boundaries.'

Suggested framework for a lesson

Jasmine Pasch emphasises that: first and foremost, the session must be an enjoyable experience, starting with brief introductions, eg games to learn the names of people in the class, ball games, swapping places.

Group activity: to increase awareness of *self*, *others*, and the *group*

Warm up to include: breathing; stretching—alone, or in a circle holding hands; massage—gentle rubbing of self and of others; mobility and identification of body parts, using students' own ideas; people-to-people game (communication and recognition); back-to-back to rest sitting; contact of body parts, eg elbow to knee, hand to foot, with self or with a partner.

Other ideas and themes: leadership — mirroring (ie couples follow or copy partners' movement), the 'magic hat' (see below); *initiating ideas* — puppets, body sculptures (statues) (see below), group fantasy sculptures (imagination) (see below); *building confidence* — moving circle, eg skip walk stop, change places as number is called.

Use of equipment: ribbons, hoops, parachutes, drawings, music (see above).

Less able groups: partner exercises, eg back to back, partner pulls, rocking, rolling, rides, tunnels (over and under), group work involving TOUCH for sensory stimulation. (Less verbal presentation).

Body exercises: (see Chapter 11)

Games: eg Dragon Tag, knots, grandmother's footsteps, name games.

Relaxation to finish.

The 'magic hat'

Aims: to develop observation skills; to explore group dynamics, particularly the leadership role; to focus attention and improve concentration; to encourage creative thinking.

Any hat can become a 'magic hat', but choose one that will stay on the head when the dancer moves and one that is brightly coloured so that it can be seen easily, eg a bobble hat.

The exercise is suitable for a group of between 8 to 16 people. The group stand in a circle and the leader takes the magic hat, puts it on and walks into the centre. The leader begins by demonstrating a simple movement, eg clicking the fingers, and if the magic is 'working' the group members will start clicking their fingers too. Other simple movements can be tried before choosing someone who would like to wear the magic hat and hence become leader. It is important to start slowly to build concentration and confidence, and to give people a chance to think of ideas of their own, gradually leading up to full body movement. Music can then be introduced, and the tempo chosen will reflect or influence the energy level of the group. The wearer/leader can pass the hat on when he/she is ready or tired, or 'rebels' may emerge from the group who snatch the hat and take over the leadership. For less active groups a variation of the exercise can be done sitting with 'magic gloves' or 'magic socks'.

Sculptures and puppets

Aims: to develop trust; to develop sensitivity towards others through the use of touch; to improve body awareness; to exercise choice and control.

Sculptures. In pairs, one chooses to be the model or sculpture, and the other the sculptor. The model can start sitting, standing or lying down. The sculptor gently moves the model's body, starting with the hands, arms and legs which are easiest, and going on to the head and trunk as trust develops between them. The sculptor sculpts the model into different shapes which the model holds in place until moved again. The model can work with eyes closed which feels very pleasant if she/he is willing.

The partners then change over and repeat the exercise.

Puppets. This is a more active development of the above exercise, and the relationship between the partners is more like that of a puppet and puppeteer. The partner playing the puppet has his/her eyes closed, and the puppeteer brings the puppet to life and stimulates it to move by touching its body, eg tapping its foot or stroking its arm. The puppeteer decides which part of the body is to move, but the puppet chooses how to respond. This offers a lot of scope for experimenting with different movement qualities with different body parts, and exploring the communication through touch between the two people. It is also fun for others to watch.

Variations, without touching:

1.   The puppeteer controls the puppet by 'imaginary strings'

from different parts of the body, using very fine control. This exercise is done with eyes open and needs concentration.

2. The puppeteer controls the puppet from a short distance away using 'gestures' to indicate how the puppet should move. It is interesting to compare the instructions from the puppeteer, and the puppet's response and interpretation.

3. The puppeteer controls the puppet by making different 'sounds' for it to dance to, using the voice or instruments.

For further information contact: Jasmine Pasch, 30 Quadrant House, Burrell Street, London SE1 0UW.

RESOURCES

Shape

Shape (London), established in 1976, is an organisation which develops the arts, including dance and creative movement, with, by and for people with physical, mental or sensory disabilities, elderly people and people recovering from mental illness. Shape organises workshops in varied locations, such as day centres, hospitals, hostels and community centres. It also organises training courses for artists, and for staff from health and social services and voluntary agency backgrounds, and takes performances and exhibitions on tour. In addition, it provides information and advice to individuals and organisations, and liaises with other arts and disability groups to establish joint projects.

The Shape Network

Since the establishment of the original Shape in London, a number of similar organisations broadly using the same approach, have been created independently to develop arts activities and events (including dance and creative movement) for people with disabilities. In 1986 these bodies federated to form The Shape Network, which now has 16 full or affiliated members, including Artibility (South Eastern England), Artlink (Eastern Scotland) and Northern Shape (North Eastern England).

For further information contact: Shape (London), 1 Thorpe Close, London W10 5XL.

Association for Dance Movement Therapy

The main aims of this Association, formed in 1982, are:

1. to facilitate the development of training in the United Kingdom;
2. to further development of theory and principles of dance movement therapy;
3. to establish regular workshops and seminars.

Further information from: The Secretary, ADMT 99 South Hill Park, Hampstead, London, NW3 2SP.

PLAYTRAC

This is a mobile play, leisure and resources centre for people with mental handicaps. Initially funded by the Department of Health and Social Security and Save the Children Fund as a two-year project, PLAYTRAC has now received guaranteed funding to continue its work from the North West Thames Regional Health Authority where it is based. The two staff describe the centre as a resource to be used any parents, voluntary organisations, and staff working in hospitals, hostels, schools and in community teams. They run training sessions for staff throughout the North West Thames Regional Health Authority and have produced information papers on a range of activities to do with play and

leisure. These include an excellent paper on practical musical activities.

For further information contact: PLAYTRAC, c/o Harperbury Hospital, Harper Lane, Shenley, Herts WD7 9HQ.

National Resource Centre for Dance

Set up in 1982 as an integral part of the development in dance at the University of Surrey, the Centre, although not yet fully operational, aims to: make information easily accessible; establish a 'living' archive; prepare and publish a variety of materials for dance; provide a liaison network between the individuals, organisations, companies and institutions involved in dance.

Therapists are among the many to whom its resources are likely to be of interest.

For further information contact: National Resource Centre for Dance, University of Surrey, Stag Hill, Guildford GU2 5XH.

Scottish Council for Movement Therapy (SCMT)

The SCMT was established in March 1987. The overall clinical remit of Movement Therapy is to establish, develop and improve inter-personal skills and communication, ie emotional and social contact through non-verbal channels of communication.

The work takes place with people who have damaged or impaired non-verbal communication systems which interfere with the quality of their relationships with other people, eg they may seem distant, cut off, display inappropriate social cues and responses, be over-active or inattentive. Movement Therapy, through the use of expressive body movements and specific movement strategies, aims to open channels of communication which allow the transmission of emotional content and help with the experience and use of these channels.

For further information contact: Ian Dick, Scottish Council for Movement Therapy, Co-ordinator at the Movement Therapy Department at Gogarburn Hospital, Glasgow Road, Edinburgh EH12 9BJ.

Disabled Living Foundation Music Advisory Service

The Music Advisory Service is available to people of all ages with any disability and everyone concerned with them. A wide range of information is available and a free newsletter *Music News* is circulated twice a year.

The Music Adviser is happy to answer individual enquiries and to offer advice on finding local music contacts, the choice and use of music and recommended background reading. Help is also available on how to introduce musical activities through games and quizzes, simple songs and instrumental work.

For further information and list of in-house publications (sae please) contact: Mrs Pam Smith, Music Advisory Service, DLF, 380-384 Harrow Road, London W9 2HU.

FURTHER READING

Creative Movement Information Pack. Vivienne Raffaele, NADMA, South Hill Park Arts Centre, Bracknell Berks RG12 4PA.

Shape News: arts opportunities for people with Special Needs. Shape, Thorpe Close, London W10 5XL.

Chapter 13

Dance

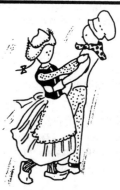

Terminology — Teaching guidelines — Hints to teachers — Formations for simple dances — Simple steps for folk/country/ national/ social dancing — Composition of simple dance-like activities — Examples of adapted simple dances - American square dancing — Music — Scottish country dancing — Displays — Parachute, ribbon, Chinese parasol and Morris dancing

Dance, however narrowly or widely interpreted, is a fundamental form of exercise, and the desire for rhythmic movement is inherent in most people.

Dance, which is both relaxing and exhilerating, is also one of the most popular of all social activities for fun and enjoyment. It can break down social barriers and provide excellent opportunities for all members of the community to share a common interest. Some people with a mental handicap have a well developed sense of rhythm and dancing can give them a feeling of normality not enjoyed to such an extent in other activities.

TERMINOLOGY

American square. A form of American folk dance originally developed in rural areas, in which a number of couples, usually in a square formation, perform changing figures with a caller.

Ballet. A classical form of theatrical dance which originally developed from Court dancing but took on its distinctive form during the 19th century. It presupposes a technique using an outward rotation of the legs which requires a lengthy training. An unusual feature is that women dance 'on the point'.

Ballroom. A social form of dance which has developed from the 19th century onwards. The English style of ballroom dancing developed during the nineteen-twenties and is famous throughout the world. Dances include the waltz, quickstep, slow fox trot and tango.

Clog. A form of tap dancing originating in Lancashire for which wooden shoes, ie clogs, are worn.

Disco dancing. A form of structured improvisation based on the current pop music. The dancers usually dance independently and the finer details of content and style are dependent on the cultural origins of the music. Although a social dance, it has recently been used for display and competition among the dancers.

Folk/community dance. A simple form of dance developed by the people of a particular country and revealing specific characteristics determined by such factors as temperament of the people, historical and geographical background, costume and musical instruments used.

Latin-American. The basic figures of the Rumba, Samba, Paso Doble, American Jive and Cha-Cha-Cha.

Modern educational dance. A method of teaching dance based on the set of principles devised by Rudolf Laban in the early years of the 20th century. This has been developed into a way of teaching creatively and is widely used in schools today.

National character dances. The steps are those used in the traditional dances. In both the music and dance arrangement, the characteristics of the country and of the particular type of dance are retained.

Both national and national character dances can be simplified to enable the non-dance specialist teacher to capture the style, quality, music and background of these countries.

National dances. Authentic traditional dances from Western and Eastern Europe, Russia and other parts of the world.

Natural movement. Natural movement is a free form of dance which trains an appreciation of beauty through the natural actions of human movement, and also lays emphasis on the importance of musical understanding. Its aesthetic appeal, and com paratively simple technique, allows pupils to respond eagerly to imaginative and creative opportunities, and develop a love of dance movement with a quality of expressiveness in interpretation which is of permanent value in their physical, musical and artistic education.

Old Time. The sequence dances were popular in the ballroom prior to the first world war. Such dances as Veleta, Boston Two Step, Military Two Step, Lancers and Quadrilles, come under this heading.

Sword and morris dancing. Sword and morris dances are danced by men only, often on village streets and green or in the market place. They are suitable for displays and festivals.

Tap. A form of dance performed with metal plates on the shoes and characterised by the rhythmic tapping of the toes and heels on the floor.

Folk, community, American square, national and old time dances seem to be the most popular with people with a mental handicap, although they also enjoy and benefit from ballet, natural movement, ballroom and modern educational dance, taught by specialist teachers.

Introducing folk or country dancing

Simple dances indigenous to many regions and counties in England, Scotland, Ireland and Wales, danced by local groups and clubs can be taught to people with a mental handicap, as can the traditional folk dances from Europe and others parts of the world.

Educational and social training

Dance is related to both educational and social training through its link with the country of origin, the music, art, history, geography, costume and customs of the people. It can also play a role in the drama production, pantomime, nativity play or musical show (maypole and country dances, national and tap dancing, for example).

TEACHING GUIDELINES

Enjoying working together and responding to the beat of the music should be established before teaching specific dances, eg sitting on chairs clapping or stamping with the leader, to the music. All can be helped to work together by following a leader in the formation with hands joined; leaders create floor patterns of their choice and finally individual groups join up in one large circle formation. Hand and eye contact help the group to gain confidence in working together, hence the value of a circle formation.

The organisation required for partner work is unnecessary at this stage. A variety of simple steps can be taught combined with easy floor patterns, eg moving towards the centre of the circle and back or travelling round the circle.

In contrast, dancers may then sit and experiment with clapping activities, at first following the leader and then creating their own clapping sequence to the music. They will now be ready to return to the simple circle movements as a climax to the session; this repetition will give the dancers confidence.

When the above dance activities can be performed with ease and enjoyment the dancers are ready to attempt simple partner dances. The teacher must assess how soon this stage is reached. Circumstances vary, the teacher with few helpers will take longer to reach this stage than one working in an integrated situation where there might be a one-to-one relationship.

When preparing a dance lesson, consider: the standard of movement and the sense of rhythm of the members of the group; the selection of dances and dance steps which can be easily learned by all; the need to repeat well known popular dances; the choice and availability of music and accompanists, eg pianists, accordionists, guitarists.

HINTS TO TEACHERS

1. Name the dance.

2. Listen to the music before dancing, talk about its characteristics.

3. Remember the gentleman *always* has his lady on his *right* unless otherwise indicated. Where there are more women than men in a class, the woman dancing 'man' should wear a band or some other identification.

4. Make sure the dancers know the formation and pattern of the dance.

5. Prompt well in advance when a change of formation or step occurs.

6. Link one phrase to the next by reminding the dancers of the steps at the end of one phrase and of those that are coming at the beginning of the next; practise these links to ensure continuity.

7. Coach good poise throughout.

8. Improve the standard of footwork even if it is a slow process.

9. Give as graphic a description as possible of the country of origin and its traditional costume.

10. **Repetition** is very important, especially when teaching links between two sequences or figures. The confidence gained by the success of learning two figures in the session far outweighs the value of attempting 3 or 4.

Adaptation and progress

Substitute easier steps for difficult ones.

Substitute or repeat a sequence of steps for ones that prove too difficult.

Delete a whole figure if necessary and repeat one of the other figures in its place, or omit it.

Simplify the formation and patterns.

Simplify the hold.

Use a longer phrase of music — 8 instead of 4, or 16 instead of 8 when teaching a step or pattern.

Although progress may be slow, improvement can be measured by:

quicker response to demonstration and verbal directions;

improved standard of performance;

improved continuity throughout the dance;

greater awareness of partner relationship and social responsibility;

ability to remember from one lesson to the next.

As dancers become more proficient, encourage those who are able, to create their own dance steps and patterns.

Steps and formations and holds

These examples of formations, steps and holds are based on traditional dances as recorded by the National Dance Branch of the Imperial Society of Teachers of Dancing, the English Folk Dance and Song Society and the Royal Scottish Country Dance Society, and have been kept deliberately simple to suit the needs of the adult person with a mental handicap whose movement, spatial awareness and feeling for direction is often limited.

Once a teacher has understood the basic formations, patterns and steps, and put them into short rhythmic phrases of 32, 16 or 8 counts it is possible without using complicated steps to choreograph a great number of dances designed to suit the abilities of any particular handicapped group. At a later stage a wider variety of steps and formations can be added

Formations for simple dances

Processional

Longways set

Casting out and its variations

Turn your partner and its variations

Right and left hand star

Circles and variations, simple or more difficult

Arches and variations

Serpentine or snake

Back to back (Do-si-do)

Sets of 2 or 4 couples.

Steps for simple dance

Walking, forwards, backwards and turning

Running, forwards, backwards and turning

Skipping, forwards, backwards and turning

Skip change of step, leading to polka

Gallop or slip step sideways and variations

Side close and its variations (chassé)

Step and hop and its variations.

Steps for more advanced dances

French runs, forward and turning

Pas de basque 1 2 3 —1 & 2

Waltz step

Pas mazurka

Step and hops, with varying numbers of hops and change of direction

Balance step (setting)

Barn dance.

Although these more advanced steps are described in detail the most effective way for a teacher to acquire them is through practical experience with other dancers.

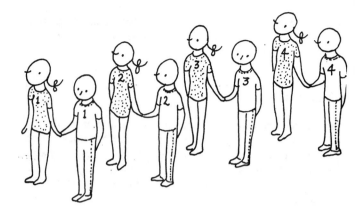

Figure 13.1 Longways set

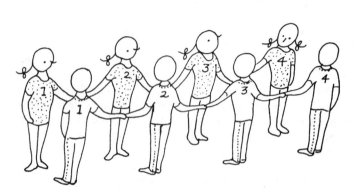

Figure 13.2 Longways set, partners facing

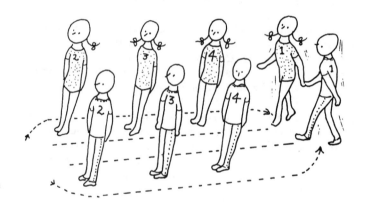

Figure 13.3 Casting out

FORMATIONS FOR SIMPLE DANCES

Processional

Line up dancers to move in anti-clockwise direction around the edge of the room. The lady is on the gentleman's right side, ie ladies on outside, gentleman on the inside.

Longways set (usually 4 couples)

Line up couples facing the teacher (thereafter referred to for this purpose as the top of the set). The lady is on the gentleman's right side, and inside hands, or right hands are joined (Fig 13.1).

In this formation the couples can move on behind each other, towards and away from the top of the set, ie moving forwards and backwards.

Alternatively the couples can turn and face each other, and move forwards and backwards — towards and away from each other. Where a group has difficulty in doing this, the gentleman's line links hands and the ladies do likewise (Fig 13.2).

Casting out and variations

Casting out and back to place. Line up without holding inside hands. Top lady and top gentleman cast outwards at the same time, the lady by turning to the right and the gentleman by turning to the left. They move to the bottom of the set, join hands, and walk to the top of the set, finishing when they reach their own places (Fig 13.3).

It might be helpful to chalk or mark the initials of the top couple on the floor in their own places, and also at the spot where they join together again.

Variations:

1. *Both lines casting out, joining hands, back to places.* Casting can be repeated with both lines moving at the same time. The ladies following the top lady and the gentleman following the top gentleman. The leaders cast out and move to the bottom of the set, with their respective lines following them. Instruct each

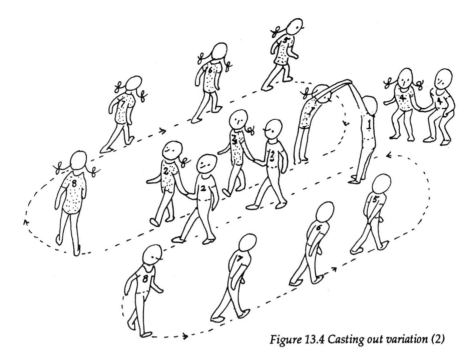

Figure 13.4 Casting out variation (2)

couple to 'find your partner, join hands and move forward to your own place'.

2. *Casting out and making an arch* (change leaders). As before, the leaders with their respective lines behind them, cast out and move to the bottom of the set. The first couple on reaching the 'joining position' face each other, join both hands, and raise them high to make an arch. The rest now join inside hands with their partners as before, and pass under the arch before returning to their own places. The first couple have now become the last, and the second couple have become the new leader at the top of ;the set (Fig 13.4). Each new couple, practise the casting out movement as before using the pattern to change leaders.

3. *Casting out and all couples make an arch*. The top couple leaders with their respective lines behind them, cast out and move to the bottom of the set. This time the first couple join hands and walk forwards to their own starting positions, where they turn and join both hands and raise their arms to make an arch. Each couple in turn following their example, except the last couple who join hands and move forwards passing under the arches until they reach the top of the set. They have now changed places and become top couple, whilst the original top couple move into second place.

Turning your partners

This movement can be performed from a procession, longways set or circle formation.

Partners face each other, join right hands or both, turn clockwise, with either a walking, running, skip or slip step for an even number of counts, eg 16. The couples stop, and turn to go the other way, ie anti-clockwise. Where a one-hand grasp is used it is essential to change hands before setting off in the other direction, ie right-hand grasp when turning clockwise; left-hand

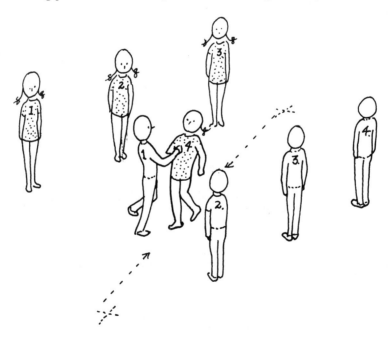

Figure 13.5 Corner couples turning

grasp when turning anti-clockwise.

Corner couples turning. In a longways set a turn can be made by: the top lady and bottom gentleman or the top gentleman and bottom lady (Fig 13.5).

The couples in a longways set turn and face each other and take one step backwards. Top lady moves diagonally forward to the centre of the set, likewise the bottom gentleman. They meet, give right or both hands and move clockwise for an even number of counts, eg 16 or 8. Walks, runs, skips or slipping steps can be used. They then change and give left hands, or keep a double hand hold and change direction and move anti-clockwise for a further 16 or 8 counts. They then fall back to their places.

Note: Practise with longer phrases of 32 counts if it helps to establish the pattern, before changing direction, and falling back to place. When this movement has been mastered, it can develop into the following turn:

meet	2	3	4
change	2	3	4 (turning anti-clockwise)
turn	2	3	4 (turning clockwise)
back	2	3	4

Right or left hand star

The last movement can develop into a right and left hand star, by 2 couples joining together. First couple extend and slightly raise their hands, at the same time turning towards the second couple. Second couple, extend and slightly raise their right hands, and turn towards the first couple. The ladies put their right hands palm down on top of their gentleman's right hand. The first gentleman puts his right hand on top of the second couple's hands. All finish standing with the right shoulders inwards, right arm extended and raised and the left arm stretched to the side to complete the star or wheel effect. The couples move in a clockwise direction, either walking, running or skipping forwards. Begin with a long phrase of 16 counts before going round the other way, with left hands joined in the centre, and the right arm stretched to the side (Fig 13.6).

Note: It is worthwhile stopping the music to make the change-over, until the group becomes competent to make a quick swing round to change arms. At first, the group will probably require talking through the change, and it may be necessary to physically correct and help with this movement.

Circle formation (simple)

Make a circle with ladies on their partners' right. The group face inwards with hands joined. All move sideways to the right, with a slipping step, ie side gallop. Keep to an even phrase before changing to move to the left, eg 32, 16 or 8.

Note: Where this proves to be difficult, make a circle and turn the left shoulder in towards the middle. 'Follow my leader'. Walk forwards in an anti-clockwise direction for 16 counts. Any marching tune can be used for this and eventually the number of steps in any direction can be cut down, or the rhythm altered, to such as slow, slow, quick, quick, slow. Introduce short phrases of varying rhythm such as 8 walks, followed by 16 runs in one direction, before turning and repeating the other way.

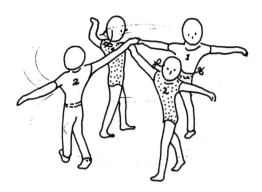

Figure 13.6 Right hand star

Variations:

1. **Forwards and backwards to the centre.** Join hands in a circle all facing the centre, 8 walks forwards to the centre and 8 walks backwards. Where the circle is too small, keep the same length of phrase but changing the movements, eg 4 walks forward, 4 claps on the spot; 4 walks backward, 4 claps on the spot. With a more advanced group, a change of rhythm can be introduced, eg slow, slow, quick, quick, slow or variations introducing claps and stamps: clap, clap, clap, wait — stamp, stamp, stamp, wait. With a more advanced group the ladies move to the centre and back whilst the gentlemen remain in their places followed by the gentlemen moving whilst the ladies remain still.

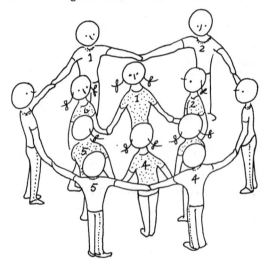

Figure 13.7 Concentric circles hands joined

2. **Concentrate circles.** Ladies join hands and make a circle on the inside. Gentlemen join hands and make a large circle round the ladies. The ladies turn left shoulder inwards and walk forwards in an anti-clockwise direction. The gentlemen turn right shoulder inwards and walk forwards in a clockwise direction. After 16 walks, both circles stop and change direction and repeat walks in the opposite direction. As the group becomes more confident, shorten the phrase to 8 counts. Running, skipping or stamps using various rhythms can be introduced.

Variations: Form two circles, one inside the other, facing the centre with hands joined. Slipping steps sideways, ladies moving to the right, and gentlemen to the left and vice versa, 16 or 8 steps (Fig 13.7).

Arches

The dancers make a circle or line, depending on the numbers with hands joined, arms raised to make arches. One dancer at a time

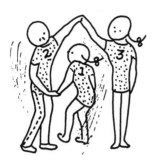

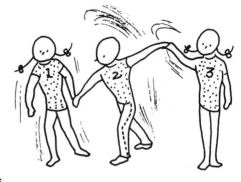

Figure 13.8 Arches

weaves in and out of the arches, until either back in her place in the circle, or to the end of the line. As soon as the first dancer is back in place or at the end of the line, the second dancer then starts to weave in and out. The dance is repeated until all have had a turn.

This sequence can be danced by a small group of dancers making a train-like formation, under the arches, as in 'Here comes a bluebird through my window' based on the Ladybird Series 'Singing Games'.

Variation: Three dancers, 1 gentlemen and 2 ladies—gentlemen in middle. The dancer on the right, No 1, passes in front of the middle dancer, No 2, and under the arch between dancers 2 and 3 and continues until back to place. The middle dancer, No 2, turns under own left arm to complete the movement, Dancer No 3 repeats the movement passing in from of dancer No 2 and under the arch between dancers No 2 and No 1 continuing back to place. The middle dancer, No 2, turns under own right arm (Fig 13.8).

Serpentine or snake

The dances line up alternately, ladies and gentlemen one behind the other. The teacher is the leader to begin with. To any popular march or rag time tune, the leader weaves a snake-like pattern from one end of the hall to the other (Fig 13.9). Many dancers tend to 'overtake' the dancers in front, but must learn to keep their place in the line. This can be danced with hands joined.

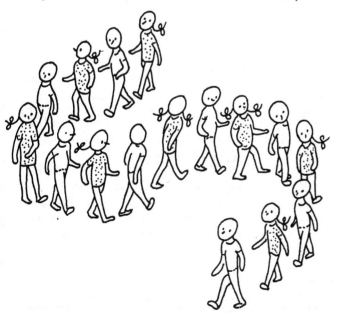

Figure 13.9 Serpentine or snake

Back to back (Do-si-do)

Start this movement in a longways set with the couples facing each other. Since each dancer walks in a square pattern, it is helpful mark the pattern on the floor. To prevent confusion use two colours, one to show the lady's track, the other the gentlemen's. Give each couple the chance to work this out under supervision. The dancers pass right shoulders as they move forwards for 4 counts. They move sideways to the right with their backs to each other for 4 counters, backwards for 4 counts passing left shoulders and finally sideways to the left to face each other again (Fig 13.10).

Ladies and gentlemen can practise separately; this means they will actually move round their stationary partner, 4 forward, 4 to the right, 4 backwards, 4 to the left. If right and left is not understood, use terms such as 'sideways towards the music/door/window'.

SIMPLE STEPS FOR FOLK/COUNTRY/NATIONAL/SOCIAL DANCING

R = Right foot
L = Left foot

The steps included in the first part of the glossary have been successfully used with older teenage and adult groups with a mental handicap. The steps described, although based on authentic footwork, have in some instances been adapted and simplified.

Walking steps 4/4 time (a light, lilting tune 4 steps to 1 bar, 2 slow steps to 1 bar)

Encourage an easy lilting walk, in time with the beat of the music, and whenever necessary indicate which foot should start. Generally work on phrases of 16, 8 or 4, and be positive about counting the correct number of steps before changing direction. Walking backwards may take time to achieve, numerous dance-like activities in lines and with partners can be practised to improve moving forwards and backwards. The ultimate aim is to dance a step called 'forward and back a double' which is 3 steps forward R L R close L to R followed by 3 steps backward R L R and close L to R.

Running steps 4/4 time (4 runs to 1 bar)

A light springing run with the weight pitched slightly forwards on the balls of the feet. Many older, heavy, adults with a mental handicap, hampered by a lack of balance and the inability to sustain a running activity for any length of time, find this move-

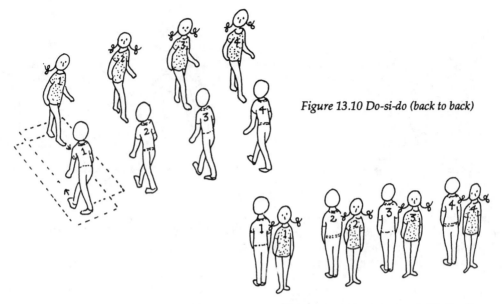

Figure 13.10 Do-si-do (back to back)

ment difficult and awkward. If a running step is used keep to even phrases of 16 or 8, and combine it with a quieter less energetic movement such as walking to ensure that the group does not tire too quickly.

French runs   2/4 or 4/4 time (2 or 4 steps to 1 bar)
A younger active group may well attempt these runs, with the weight of the body pitched slightly forwards and the toes kicked up as high as possible behind. (Think of the feet touching the seat whilst running.)

Skipping   2/4 or 6/8 time (2 steps to 1 bar)

Many adults find this difficult, because of their weight and a lack of resilience. A skip is simple:

'Step forward, hop, bring the other leg to the front'. Repeat continuously.

Turn on the spot   4/4 time (4 steps to 1 bar)

Short walking or running steps in a small circle to the right or left to 8 or 4 counts.

Chant: 'Turn 2 3 4 or right 2 3 4, left 2 3 4'.

Gallops forwards   2/4 or 6/8 time (2 steps to 1 bar)

A light springy step taken forwards, normally in phrases of 8 or 4, ie the R leads for 8, then change and bring the L through to lead for 8.

A gallop is a step forward on the right, followed by the L immediately closing with a spring so releasing the R forward again.

Simple version: Step R forward, close L to R hop on the L and lift R up.
Chant: 'step,   close,   hop'   1 & 2.
Chant: 'step,   close,   hop'.

Skip change of step   2/4 time (1 step to 1 bar)

This is a development of the forward gallop, and may well prove to be too difficult for some groups, because of its short phrasing (and 1 and 2). It is a lilting step that travels forwards, the leading foot changing at the beginning of every phrase. Start with the

weight on the L, and the R free just off the floor. Hop L and step forward R quickly close L foot to R and step forward again R. Hop R and bring L foot through and step forward, close R to L and step forward again L.

Chant:	'Hop,	step,	close	step'
	and	1	and	2

Polka   2/4 time (1 step to 1 bar)

A springy step similar to the 'skip change of step' which has a rhythm of ' and 1 and 2', ie hop, step, close, step. Polka steps can be danced forwards, to one side or turning. Polka steps can be combined with skips, slips or runs, eg 2 polka steps followed by 4 skips.

Slip step or gallops sideways   2/4 or 6/8 (2 steps to 1 bar)

A bouncy step that travels sideways, normally in phrases of 16, 8 or 4. Encourage a good 'lift'. Step sideways with R to the R. Quickly close the L foot to the R with a feeling of knocking the R one out of the way. Immediately release the R to the side and repeat the movement.

Chant:	1	and	2	and
	R	close	R	close
	1	and	2	and
or	step	close	step	close

This gallop step can be performed in circles, concentric circles, in lines or with partners, or by a solo dancer. It can be taken at a galloping tempo resembling the rhythm of horses hooves or more slowly and strongly, so that it is akin to the straddle step of men's morris dancing.

Many of the more advanced steps may be unsuitable for some groups, but teachers can modify the steps and use the original folk tunes and rhythms to compose a variety of dances.

Step and close in different directions

If this can be mastered it provides a movement which is the basis of many central European dances, Afro/Carribbean and Disco dancing, as well as the beginnings of slow rhythm and social dancing.

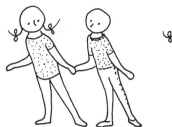
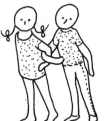
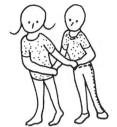

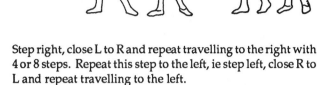

Figure 13.11 Holds (side by side)

1. Step right, close L to R and repeat travelling to the right with 4 or 8 steps. Repeat this step to the left, ie step left, close R to L and repeat travelling to the left.

    The steps can be repeated 8, 4 or twice as required.

2. Step R, close L to R without weight, ie step right rest L, step left, rest R.

    Chant: 'step right, rest L, step left, rest R'.

    This develops into a swaying movement alternately to the right and left and can be further developed into a forward and backward movement taken slowly or quickly.

3. Step R forward, rest L in behind, step back, L and rest R in front.

    Chant: 'forwards 2 3 4 back or front 2, back 2'.

Step and hop

A springy movement that can be performed in a variety of ways with or without a turn and or change or direction. Since it entails balance, co-ordination and control, it may take some time to achieve.

1. Simple step and hop.
    Step R to right. Swing L up and across in front. Repeat to the L.

    Chant: 'Step, lift, step, lift'.

    Later hop as the second leg swings up and across in front. Step, hop, step, hop (R hop L hop).

2. More difficult version.
    If and when this is mastered a variety of rhythms can be introduced, eg

    (i)   Step R swing L across and make 3 hops on the R.

          Chant: 'step, hop, hop, hop'.

          Repeat to the left.
          This movement and rhythm is to be found in the tarantella (6/8 rhythm) and other Italian dances.

    (ii) Glide, hop, hop (skating step) as in some Dutch, Danish and Swedish dances, 3/4 time (1 skating step to 1 bar). In couples, hands joined in front of the body right with right and left with left. Glide diagonally forward on R, 2 hops on R repeat with L.

          Chant: Glide, hop, hop. (Skate, hop, hop).

Pas mazurka   3/4 time (1 step to 1 bar)

This is a graceful step in 3/4 time, as in many Polish and Swedish dances.
Stamp, close, hop.
Teach it moving forward altogether.
Stamp, R forward, close L to R, hop L raising R in front.
It repeats with the same foot leading and will combine well with

runs or stamps eg Stamp R, close L, hop L. Stamp, close, hop. Stamp, step, hop. 3 runs R L R.
Repeat this starting on the L foot.

Pas de basque   2/4 or 3/4 (1 step to 1 bar)

This step is taken from side to side, it is found in dances from Russia, Central Europe and in English and Scottish country dancing. One step has 3 beats and 3 changes of weight and is performed to a rhythm of 1 and 2.

Simplified version: Step R to the right side. Quickly close L into the R and immediately stamp on the R—in place. This whole movement repeats to the left. It is easier to chant: step, mark time, or R mark time, L mark time.

Note: This step requires a quick change of balance. It is however, with a change of rhythm and tempo into a slow 3/4 (waltz), an effective simple way of teaching a step in waltz rhythm.

Waltz   3/4 time (1 step to 1 bar)

A gentle swaying movement in 3/4 time that can be danced with a partner. At a later stage, if this is mastered, it is possible to introduce a simplified close, change step, or 3 passing steps, long, short, short.

Basic waltz rhythm step

1. Step R to right.
2. Close L to R.
3. Transfer weight back to R.

Holds

Holds can be varied to suit the ability of the class members. The following are some simple examples.

Partners stand side by side facing the same direction

1. Link inside hands
2. Link inside elbows
3. Cross arms in front, hold hands R with R and L with L (promenade hold) (Fig 13.11).

Partners face each other

1. Shake right hands 'as if to say hello' and then turn side by side to move round the room (anti-clockwise).
2. In couples, the gentleman puts his hands on the ladies' waist and the lady puts her hands on the gentleman's shoulders (lean away). They turn on the spot together. Gentleman starting with R and the lady with L.

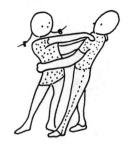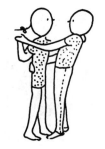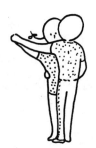

Figure 13.12 Holds (facing)

3. The gentleman puts his right arm round the lady's waist and grasps her right hand with his left hand. Keep arms at shoulder height. The lady places her left hand on the gentleman's shoulder from behind (ballroom hold) (Fig 13.12).

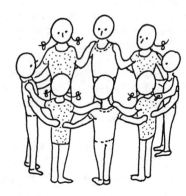

Figure 13.13 Holds (facing into circle)

4. In a circle, the gentlemen put their arms round the ladies' waists and the ladies put their hands on the shoulders of the gentlemen on either side of them (Fig 13.13).

COMPOSITION OF SIMPLE DANCE-LIKE ACTIVITIES

When practising the steps of a particular dance, it helps to compose a simple dance-like activity to an 8 or 16 bar phrase of 2/4, 4/4, 6/8 or 3/4 music according to the nature of the step(s). Keep the activities simple using one or two different steps only. The following are some examples.

Walking (promenade) 4/4 time (4 steps to 1 bar)

Music   Any lively marching or walking tune (4 steps to 1 bar).

Formation   In couples.

Activity   Practise walking to the music (a light lilting step). With inside hands joined partners walk anti-clockwise, round the room — 8 steps.
                                              (Bars 1 - 2)

              With right hands joined (or right elbows linked) turn partner clockwise on the spot — 8 steps.
                                              (Bars 3 - 4)

              Repeat Bars 1 — 2   *(Bars 5 - 6)*

              Repeat with left elbows linked turn anti-clockwise on the spot.   *(Bars 7 - 8)*

              Repeat all.

Variation   Instead of bars 7 — 8, walk 8 steps to find a new partner: this makes the dance progressive and changes partners in a simple way.

Slipping and skipping   (in a circle)

Music   Jig or reel. 2/4 or 6/8 time (2 steps to 1 bar).

Formation   Couples in a circle hands joined.

Activity   8 slipping steps (gallops) anti-clockwise
                                              (Bars 1 - 4)

              Repeat clockwise.   *(Bars 5 - 8)*

              4 skips into centre raising arms, 4 skips back to places lowering arms.   *(Bars 9 -12)*

              4 stamps and 4 claps on the spot. *(Bars 13 - 16)*

              Repeat all.   *(Bars 17 - 32)*

Variation   Instead of bars 13 — 16, drop hands, turn to face partner. 4 stamps, clap own hands, partner's hands twice.

Gallops and walks   (in longways set)

Music   2/4 or 6/8 skipping tune (2 steps to 1 bar).

Formation   Longway set of 4 couples, gentleman facing ladies.

Activity   Gentlemen and ladies walk forward towards each other and back — 8 steps.   *(Bars 1 - 4)*

              Gentlemen and ladies turn each other with right hands.   *(Bars 5 - 8)*

              Repeat from beginning.   *(Bars 9 - 12)*

              Repeat turn giving left hand,   *(Bars 13 - 16)*

              Top couple gallop down to the bottom of the set (both hands joined).   *(Bars 1 - 4)*

              Repeat back to place.   *(Bars 5 - 8)*

              Top couples cast right and left skip of walk to the bottom of the set.   *(Bars 9 - 16)*

              Repeat all with the new top couple leading the dance.

Variation   The other dancers clap while the top couple slip down and up the set.

Polka   (Hop step close step = Hop 1 and 2)

Practise polka step round the room.

Music   Any lively polka tune 2/4 (1 polka step to a bar and 2 skips to a bar).

Formation	In two's facing counter clockwise. Inside hands joined.
Activity	4 polka steps forward. *(Bars 1 - 4)*
	8 skips forward finish facing partner. *(Bars 5 - 8)*
	Lady 4 polka steps round gentleman while he claps. *(Bars 9 - 12)*
	4 polka steps round the lady while she claps. *(Bars 13 - 16)*
	Finish side by side ready to start again.

Waltz or triple run

Music	Any waltz 3/4 time (1 waltz step to a bar).
Formation	Sets of 6. Two lines of 3 facing each other: 1 gentleman and 2 ladies in each line
	L G L
	L G L
Activity	Lines waltz towards each other 2 steps. Lines waltz away from each other 2 steps. *(Bars 1 - 4)*
	No 1 lady cross diagonally 4 steps. *(Bars 5 - 8)*
	No 2 lady cross diagonally 4 steps. *(Bars 9 - 12)*
	The gentlemen change places - 4 steps. *(Bars 13 - 16)*
	Repeat all back to places. *(Bars 17 - 32)*

A musical medley

Use tunes suitable for different steps, skipping, polka, slipping, waltz walking etc. The dancers listen to the music, identify the step(s) verbally and then dance them.

EXAMPLES OF ADAPTED SIMPLE DANCES

Shepherd's hey

Music	'Shepherd's hey' 4/4 time (4 runs to 1 bar).
Formation	All dancers stand facing the teacher with hands by sides.
Dance	4 runs forward, 4 runs backwards. *(Bars 1 - 2)*
	Jump feet apart rebound, jump together. *(Bar 3)*
	Repeat jump. *(Bar 4)*
	Chant: 'Out — wait — in — wait — out — wait — in — wait'
	Repeat Bars 1 - 4 *(Bars 5 - 8)*
	Clapping pattern
	Clap, clap, 'slap' slightly raised right knee
	Chant: '1 2 3, wait' *(Bar 9)*
	Chant: '1 2 3, wait'. *(Bar 10)*
	3 claps under right knee 1 2 3 wait. *(Bar 11)*
	Repeat claps under left knee 1 2 3 wait.*(Bar 12)*
	Repeat the clapping pattern. *(Bars 13 - 16)*

Country gardens

Music	'Country gardens' 4/4 time (4 steps to 1 bar).
Formation	The couples line up one behind the other in longways set formation with the lady on the gentleman's right.
Dance	The ladies following the top lady, cast out to the left and walk round the gentlemen's line and back to their places. *(Bars 1 - 4)*
	The gentlemen following the top gentleman cast out to the right and walk round the ladies' line and back to their places. *(Bars 5 - 8)*
	Casting out
	Both leaders cast out simultaneously, the ladies to the right and the gentlemen to the left. *(Bars 9 - 12)*
	The first couple meet join hands and walk forward to their starting positions. They face each other. They raise their arms to make an arch, 1st and 2nd couples follow and do likewise. *(Bars 13 - 16)*
	4th couple meet and join inside hands and pass under all the arches until they reach the top of the set. *(Bars 17 - 20)*
	They have now become the top couple, and the former top couple become the 2nd couple.
	The new top couple turn on the spot 8 steps clockwise — 8 steps anti-clockwise. *(Bars 21 - 24)*
	Repeat the dance sufficient times until all the couples have led the dance.

Here comes a bluebird   (based on the song in the Ladybird Series Dancing Rhymes)

Music	'Here comes a bluebird' — 3/4 time (1 waltz step to 1 bar).
Formation	All the dancers form a circle or line with hands joined and arms raised to make arches. A dancer at the end of the line dances with the teacher with the waist hold.
Dance	The teacher and dancer weave in and out through the arches. *(Bars 1 - 8)*
	They separate and join hands with the nearest dancer to them and each couple turns his new partner on the spot. *(Bars 9 - 16)*
	At the end of this phrase, the dancers left in the line make their arches, and the 2 couples now make a line one behind the other and weave in and out of the arches. *(Bars 17 - 24)*
	Each time the dance is repeated the number of couples dancing doubles and the number in the line decreases. *(Bars 25 - 32)*
	This is a simple dance in which everybody can join. It can also be danced in a circle formation.

A-hunting we will go

Music	'A-hunting we will go' — 2/4 time (2 gallops to one bar).

Dance

Formation	Longways set (4 couples)
Dance	1st couple gallop down the set. *(Bars 1 - 4)*
	Repeat back to places. *(Bars 5 - 8)*
	First gentleman and lady cast out right and left to the bottom of the set followed by the rest (skipping or walking step). *(Bars 9 - 12)*
	1st couple make an arch — all dancers pass through ready for 2nd couple to become the new 1st couple and lead the dance.
	Repeat until each couple has led the dance. *(Bars 13 - 16)*
	It may be necessary to lengthen the phrases to 8 bars = 16 gallops or skips at first.

Handkerchief dance

Music	6/8 time (2 steps to 1 bar).
Formation	Couples linked by large handkerchief or scarf held in right hands throughout.
	Do not break the hold.
	1st lady stands between and below the second couple.
Dance	Star clockwise (right hands raised). *(Bars 1 - 4)*
(skips or	Star anti-clockwise (right hands raised) *(Bars 5 - 8)*
	1st man under 2nd couple's arch. *Bars 9 - 10)*
	2nd couple under 1st couple's arch. *(Bars 11 - 12)*
	1st couple under 2nd couple's arch. *(Bars 13 - 14)*
	End couple under 1st couple's arch. *(Bars 15 - 16)*
	Swing and change 1st lady under 2nd couple's arch. *(Bars 1 - 16)*

Pop goes the weasel

Music	'Pop goes the weasel' — 2/4 time (2 skips to a bar).
Formation	Circles of 3 dancers with hands joined. 1 dancer in the centre of each circle (the weasel). 1 free dancer (Fig 13.14).
Dance	Skip round clockwise singing:
	'Half a pound of tuppenny rice

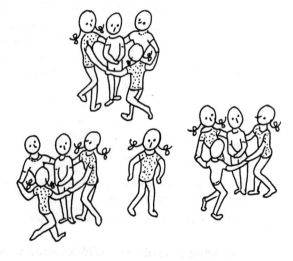

Figure 13.14 Pop goes the weasel'

Half a pound of treacle

That's the way the money goes

'Pop' goes the weasel'. *(Bars 1 - 6) (12 skips)*

On 'Pop' the dancers lift their arms high and the 'weasels' 'pop' out and run into another circle. *(Bars 7 - 8)*

The free weasel runs into a circle leaving another weasel free.

Repeat skipping anti-clockwise.

Walking steps or slip steps can be substituted for skips.

Two circles

Music	Barn dance — 4/4 time (1 barn dance step to 1 bar, 4 walks to 1 bar).
Formation	Two circles — gentleman outside, with hands joined, ladies inside facing the gentlemen with hands joined.
Dance	8 barn dance steps to left (1 - 2 - 3 hop). *(Bars 1 - 8)*
	Gentlemen grab a partner from the other circle and promenade her towards the teacher (8 walking steps). *(Bars 9 - 10)*
	Promenade away into a space. *(Bars 11 - 12)*
	All swing partners. *(Bars 13 - 15)*
	Reform 2 circles and start again. *(Bars 16)*

Promenade dance

Music	'Waltzing Matilda' — 4/4 time (4 steps to 1 bar).
Formation	In two lines facing each other, hands joined down the line partners side by side (not opposite).
Dance	Top and bottom gentlemen lead their lines up or down the room with 8 walks, turn, ladies lead lines back to places, 8 walks. *(Bars 1 - 4)*
	Each gentleman stamps to the lady opposite to him to attract her attention, then turns and walks away from her across the room while she follows —8 steps: turn, and the lady leads back to places, 8 steps. *(Bars 5 - 8)*
	Partners link right arms and turn with 8 walks: link arms and turn with 8 walks. *(Bars 9 - 12)*
	'Thread the needle'. Top gentleman and lady lead the others with 8 polka steps or 16 walking steps down the inside of the set under an arch made by bottom couple, and divide back to places. *(Bars 13 - 16)*

Teddy bear's picnic (walking step)

Music	'Teddy bear's picnic' — 2/4 time (2 steps to 1 bar).
Formation	In three with elbows linked, or hands joined, facing counter-clockwise. One gentleman between two ladies.
Dance	Eight walks forward *(Bars 1 - 4)*
	Eight walks backward *(Bars 5 - 8)*

Eight walks forward *(Bars 9 - 12)*

Gentleman turns the lady on his left under his left arm, then the lady on his right under his right arm *(Bars 13 - 14)*

All clap hands 4 times *(Bars 15 - 16)*

Ladies four walks forward to the gentleman in front to make the dance progressive.

Skipping dance (based on a French folk dance)

Music Any 6/8 skipping tune, eg 'Girls and boys come out to play', 'Sur le pont d'Avignon'.

Formation 6 or 8 dancers — the couples stand facing each other holding right hands.

Dance Fig 1. The outside dancers skip back leading their partners away from the centre. *(Bars 1 - 4)*

Repeat skipping back to original places. Repeat all. *(Bars 5 - 8)*

Fig 2. All join hands in one circle, skip round to the right - 16 skips. *(Bars 9 - 16)*

Fig 3. The two dancers at the front of the circle break hands while the two at the back of the circle make an arch. The front two turn inwards and lead through the arch turning to left and right respectively, skipping round to the front to re-form the circle, the rest all following, hands joined. The two forming the arch turn under their own arms. *(Bars 1 - 8)*

Fig 4. Repeat Fig 2, end divided into 2 lines facing each other. *(Bars 9 - 16)*

Fig 5. 4 skips forward, 4 skips backward, 8 skips forward across to opposite side passing right shoulders. *(Bars 1 - 8)*

Fig 6. Repeat Fig 2. *(Bars 9 - 16)*

Fig 7. Repeat Fig 3. *(Bars 1 - 8)*

Fig 8. Dance in one long chain in any direction and back to original places to start the dance again. *(Bars 9 -16)*

Adaptations Use a lilting walking step at first until the formations are known. Use longer phrases of music, eg 16 bars for Fig.3. Slipping step sideways can be substituted for skipping in Fig 1. Dancers would stand sideways to the centre to do this. Slipping step sideways can be substituted for skipping in Fig 2.

Polka

Music Any polka tune ('See me dance the polka') — 2/4 time (1 polka step to 1 bar or 2 skips to 1 bar of music).

Formation In couples with inner hands joined, facing anti-clockwise.

Dance Starting with foot away from partner 4 polka steps forward, finish facing partner. *(Bars 1 - 4)*

With both hands joined, 8 skips round clockwise. *(Bars 5 - 8)*

Repeat 1 - 4 *(Bars 9 - 12)*

Repeat 5 - 8 skipping round anti-clockwise. *(Bars 13 -16)*

Repeat all.

Variation Instead of 13 — 16, spin partner on the spot arms straight, pulling away from partner (very small steps).

Circle walk

Music 4/4 gay walking tune (4 steps to 1 bar)

Formation In threes with elbows linked, facing counter-clockwise. One gentleman between two ladies.

Dance 16 walks forward, ie counter-clockwise. *(Bars 1 - 4)*

4 step-hops, stepping on left foot and swinging right leg across. *(Bars 5 - 6)*

Gentleman joins hands (cross grasp) with outer lady and they spin round on the spot, leaning away from each other and taking very small steps. *(Bars 7 - 8)*

Repeat 5 - 6 and 7 - 8 starting the step-hops on the right foot, and gentleman spinning with inner lady. *(Bars 9 - 12)*

Join hands in circle of three 8 skips to left and finish in a line. *(Bars 13 - 14)*

Gentlemen, 8 walks forward to the next toe ladies, join elbows ready to repeat dance *(Bars 15 - 16)*

Four meet

Music Walking — 4/4 time (4 steps to 1 bar).

Formation In twos, side by side. An even number of couples, in circle formation, alternate couples facing counter-clockwise. One longways set is a better formation for an uneven number of couples.

Dance 4 walks forward to meet the opposite couple, 4 walks backward to places. *(Bars 1 - 2)*

Join right hands in a star and walk halfway round with 6 steps, falling back to the other couple's places on 7 and 8. *(Bars 3 - 4)*

Giving left hands, ladies change places; gentlemen do likewise giving right hands. *(Bars 5 - 6)*

Join in circles of four. 6 slips clockwise (one and a half times round), drop hands with opposite couple (partners keep hold) and move on to meet new couple . *(Bars 7 - 8)*

Circle waltz

Music Valeta or any quick waltz — 3/4 time (1 waltz step to 1 bar) (3 running steps to 1 bar).

Formation One circle, hands joined, gentlemen and ladies alternatively, four couples.

Dance All 'balance' toward and away from centre. *(Bars 1 - 2)*

Gentleman hands the lady on his left across to his right side. Lady moves counter-clockwise in

front of gentleman with 6 small runs or 2 waltz
steps. *(Bars 3 - 4)*

Repeat 1 — 2 and 3 — 4 three times, finish holding
both hands with a partner, gentleman back to
centre, lady facing him (on the last handing the
lady is handed from left to right and further to
form an outer circle — she faces the gentleman)
(Bars 5 - 16)

'Chassé anti-clockwise step close, step close.
(Bars 17 - 18)

Repeat clockwise. *(Bars 19 - 20)*

Repeat 17 - 18 and 19 -20. *(Bars 21 - 24)*

Waltz in two's counter-clockwise; all finish in a
circle with hands joined. `*(Bars 25 - 32)*

Repeat all.

If the above dance is performed with five or more couples in
a larger circle, different partners will be secured each time. This
is useful as a 'mixer'.

American Square dancing

With a basis of folk dancing steps, formations and holds, people
with a mental handicap will develop confidence to respond to
American square dancing where there has to be a quick response
to a caller.

People from all parts of the British Isles who settled in
America not only kept alive traditional dance music (jigs, reels
and hornpipes), but also developed a modern form of community dancing in true country style.

Cecil Sharp discovered this American dance from collecting
folk songs of English origin in America. At a 'Frolic' in the
Southern Appalachian Mountains songs like 'Billy Boy' and 'On
Top of Old Smokey' and others were being sung by the mountain
folk and they were dancing 'sets' similar to those still danced in
English country villages. Square dancing, with other forms of
community dancing, should be included in the physical activity
programme. It is fun, social and useful as a display item. It can
fit into a composite lesson as a final dance or form part of a social
evening of dancing and games. In some places square dance
groups meet frequently. These groups often welcome new
members and might, if asked, give a demonstration of simple
dances with a 'join in session' to follow.

Square dancing is particularly suitable for people with a
mental handicap because the steps are simple and because of the
way it is presented; the calling (promoting) is a continuous
reminder of what comes next and the repetition in the various
figures and choruses provides opportunity for practice.

Presentation

Steps and style. The steps and style of square dancing are
adapted to suit the local people, local music and conditions. In
some areas it is danced more vigorously using the country polka
step. When introducing these dances to beginners, start with the
single 'dancy-walk' step (when covering the ground): an occasional shuffle or double step can be used to cover less ground or
the balance or setting step on the spot.

Dance — walk step. Although this is simply a movement from

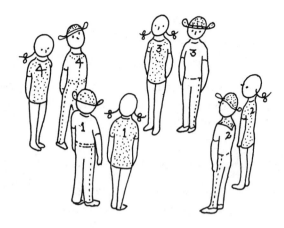

Figure 13.15 American square set

foot to foot like a walk, it is very different from the everyday street
walk. There is a lilt in the movement and the steps are shorter.
The heel is not dropped. Swings can be modified at first by using
a flat walk step from foot to foot and the propelled pivot introduced at a later stage.

Traditionally the dancers carry themselves upright with
arms relaxed at the sides.

Gentlemen always look after their partners and often dance
more vigorously than the ladies. Good dancers appear to be on
skates as they move smoothly round. Skipping and the pedes-
trian walk or march should not be used.

Calling. The caller is the person who directs the dance either by
warning, 'prompt calls' or singing calls. The dancers should
always know beforehand what figures they are going to perform.

'Warning or prompt calls' are used to prepare the dancers
and action calls give them the actual moment of starting. The
singing calls fit in with the rhythm of the music and the words
synchronise with the movements as they are being danced.
Singing calls should only be used when the dancers are more
experienced.

Music. Square dance music is usually jigs, reels hornpipes or
waltzes. 2/4, 4/4, 6/8, 3/4 time. Piano and square dance band
records are obtainable. (See Further Reading p. 138).

Square sets. The set is made up of four couples numbered
counter-clockwise from couple No 1 (Fig 13.15).

Remember: the gentleman always has his partner on his
right; the gentleman has his **corner partner** on his left; the lady
facing him is his **opposite**; the lady has her own **partner** on her
left; the lady has her **corner partner** on her right; the gentleman
facing her is her **opposite**.

Big set. Some simple figures can be practised in a circle of more
than four couples, eg:

Circle right

Circle left

Forward and back

Promenade

Break the chicken's neck

London Bridge

Single file Indian style

Swing.

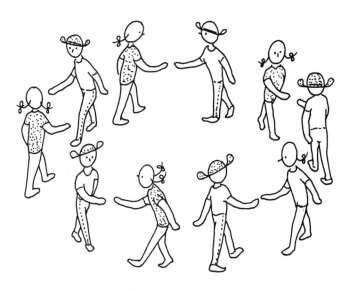

Figure 13.16 Grand Chain

Glossary of simple square dance terms and figures

Allemande left. Corner partners join left hands and walk round each other in an anti-clockwise direction. One complete turn and back to own places.

Allemande right. Partners join right hands and walk round each other in a clockwise direction, one complete turn and back to own places.

Circle left. All join hands in a ring and walk round in a clockwise direction.

Circle right. All join hands in a ring and walk round in an anti-clockwise direction.

Do-si-do corners. Corner partners walk forward passing right shoulders, step sideways back to back. Walk backwards to places passing left shoulders.

Do-si-do partners. See do-si-do corners.

Grand chain. Partners face each other in a circle and join right hands. They move forwards round the set giving left and right hands alternately to the oncoming dancer. Gentlemen move anticlockwise and ladies clockwise (Fig 13.16).

Honour. Gentlemen bow, ladies curtsey.

Left hand star (for two couples). Gentlemen join left hands and ladies join left hands, forming a star and move round in an anticlockwise direction.

Right hand star (for two couples). As left hand star but join right hands and move in a clockwise direction (Fig 13.17a).

Promenade. Partners join hands in a skating position and lead round the set in an anti-clockwise direction (unless otherwise directed by the caller (Fig 13.17b).

Top or head couples. Couples 1 and 3.

Side couples. Couples 2 and 4.

Swing. Step towards partner with right foot, join crossed hands, right hand to right hand and left hand to left hand. Keep the weight on the right foot and propel round with short pushing steps with left foot which is kept slightly behind and to the side of the right foot. Lean away from partner (Fig 13.17c).

Examples of big set figures (any number of couples in a circle)

Music   'Yankee Doodle' — 4/4 (4 steps to 1 bar)
'John Brown's Body' — 6/8 (2 steps to 1 bar)
'White Cockade' — 2/4 (2 steps to 1 bar).

Linking figures

All join hands and circle right 8 steps   *(Bars 1 - 4)*
Turn round and come back left 8 steps   *(Bars 5 - 8)*
Call: 'Back track, back track, circle back on the same old track'

All to the centre and fall back twice

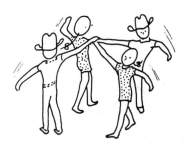

a Right hand star (for two couples)

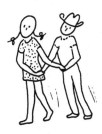

b Promenade

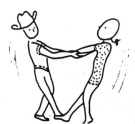

c Swing

Figure 13.17 American square — star — promenade — swing

4 steps into the centre	*(Bars 1 - 2)*	Circle left	*(Bars 1 - 4)*
4 steps back to places	*(Bars 3 - 4)*	Circle right	*(Bars 5 - 8)*
Repeat	*(Bars 5 - 8)*	All promenade	*(Bars 9 - 16)*

Call: 'Advance and retire, forward and back,

Make those feet go whichetty whack'

'Everybody Swing'. Swing your partner   *(Bars 1 - 8)*

Call: 'Swing your partner round and round

till the hollow of her foot makes a hole in the ground'

Promenade your partner round the set   *(Bars 1 - 8)*

Call: 'All promenade your honeys, take them around the green,

Be sure you take them home again,

no matter where you've been'.

1st couple London Bridge	*(Bars 17 - 24)*
Promenade	*(Bars 25 - 32)*
2nd couple London Bridge	*(Bars 1 - 8)*
Promenade	*(Bars 9 -16)*
3rs couple London Bridge	*(Bars 17 - 24)*
Promenade	*(Bars 25 - 32)*
4th couple London Bridge	*(Bars 1 - 8)*
Promenade	*(Bars 9 - 16)*
Swing your corner	*(Bars 17 - 24)*
Swing your partner	*(Bars 25 - 32)*

These figures can be danced in square sets of 8.

Examples of figures and calls

Break the chicken's neck

While hands are joined in a ring, the leading couple moves

under an arch made by the opposite couple, they break hands,

separate left and right taking the two ends of the ring round

until it joins again. The couple who made the arch finish by

turning under their own arms. 16 steps   *(Bars 1 - 8)*

Call: 'John and Joan break the chicken's neck

Break to the right and break to the left'.

Repeat until all dancers have led the dance.

Displays

Simple American square set dances can be used for display purposes.

Suggested costume* for a display team

Ladies. three-quarter length brightly coloured skirts, plain or patterned gathered into a waistband; pretty white cotton blouses with short puff sleeves and round drawstring neckline; low heeled shoes and stockings. Gentlemen: slacks all the same colour navy; brightly coloured shirts to tone with the girls' skirts; red, green, yellow or blue; low heeled shoes and socks.
*(See also **Costume**, p. 137).

London Bridge

This is called when all couples are promenading in a circle. The first couple make an arch and turn back on their tracks, and each couple makes an arch in turn and follows the first couple. These figures and calls can be put together in any order as the caller directs, but each couple should should lead the figure in turn,

for example:	*(Bars 1 - 16)*
1. *Hold your partner*	*(Chord)*
Honour your opposite	*(Chord)*
Circle right and left	*(Bars 1 - 8)*
1st couple Break the Chicken's Neck	*(Bars 9 -16)*
All to centre and fall back twice	*(Bars 17 - 24)*
2nd couple Break the Chicken's Neck	*(Bars 25 - 32)*
3rd couple Break the Chicken's Neck	*(Bars 1 - 8)*
Promenade your partner	*(Bars 9 - 16)*
4th couple Break the Chicken's Neck	*(Bars 17 - 24)*
Everybody swing.	*(Bars 25 - 32)*

If there are more than 4 couples, repeat until all have had a turn to lead the dance.

2. *Honour your partner.*	*(Chord)*
Honour your opposite.	*(Chord)*

Set figures

Suitable set figures are:	*Music*
1. Hinky Dinky Parlez Vous	'Mademoiselle from Armentiers'
2. Solomon Levi	'Solomon Levi'
3. Circle All	'Oh dem Golden Slippers'
4. Texas Star	'Camptown Races'.

Once the lilting walking step is mastered and the group understand the square set, many simple patterns can be made up by the teacher and class members from the glossary of square dance terms (see p. 129).

Phrases of music can be lengthened to give more time. The call 'promenade your partner' can overcome problems such as couples losing their places or dancing out of time with the music, by bringing the phrase or dance to an end or continuing until dancers are back in their own places.

Hinky Dinky Parlez Vous

Music	'Mademoiselle from Armantiers' or other 6/8 tune.
Introduction	Honour partners	*(chord)*
	(Honour corners)	*(chord)*

(Circle left)   *(4 bars)*

(Circle right)   *(4 bars)*

(All promenade)   *(8 bars)*

Dance   1.   1st and 3rd ladies advance to the centre and back 4 steps in, 4 steps out.   *(4 bars)*
Call: 'Two head ladies forward and back parlez vous'.
Repeat.   *(4 bars)*

2.   1st and 3rd ladies advance, join hands, turn once round and back to places.   *(4 bars)*
Call: 'Two head ladies turn around parlez vous'.

3.   All swing partners   *(4 bars)*
Call: 'All swing partners round and round parlez vous'.

4.   All promenade partners anti-clockwise.   *(8 bars)*

Call: Promenade her up and down —promenade her round the town'.

Chorus   As introduction without honours   *(16 bars)*

Repeat the dance 3 times starting with side ladies (2nd and 4th) followed by head gentlemen (1st and 3rd) then side gentlemen (2nd and 4th) in turn.

The Chorus can be used after each pair has danced as indicated buy the caller.

Solomon Levi

Music   'Solomon Levi' or any 6/8 tune.
Introduction Honour partners   *(chord)*
Honour corners   *(chord)*
Do-si-do corners   *(4 bars)*
Do-si-do partners   *(4 bars)*
Promenade round the set back to places   *(8 bars)*

Dance   1.   1st couple divides and walks round outside the set passing each other behind 3rd couple back to place.   *(8 bars)*
Call: 'First couple separate out around the ring, pass your partner going out, meet her coming in.'

2.   When they reach their own place they pass and honour the corner girl.   *(4 bars)*
Call: 'Pass right by your partner salute (honour) your corner girl'.

3.   Turn and swing partners.   *(4 bars)*
Call : 'Turn your partner round and round and promenade the set.'

Promenade round anti-clockwise.   *(8 bars)*

Repeat the danced 3 times, 2nd, 3rd and 4th couples starting inturn.

After the 4th couple have led the dance the call can be 'promenade the hall' — the gentlemen lead the ladies off to a chair.

Circles All (pick up two, four and six)

Music   'The Irish Washerwoman' or any 6/8 tune.

Introduction Honour partners   *(chord)*
Honour corners   *(chord)*

Dance   1.   1st couple walks to 2nd couple, joins hands in a circle and circles once round left (clockwise).   *(8 bars)*

Call: '1st couple to the 2nd couple, circle four circle four around the floor'.

2.   1st gentleman breaks hands and leads the line of 4 to 3rd couple, all join hands and circle once round to the left.   *(8 bars)*
Call: 'Pick up next couple and circle six, circle six around the floor'.

3.   1st gentleman breaks hands and leads line of six to 4th couple and circle round to left.   *(8 bars)*
Call: 'Pick up the last couple, circle left'.

4.   Back to back with corner girl.   *(4 bars)*
Call: 'All do-si-do with your corner girl, back to back'.

5.   Back to back with partner.   *(4 bars)*
Call: 'Do-si-do with your own back to back till you reach home'.

6.   Swing with corner girl.   *(4 bars)*
Call: 'Turn and swing your corner girl'.

7.   All promenade with partners.   *(12 bars)*
Call: 'Promenade your partner

promenade your own
promenade around the track
promenade till you get home'.

Repeat the dance 3 times with 2nd, 3rd and 4th couples leading in turn.

Texas Star

Music: 'Camptown Races'

Introduction Honour your partners   *(chord)*
Honour your corners   *(chord)*
All forward to the centre and back *(4 bars)*
All swing partners.   *(4 bars)*

Dance   1.   Ladies advance to the centre and back to place.   *(4 bars)*
Gentlemen to the centre join right hands in star.   *(4 bars)*
Call: 'Ladies to the centre and back to the bar
Gents to the centre with a right hand star'.

2.   Gentlemen walk round in star formation clock-wise; on the last beat they turn about and form a left hand star.   *(4 bars)*
Call: 'Right hands round don't be slow
Now with the left and home you go.'

3.   Gentlemen walk round in star formation anti-clockwise, ladies turn with left shoulder to centre; as the gentlemen pass they

give their partners a little push on the shoulder causing them to spin once round on the spot. Gentlemen then link arms with the next lady (new partner). *(4 bars)*
Call: 'Pass your partner give her a whirl
Now link up with the next wee girl'.

4. Gentlemen walk on with a new partner, then drop left hands and move back, with arms still linked, they swing the ladies into the centre. The ladies join right hands and form a star. *(4 bars)*
Call: 'Ladies swing in and gents swing out
Turn the Texas Star about'.

5. Ladies move round the set clockwise back to the gentlemen's home. *(4 bars)*
Call: 'Keep the new one and circle back'.

6. All swing partners *(4 bars)*
Call: 'Swing your little girl round and round,
Swing her up and swing her down'.

7. All promenade partners *(4 bars)*
'Then promenade away you go,
Chicken in the bread pan
Kickin' up the dough
Promenade with a whickety-whack
All around till you get back'.

Repeat the dance 3 times until gentlemen get their own partners back.

The Texas Star can be danced with your own partner throughout. In 3. the gentlemen return from the star with their **own partners.**

MUSIC

Selection

Music needs to be carefully selected. Most traditional folk dance records and tapes are recorded at the proper tempo for folk dance groups. As these records appear to be the only ones available, many of the steps and sequences will require twice as much music as normal when taught to people with a mental handicap, eg if a step takes 2 beats normally, allow 4 beats at first to complete it. If a sequence of steps takes 4 bars, allow 8 bars, or 8 bars allow 16 bars.

Live music

The ideal situation is to have a musician, a pianist, violinist, accordionist or guitarist either paid or voluntary. The accompanist can contribute so much to a dance lesson not only musically but as a person and friend to both class members and teacher.

A musician can help in the selection of tunes, quicken or slow down a phrase as necessary, repeat a phrase over and over again for practising steps or sequences, and slow down the end of one phrase and the beginning of the next phrase to enable the linking of one sequence of steps with the next.

Cassette tapes

If live music is not available, try to find a musician who can make a cassette tape with tunes for walking, skipping, running, clapping, side slipping 16 or 32 bars of 4/4, 2/4, 6/8 time followed by a short sequence of steps based on these steps; eg

in couples — round the room
8 walks forward — 8 walks backward
8 claps — 8 walks round partner clockwise.

Progress by substituting skips or runs for the walking steps. Clap own hands, different parts of the body or partner's hands. The turn can be made by crossing one or both hands with a partner and either walking, running or skipping.

Count a steady beat, which one of the group can maintain, and ask the accompanist to play a tune suitable for steps chosen and record it at the right tempo. A slow version should be made for practice and a further one for the better performers.

It is advisable to leave **spaces** on the tape between the practices to give time for the teacher to prompt and coach without having to switch the tape on and off.

Tapes can be made of all the other steps and dances recorded in the same way.

Note: Although there is some repetition in the Dance and Movement Training music sections, it is necessary to emphasise the special use of music in both.

Music for relaxation

For details of 'Tape Tranquility' by David Sun see Appendix 6.

SCOTTISH COUNTRY DANCING

Scottish Country Dancing is another popular form of dance. A Scottish Country Dance teacher has taken classes in Hansel Village, Ayrshire — a happy well balanced community for people with a mental handicap where young people are trained to reach their full potential in living and working.

Development

Since starting as a one night week recreational evening of country and pop dancing, the class has flourished. In 1973 a mixed team of dancers entered the Ayrshire and Edinburgh Music Festivals winning certificates (with merit) on both occasions. The team danced against Branch teams but as no other mental handicap teams entered, the judges judged them for their overall ability. In 1978 there were three teams, mixed, ladies and a demonstration team all correctly dressed. These teams compete in festivals, give displays and help the less able dancers in the classes.

Once a year other groups come to a dance in the village. The less able dancers look forward to this occasion as they never dance outside the village. The guests are happy to dance simple dances with them.

Presentation

Years of interest and patient teaching has produced this development and the standard is still improving. The teacher has built a team of helpers round her — an assistant teacher, a pianist and an accordionist. The age range of her class members is 16-55 years.

She starts her beginners by getting them moving. She says,

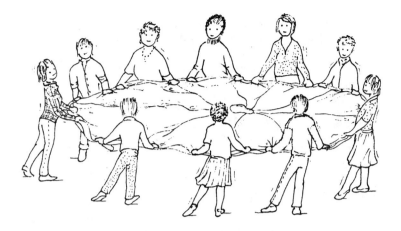

Figure 13.18 Party Valeta

'Moving around is more important initially than actual step learning — let them "skip" round to the music'.

Gradually skip steps, skip change of step and pas de bas are introduced — some take a very long time to perform them and others never seem to quite manage it. Nevertheless many do reach a reasonable standard. Only team members dance Strathspeys.

Once the simple steps are known, the teacher makes up her own very simple dances before using those from Scottish Country Dance books, often adapting the formations to suit the ability of the dancers.

During the class, some 'pop' music is played by the accordionist — they sing and dance to this which adds variety. The more severely handicapped people who cannot country dance can join in the pop.

The teacher finds it is necessary to be firm and make them change partners from time to time or they will always dance with their 'best friend'. She also dances with them herself. Having an assistant and live music makes this possible. Dancing with the class members is specially important when training the teams.

Simple dances

The following dances have been taught successfully — all are from the Scottish Country Dance book series.

Book	1	Petronella
	1	Rory O'More
	1	Cumberland reel
	2	Soldiers joy
	3	Blue bonnets
	5	Linton ploughman
	9	More Lady Catherine Bruce
	21	My only Jo and Dorrie O.

The team's dances in 1978 were:

Montgomeries fant (mixed)
Strathglass house (mixed)
Durham ranger (ladies team)
The Earl of Home (ladies team)
Bonnie Ann (demonstration team).

The teacher and her helpers hold the opinion that if anyone contemplates teaching people with a mental handicap to dance, it is worth 'having a go', 'little by little you will see your efforts

bearing fruit and the pleasure and enjoyment it brings to handicapped people is ample reward at the end of the day'

DISPLAYS

Simple folk, national and national character dancing, parachute, ribbon and Chinese parasol dancing can be used effectively for display purposes.

PARACHUTE DANCING

The silk canopy of the parachute has an aesthetic appeal to the dancers which greatly assists concentration. This type of dancing is an ideal activity for integrating a wide range of abilities and can be enjoyed as much by the helpers as the clients.

Party Veleta

All face the centre holding parachute waist height with both hands (Figure 13.18).

Bars

1	Step to the side on the R F	*(count 1)*
	Swing L F across R F	*(count 2 3)*
2	Step to the side on the L F	*(count 1)*
	Swing R F across L F	*(count 2 3)*
3	Step to the side on R F	*(count 1)*
	Close L F to R F	*(count 2 3)*
4	Step again to the side with R F	*(count 1)*
	Close L F retaining weight on R F	*(count 2 3)*
5-8	Repeat these 4 bars in the reverse direction	

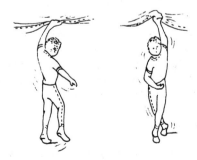

Figure 13.19 The St Bernard's Waltz — turning under

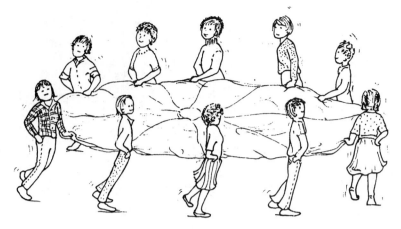

Figure 13.20 Gay Gordons

9 & 10	Inflate the parachute
11 & 12	Let go with one hand and turn under the other arm (*Figure 13.19*)
13-16	Watch the parachute come down and prepare to repeat the dance.

St Bernard's Waltz

All face the centre holding the parachute waist with both hands.

Bars

1	Step to the side with R F	(*count 1 2*)
	Close L F to R F	(*count 3*)
2	Step again to the side with R F	(*count 1 2*)
	Close L F to R F	(*count 3*)
3	Step again to the side with R F	(*count 1 2*)
	Close L F to R F with a little stamp	(*count 3*)
4	Replace weight on R F with a stamp	(*count 1 2 3*)
5	Step to the side with L F	(*count 1 2*)
	Close R F to L F	(*count 3*)
6	Step again to the side with L F	(*count 1 2 3*)
7	Step forward with R F	(*count 1 2 3*)
8	Step forward with L F	(*count 1 2 3*)
9	Step backward with L F	(*count 1 2 3*)
10	Step backward with L F	(*count 1 2 3*)
11	Inflate parachute	(*count 1 2 3*)
12	Let go with one hand and turn under other arm	(*count 1 2 3*)
13-16	Watch the parachute come down and prepare to repeat the dance.	

Gay Gordons

All have left side nearest the parachute and hold it waist height in the left hand (Fig 13.20).

Bars

1 & 2	Walk forwards round the circle 4 steps	(*count 1 2 3 4*)
	On the last step turn about and change to right hand holding the parachute.	
3 & 4	Walk backwards round the circle 4 steps	(*count 1 2 3 4*)
5 & 6	Walk forwards for 4 steps	(*count 1 2 3 4*)

	On the last step turn about and change to left hand holding the parachute	
7 & 8	Walk backwards round the circle 4 steps	(*count 1 2 3 4*)
9 & 10	Hold parachute with both hands and inflate	
11 & 12	Turn underneath one arm	
13-16	Watch the parachute come down and prepare to repeat the dance.	

Two-step

Many recordings of Two-steps are most useful when dancing with a parachute. Steps from the Boston Two-step and the Military Two-step can be used. The starting position would usually be as for the Gay Gordons, for example;

1. Pas de Basque outwards, away from the parachute and towards the parachute followed by 4 walking steps repeat *ad lib;*

2. Outer foot point forwards, point backwards followed by 4 walking steps forwards . . . repeat *ad lib.*

Gradually make up your own dances and introduce changes of direction.

The Lambeth Walk

Two walking steps towards the centre, three steps backwards, away from the centre, repeat (8 beats).
Slow slow, quick quick slow, repeat.
Eight walking steps going round the circle, counter clockwise and finish facing the centre to repeat the dance.

Music

Sydney Thompson and his Olde Tyme Dance Orchestra — several tapes are available in cassette form in shops.

We won't go home till morning (adapted)

Hold parachute waist high with one hand or in both hands.

Figure 1   Walk/skip to the left (16)

Face the centre and stamp this rhythm

6/8 ♩.♩.♩. / ♩.♩.♩./ (quick quick slow, twice)

Repeat this figure moving to the right.

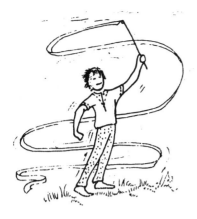

Figure 13.21 Moving many ways

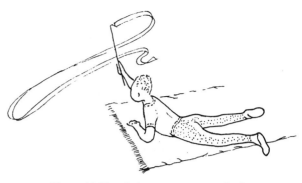

Figure 13.22 a. Lying on tummy on the floor

Figure 2   All face the centre. Shake parachute (16).

Swedish Masquerade (adapted)

Each figure has its own distinctive dance rhythm.

Hold parachute in left hand as in the Gay Gordons.

Figure 1   Promenade (16)

Figure 2   (Waltz rhythm) Face the centre holding parachute in both hands.

                Slowly lower the parachute down (1 2 3 4 5 6), (1 2 3 4 5 6)

                Progression: Let knees give as the parachute is lowered, keeping the back straight.

Figure 3   Shake the parachute in vigorous, jocular rhythm.

Repeat dance holding parachute in the right hand.

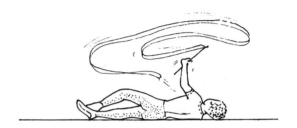

Figure 13.22 b. Lying on side on the floor

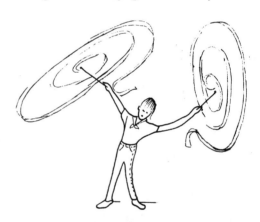

Figure 13.23 Working with a ribbon in each hand

RIBBON DANCING

Modern Rhythmic Gymnastics is a feature of International Gymnastics Competitions for women. It is promoted by the Olympic Gymnastics Association. One aspect of this work uses ribbons and wands.

These notes are intended for leaders wishing to initiate this activity with disabled people. It is enjoyed equally by men and women.

Points for leaders

1. Ensure adequate space for each performer.

2. Be ready to help undo knots in the ribbon as soon as they arise, otherwise they quickly become very tight.

 Train the more able to cope with their own knots!

3. Encourage performers to listen to the music by not having it too loud.

4. Constantly invite onlookers to try and join in, they are often waiting for an opportunity to participate but are shy.

5. Encourage the more inventive performers by asking the group to watch them. This helps everyone to extend their repertoire.

6. Take care of apparatus at all times. Each leader must establish the routine to be followed.

Progressions

1. Ability to change hands.

2. Travel while swinging the ribbon.

3. Keep the ribbon moving while changing body stance, eg stand — kneel — lie down then return to standing. (Fig 13.21).

4. Work the ribbon while lying or rolling (Fig 13.22 a and b).

5. Work with a senior length ribbon (see page 141).

6. Work with a ribbon in each hand (Fig 13.23).

7. Make up a sequence with a partner.

8. Respond to music of varying tempos (Fig 13.24).

9. Make up a dance co-operating in a small group.

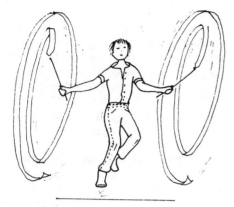

Figure 13.24 Skipping action

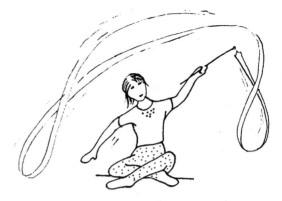

Figure 13.26 Using a ribbon sitting on the floor

Value of the activity

1. It provides an integrated recreational activity which is ideal because all derive enjoyment from it.

2. The 'loner' enjoys it as well as the gregarious.

3. It encourages experimentation and concentration.

4. It appeals to all ages including the over sixties.

5. It exercises the whole body and can be very energetic.

6. Those in wheelchairs can participate if encouraged by having a shorter ribbon (Fig 13.25).

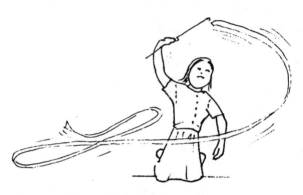

Figure 13.27 Using a ribbon kneeling up

ribbon, 4-6 cm wide (1^1/2-2^3/8 "). The ribbon is folded and doubled for 1 m (3'3") at the end where it is attached to the wand by a button-hole loop. This makes the finished length 4.5 m (1 m double plus 3.5 m (11'7" single).

The ribbon must be of the best quality so that it is washable and has adequate weight. This quality ribbon may be bought at a John Lewis store.

A standard senior length ribbon is made from 6.5 m of ribbon making the finished length 5.5 m long.

A person in a wheelchair will find a shorter ribbon on a mini wand easier to manage (see page 141).

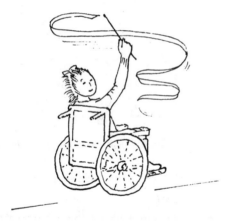

Figure 13.25 Ribbon dancing in a wheelchair with a short ribbon

7. Active non-ambulant youngsters enjoy using the ribbons when sitting on the floor (Figure 13.26): they often change their position to kneeling in order to get the ribbon higher and start walking on their knees with **extended** hips which is a vital preparation for becoming ambulant (Fig 13.27).

Music

It is possible to use a wide range of modern and traditional dance music which is obtainable on cassette. Some selections which include popular songs are also appropriate, eg 'Herb Albert and Tijuana Brass — Greatest Hits' (AM Records CM1 D 111).

Equipment

Standard junior length ribbons are the most useful for this type of dancing (Fig 13.28). They are made from 5.5 m (8'1") of satin

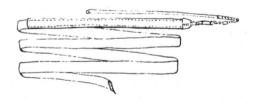

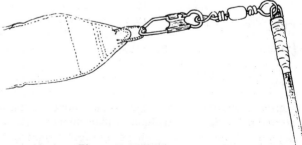

Figure 13.28 Ribbon — detail

Wands

Wands are made from tapered fibre glass. The local fishing tackle shop may be able to help if shown a sample.

Firms supplying this equipment

BAGA, 95 High Street, Slough, Berks. SL1 1DE.

Carita House, Stapeley, Nantwich, Cheshire, CW5 7LJ.

CHINESE PARASOL DANCING

A Gateway Club in West London took a group of its members to a Chinese theatre production which included parasol dancing. The members were keen to experiment, so the club leader purchased some Chinese parasols and encouraged their interest with the provision of appropriate music.

This led to a variety of imaginative responses. Some experimented with a dramatic interpretation of their use by hiding behind an open parasol placed on the ground, others chose to walk down the High Street displaying their beautiful parasol. Some concentrated on the manipulative skills needed to open and close a parasol and twirling it, while others tried their skill at dancing round a spinning parasol. The colourful display of parasols which they were able to control helped their concentration. They became very absorbed in their dancing and gave great pleasure to spectators.

MORRIS DANCING

The Gainsborough Gateway Club has developed a Morris Dance team which gives displays in various parts of the country. The Chairman of the Gainsborough and District Society for Mentally Handicapped Children and Adults, Geoff Layne, describes how the team came into being.

Gainsborough Gateway

'Knowing how to start anything is often the most difficult part of any exercise, so I will start by explaining how and why I became involved with Gateway. Around 1978 my Down's Syndrome daughter attended Gainsborough Gateway which met once a week at the Adult Training Centre. Arriving early to pick her up one evening I was asked what I thought of the Club. "Rubbish", I replied, "no effort, no ambition, staid 1960s activities". I was told "if you can do better have a go". So I did.

'I immediately started trying to convince the members that their club could become one of the best and most progressive in the UK, but that, to prove it, they had to do something to make people "take notice" and see the club as part of the community — givers as well as takers. Pub teams were challenged to darts and pool, and barn dance and folk dance were introduced into club activities. In early 1980, I asked my nephew a member of a Morris Team, if some of his team would try to teach Gateway members a dance. They agreed, and soon after 18 or so members joined in a practice night. Such was the interest that eventually a dance team was formed. Gateway also branched out into many sports and activities, previously looked upon as out-of-bounds. However, since the Club felt it needed more independence, it started to look for a club room. An old chapel was found right in the centre of the community. This was renovated and furnished.

'After much discussion it was decided to open the new club room in style in December 1981, during the International Year of the Disabled. It was to be a full day of activities attended by Yorkshire Television and press from all over Lincolnshire. But most important of all, the day would see the launch of "The Gainsborough Gateway Morris Team". The impact was tremendous, and bookings rolled in from garden fêtes, Lord Mayors' Shows and garden festivals. The Club had proved the point that people with a mental handicap can do anything that other people can do — it just takes a little bit longer.

'The Morris Team activity has given not only the dancers but all Club members a pride in themselves and in the Club. It has also encouraged them to 'have a go' at anything, so that now the Club boasts quite accomplished cavers, pot-holers and absailers. In addition, the Club finds that it joins in an increasing number of community-based activities. However, the main benefit is that people now recognise club members as people, treat them as equals and often as superiors. And all this happened because I "gave them a chance".'

COSTUME

As many characteristics of the dance are related to the costume and because it helps to create an atmosphere it is important that the costume is as authentic as possible. It would be unrealistic to provide a costume for each nationality but the following simple basic costume can be made — authentic headdresses, waistcoats, aprons and footwear can then be added, appropriate to the country.

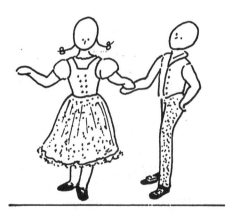

Figure 13.29 Basic costume

Ladies' basic costume

Skirt : three-quarter length brightly coloured skirts, plain or patterned, gathered or pleated into a waistband. *Blouse:* white blouse, with short or long puff sleeves and a round drawstring neckline. *Bodice (waistcoat):* this can be made with a side opening made with an open-ended zip; 6 small brass or silver buttons sewn in a double row down the front will give the effect of a double-breasted fastening. *Petticoat:* stiff taffeta or paper nylon — frilled to suggest petticoats (Fig 13.29).

Gentlemen's basic costume

Trousers: slacks or jeans all the same colour. *Shirts:* white or brightly coloured shirts. If coloured, to tone with or contrast with the ladies' skirts. *Waistcoat:* as for the ladies but with a high neckline. *Collar and cravat:* white plastic collar. Large soft bow with ends like a cravat to be worn outside waistcoat.

Footwear

Stockings: white stockings or socks. *Shoes*: black leather low-heeled shoes. The same for lady and gentleman. The gentleman should wear a wide elastic garter round the foot and the shoe with a large buckle attached to the top. *Boots*: these can be improvised by making a black gaiter in felt or canvas with a zip side fastening and elastic straps worn under the shoes.

For illustrations and descriptions of costume see Mann, Further Reading (below).

FURTHER READING

Carroll, J and Lofthouse, P. *Creative dance for boys.* Northcote House, London, 1969.

Haylor, P Spencer, P and Walshe, G. *Teach yourself dancing — ballroom, Latin-American, social.* London, Imperial Society of Teachers of Dancing, 1977.

Know the Game Series. *Dancing: English folk dancing; Scottish country dancing; Sequence dancing.* London, A & C Black.

Ladybird Series. *Dancing rhymes; Action songs; Singing rhymes.* Loughborough, Ladybird Books.

Lavelle, D. *Discotheque dancing.* London, Imperial Society Society of Teachers of Dancing, 1970.

Lavelle, D. *Latin and American dances.* London, A & C Black, 1983.

Lingarde, A ed. *Party dances and games.* London, Imperial Society of Teachers of Dancing, 1972.

Lofthouse, P. *Dance activity in the primary school.* London, Heinemann Educational, 1970.

Mann, C. *European peasant costume.* London, A & C Black, 1968.

Slater, W. *Teaching modern educational dance.* London, Northcote House, 1987.

Smedley, R and Tether, J. *Let's dance country style.* London, Granda, 1981.

EMI Records RLS 7 20.20 European dances mostly from Scandinavia — *Dances and folk dances from many lands.* English Folk Dance and Song Society (2 Regent's Park Road, London NW1 7A) publishes catalogues of dances and records also 'Folk Mail', a bulletin of folk song, dance and music.

Information on dances, records and music can be obtained from the following:

Royal Scottish Country Dance Society, The Secretary, 12 Coates Crescent, Edinburgh EH3 7AF.

Society for International Folk Dancing, The Secretary, 16 De Vere Walk, Eatford, Herts. WD1 3BE.

Welsh Folk Dance Society, The Secretary, Dolawenydd, Betws Ammanford, Dyfed SA18 2HE.

Chapter 14

Physical Activities for People with a Severe or Profound Mental Handicap

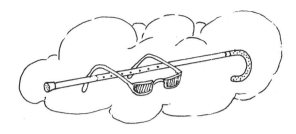

In this chapter the recreational needs of people with a severe or profound mental handicap are considered. It is difficult to define very precisely those who should be included under this heading.

The majority are so severely handicapped that many are either non-ambulant or so lacking in motivation that their walking ability can only be maintained by constant stimulation. In addition, their ability to communicate is often severely impaired. These factors determine the type of activities that can be attempted.

STAFFING

Whatever activity is undertaken, it is going to demand a certain amount of energy, interest and enthusiasm from the care-giver. Without any of these qualities, even the best ideas in the world will be dismal failures. For profoundly handicapped people work must be done on a one-to-one basis and, in the case of severely handicapped people, the nearer this ratio can be reached the greater will be the chances of developing potential and making progress. It is important to recognise the difference between custodial care, where staff oversee a group, and the need for a one-to-one ratio when developing potential. Group teaching has no relevance when working with people who have this degree of disability.

Both staff and clients experience a much more stimulating environment when the whole group can receive individual teaching at the same time. This can only be provided if it is recognised that volunteers have an important role to play.

Aides/volunteers

It used to be thought that professionals were in danger of losing their status if 'aides' or volunteers were employed to do some of their work. However, the importance of the role of helpers in improving the quality of life for many in the community needing support and individual attention is now generally recognised. It is the work of the professional to head a team of carers each with their clearly defined role. Where volunteers are used, bridges can be built between handicapped people and the community which is of mutual benefit and of long term significance.

It is important that those with special responsibility for people with a severe mental handicap regard it as part of their professional work to explore every avenue open to them to recruit volunteers. Having recruited such helpers it is equally important to structure their programmes carefully so that their interest is maintained and that their contribution is effective.

'Management' needs to support staff who use their initiative to develop such programmes. It is a method of working which enhances the role of the professional and greatly benefits the client.

Examples of good practice

Some schools which specialise in teaching children with severe learning difficulties have found it beneficial to develop a team of volunteers to assist staff. A school in Norfolk has had such a team for several years. The team works on a weekly basis with a group of children for about a term and then moves on to help another group. The children are so stimulated that it enables them to know the day of the week when they are due for a session with their special visitors. The volunteers are mostly young mothers who have found the experience one which has enhanced their understanding of the needs of their own young family for play and individual attention.

Another way in which one-to-one help can be achieved is for the less severely handicapped people to be invited to assist staff working in the 'special care unit'. In one London ATC a visiting teacher asked for some volunteers; the most able were not available and the management had grave misgivings about accepting some other students who learnt of the need and were determined to help. Finally, their offer was accepted, and their good motivation proved of far greater significance than their limitations. As they related to their individual 'charge' in the special care unit their own self-esteem was enhanced and the staff were amazed at the goodwill generated and the stimulus given to the group as a whole through the experience.

Multi-disciplinary teams

Whenever possible programmes should be devised by a multi-disciplinary team. Each member of the team has a contribution to make and each member can be stimulated by the observations and expertise of others. The morale of staff can be greatly improved when multi-disciplinary co-operation is a regular feature of in-service training.

Working with this client group brings staff into contact with a very wide range of physical complications. The physiotherapist can help them to be aware of all the 'do's and 'dont's'. Furthermore they will all need training in the correct techniques of lifting. This training needs to be constantly re-inforced if standards are to be maintained and staff are to be protected from back injuries. Senior nursing staff should also be able to assist in providing this training on a regular basis. It must be remembered that many members of a multi-disciplinary team who have had excellent professional training may not have been specifically prepared for working with non-ambulant people.

One of the problems of working with profoundly handicapped people is having to work with their 'equipment'. In this context a practitioner says 'I refer to all those items of support that are permanent fixtures to enable the correct body position and posture. It is important to realise that work and play can take place without them. If we just take body braces as an example, there are many times of the day when these have to be removed — for dressing and changing. Rhyming games can take place anywhere — in the toilet, in bed or in the swimming pool. Rhyming games can be invaluable in creating greater body awareness'.

When working on vocabulary and language development the formula can be used as the base for introducing new and not-so-new concepts. If the teacher places his hands on the legs or arms of the client, he can use some of the following:

'Rub, rub, rub'

'Stroke, stroke, stroke'

'Pat, pat, pat'.

Experience shows that, to conclude this type of session, by far the most popular formulas are:

'Hug, hug, hug'

'Cuddle, cuddle, cuddle'.

Aims and objectives

These are broadly the same as when working with less severely impaired people but it is worth remembering that their degree of isolation may be greater. This fact should lead to an emphasis on activities where communicating and having fun at any level relevant to the client has priority. It is necessary to safeguard the dignity of the client and to ensure that clothing is appropriate to the activities being undertaken. The value of physical activities presented in a stimulating and interesting way is now being more universally accepted as a part of life for people with a severe mental handicap.

ACTIVITIES SUITABLE FOR MORE SEVERELY MULTIPLY HANDICAPPED PEOPLE

Blanket play

(See also page 62.)

Playing in a small group with a blanket as the centre of interest helps to establish relationships through the fun it can create and through the acceptance of body contact as people tumble, roll, crawl and hide in and under the blanket (Fig. 14.1). Conversation is also stimulated within the group. These group activities can also stimulate movement when balls are tossed up and down on the blanket or when games of tug-of-war are introduced as the participants sit in a circle holding the blanket.

For those with very limited capacity for movement, blanket play can help to create the sensation of movement. How this is done depends to a large extent on the size and weight of the handicapped person. The safest way for the care-giver is to take the client for a slide on the blanket, adapting the speed and

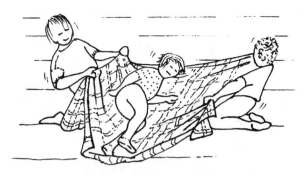

Figure 14.1 Blanket play

direction to the client so that at all times he feels safe. Some children or small adults can enjoy being swung in the blanket. By watching the facial expression of the client the care-giver can usually gauge how energetic the play should be.

Parachute play

(See also pages 58-61.)

The canopy of a parachute is a most versatile piece of equipment and can be used to great effect with people of all abilities and on occasions when the object is to integrate a wide ability range. The canopy can create a colourful and stimulating environment for those with very little capacity for movement. Many enjoy lying on mats under the parachute accompanied by care-givers (Fig 14.2) while others enjoy playing and dancing with it (Figs 14.3a, 14.3b). Enjoyment gradually builds up and this can be detected from the facial expressions of those taking part. Even the draught of air the parachute creates is pleasurable because those with this degree of disability often spend much of the day indoors where it is very warm. They seldom experience the stimulation of an out-of-doors environment.

For those able to sit on the floor in a circle holding the parachute beside their care-givers quite a range of activities can be introduced.

1. Shaking the parachute:

    (i) shaking it in rhythm to a client's name with all those who are saying the name looking at the client so named;

    (ii) an attention game using music so that they start and stop with the music. This can be varied so that it is a very gentle and calming activity when the music is soft but vigorous and energetic when the volume is increased; the latter should always be for a much shorter space of time to prevent over-excitement;

    (iii) shaking the parachute to make foam balls of varying sizes bounce up and down. In contrast, a calming activity is to gently roll the foam balls across or around the parachute. This activity requires a much greater degree of control and concentration.

2. Inflating the parachute canopy and then encouraging participants to crawl underneath to the other side of the circle. Provided the care-givers lead the way, many participants will be prepared to do a lot of crawling and playing in the enclosed area (in a more open space, they would be disinclined to move about).

3. In a group with a wide ability range and a generous number of helpers, those in wheelchairs enjoy being taken for a ride across the circle when the parachute is being inflated — especially if it is in the context of a dance sequence (Fig 14.4).

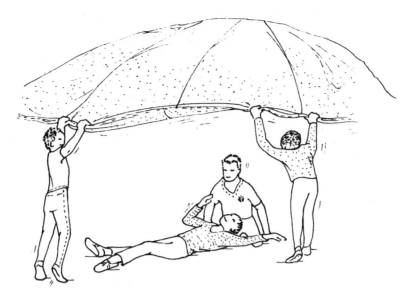

Figure 14.2 Canopy lifted over

4. All enjoy watching a 'fly away' — when all those inflating the parachute let go simultaneously just as the chute is rising. (Note: this cannot be done when the ceiling or the light fixtures are low and unprotected.)

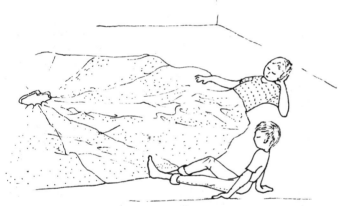

Figure 14.3a Feeling the parachute silk

Ribbon dancing

(See also page 135.)

For those who are non-ambulant or of very low motivation, success is more likely if the wands are fairly short — about 38 cm (15"). Some people make wands of wooden dowel rather than glass fibre so that they are easier to grasp.

Ribbons should be correspondingly shorter, between 1 to 3m (3'3" to 10'). Initially the care-giver may provide most of the action (Fig 14.5) but gradually the client becomes involved and some are able to take a real delight in controlling the movement of the ribbon from a lying or sitting position (Fig 14.6). A variety of starting positions should be encouraged once some confidence in the activity has been established.

Wheelchair games

Dancing with wheelchairs can be great fun and need not entail a cassette player or extra staff. All that is needed is space and a bit of imagination:

On one occasion, a teacher, investigating what she thought was squeals of laughter coming from an apparently empty room, found a member of staff pushing a wheelchair-bound girl backwards and forwards across the room, American style, singing:

'Take your partners and their chairs
Cross the room and away you go
Turn around and say hello
Cross the room as fast as you can
Say hello and do it again'.

The fact that it didn't quite rhyme was entirely beside the point.

(See Chapter 11, page 110 for ideas on adaptations for wheelchairs.)

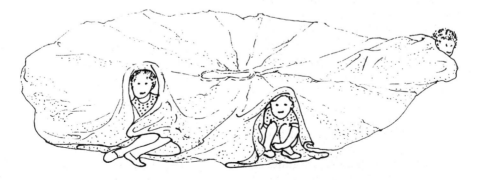

Figure 14.3b Feeling the parachute silk

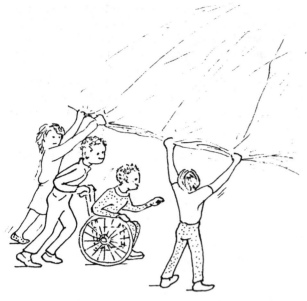

Figure 14.4 Wheelchair under the parachute

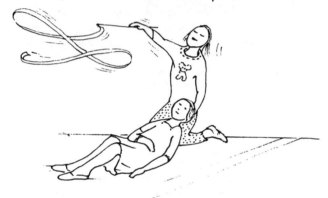

Figure 14.5 Ribbon work (trying to get through)

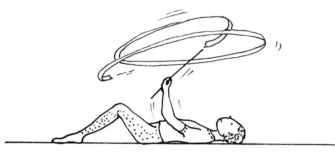

Figure 14.6 Controlling the ribbon lying on the floor

Obstacle games can be played in wheelchairs. If clients have the use of hands or arms, a course can be arranged so that objects have to be placed in designated areas, eg drop a ball into a bucket, or place a hoop over a skittle. Objects can also be 'carried' on people's feet. This will develop an awareness of parts of the body and encourage movement.

Kites

Kites are relatively inexpensive and their use can be adapted for people with profound mental handicap. They are fascinating to watch as the wind catches them and tosses them about in the sky. They can be attached to wheelchairs, standing frames, and even to arms and legs. And if this is impossible, a great deal of pleasure can be derived from just watching other people flying them.

Sitting down games

It is important to build into any activity as many teaching variables as possible. It is never enough just to play a game for its own sake.

A number of rhyming games can be played with a client in a wheelchair sitting at a table or sitting on the floor. As well as being good fun, these games also encourage hand/eye co-ordination, body awareness and improve the span of concentration.

There are many games to choose from, a number of which have been improvised or adapted from more complex rhymes, but two of the best are:

1. Sitting opposite your client, with either a table or board between you, 'sing' the following, matching the action to the words:

    'We can clap with our two hands

    Clap clap clap

    We can knock with our two hands

    Knock knock knock

    We can tap with our two hands

    Tap tap tap

    We can stroke with our two hands

    Stroke stroke stroke.

This can be adapted to one hand only. Practitioners can hold clients' hands and sing the rhyme — or just demonstrate it and then ask the client to repeat it. Any action can be used, so that the game can be pitched at the most appropriate level according to individual needs. Two clients can do this together — as can 4 or even a group of 20.

2. The next game is probably best played on the floor, although each person must decide on the most suitable position for them.

    Again, sitting very close, and preferably opposite your client, 'sing' the following, using the appropriate action, ie hands on parts of the body:

    'Head head head

    Hair hair hair

    Eyes eyes eyes

    Ears ears ears

    Nose nose nose

    Mouth mouth mouth

    Chin chin chin

    Neck neck neck

    Chest chest chest

    Arms arms arms

    Hands hands hands

    Tummy tummy tummy

    Knees knees knees,

    Toes toes toes.'

Using this as a simple base, the variations are innumerable. Clients' hands can be placed either on different parts of their own body or those of the practitioner. With practice, clients can do this on their own; in unison with the practitioner's actions; copying the practitioner, and so on. Once again, a basic formula can be adapted to suit individual needs.

Depending on the ability of the person concerned, added variations can easily be built in:

'Stretch stretch stretch
Push forward push forward push forward
Lean back lean back lean back.'

Music and movement

Both passive and active movements on a one-to-one basis can be enjoyed when accompanied by music (Fig 14.7). With the proviso that this type of structured programme should be devised and monitored by physiotherapists or other senior para-medical staff, there is no reason why aides and volunteers cannot implement such programmes on a daily basis wherever the client may be — in a hostel, at home, in a special care unit or in hospital.

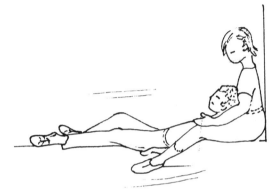

Figure 14.7 Floor-based activities to music — rocking leaning back on wall

Cassette tapes to encourage staff to begin such a programme are available: *Chair-based activities* — Tape 1; *Floor-based activities* (See Appendix 6).

For further activities, see swimming and movement in water (page 69), horse riding (page 163), games skills (page 26), the work of Veronica Sherborne (page 94), adventure playgrounds (page 167).

SOFT PLAY AREAS

How can children who are unable to run about, see or hear, or find it difficult to learn to experience 'play'?

One of the ways to help children who have all, or many, of these problems is to provide a soft play environment. This involves choosing soft, bright, visually stimulating shapes and apparatus to encourage responses that most parents probably take for granted.

A room or an area can be set aside to give children a great deal of fun and at the same time help them experience physical activity in a safe stimulating environment. The colour of the modules helps to direct the children's vision — the sound that the soft plastic material makes means that they are getting auditory feed back. The smell of the material is obviously different and the texture is also important.

The module that provides a sloping surface means that children can roll or slide freely without adult intervention and experience the sensation of gently being pulled through a short tunnel, the resistance felt when moving through 'soft pillows', and trying to bounce or being bounced on an air-filled cushion.

By using the soft play environment to stimulate all the senses — olfactory, auditory, visual and tactile — the children can begin to experience physical/play activities and subsequently gain the related learning experiences of their peers.

Catalogues for special physical education equipment can be obtained from:

Rompa Pressure Sealed Plastics Ltd, PO Box 5, Wheatbridge Road, Chesterfield, Derbyshire S40 2AE (inflatables);

Jim Friend, Supabounce Ltd, Newton Road, Harrowbrook Industrial Estate, Hinkley, Leicestershire LE10 3DS (ball pool and bouncing equipment).

FURTHER READING

Lambert, Michael S. *Using soft play environment for pupils with severe or profound multiple handicaps.* Victoria School, Birmingham, 1984 (tel: 021 476 9478).

Chapter 15

Outdoor Pursuits

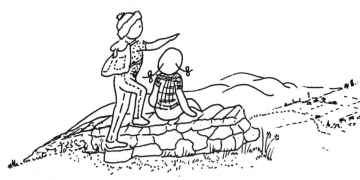

Facilities — Types of activities — 1. Individual outdoor activities and water sports — camping — canoeing — rambling — route-learning — sailing — walking — 2. Guidelines to planning an outdoor activities course — 3. Schemes of training in outdoor pursuits combining several activities — Sheffield training centres — Churchtown Farm Field Studies Centre — Outward Bound — Calvert Trust Adventure Centre — Katherine Elliot Cottage Project — 4. Holidays providing an introduction to outdoor pursuits — 5. Eight years on (1989).

Outdoor pursuits make a valuable contribution to the social and educational training and to the health of people with a mental handicap. Fresh air alone is health-giving and outdoor activities offer opportunities for integration and place the individual in situations which can never be simulated in the hospital, classroom or workshop.

Since the first edition of the book was published, many developments have taken place. Some of the outdoor pursuit centres mentioned have now closed and many new establishments, such as Brendigg Lodge, Keilder Centre, Penzance Wharf, Loseley Campsite, have been opened. As it is impossible to check all the centres, readers are reminded that they should ask for details of safety arrangements and insurance before making a booking and thus avoid problems or disappointment (see 'Choosing an outdoor pursuits centre', page 151).

FACILITIES

Many hospitals have extensive grounds — some have natural sites for camping within easy reach of the buildings yet out of sight, most have wooded areas, paths and playing fields where simple orienteering games, route-finding and nature trails can be organised. Few adult training centres, on the other hand, have suitable on-the-spot facilities but the staff of some centres have investigated their environment and found fields, woods, country walks, hills, mountains, the sea, inland lakes, lochs or canal and rivers, and also co-operative farmers and qualified coaches expert in a variety of outdoor pursuits and water sports. Further afield, they have found outdoor pursuit or adventure training centres which have been used successfully for adventure training and holidays. These centres are usually run by national and local voluntary organisations or local authorities.

TYPES OF ACTIVITIES

The following activities are being practised in one or more areas in England, Northern Ireland, Scotland and Wales:

angling (see p 160)

camping (see p below)

canoeing (see p 145)

caving (see p 154)

expeditions (see p 153)

map reading and compass work (see p 157)

mountaineering (see p 152)

orienteering (see p 149)

potholing (see p 154)

rambling (see p 147)

rock climbing (see pp 153 and 155)

route learning (see p 147)

sailing (see p 149)

water-skiing (see p 150)

youth hostelling (see p 150).

Other activities such as boating, go-karting, grass skiing, sail boarding, skiing and tobogganing can be practised when facilities are suitable and equipment available for the few who show an interest and have the capacity. Details of these activities can be obtained from the Sports Councils or the leisure departments of local authorities.

This chapter gives details of the ways in which local authorities, managers, instructors, recreation officers and nurses have pioneered their schemes. It is hoped that many others will feel inspired to examine the possibilities of encouraging people with a mental handicap to take part in outdoor pursuits and to make use of existing facilities and expertise. It is also hoped that parents and other members of the family will find ways of participating in some form of outdoor activity in which the handicapped person can be involved and be more ready to consent to their son or daughter joining in planned outdoor pursuits be it in hospital, centre or Gateway Club.

Although at first sight some of these activities might appear dangerous, with expert knowledge, co-operation and total attention to the details of safety and prior preparation, they are being enjoyed by and are challenging to many people with a mental handicap.

This chapter has been divided into five sections — listed at the beginning of the chapter.

1. INDIVIDUAL OUTDOOR ACTIVITIES AND WATER SPORTS

CAMPING

Several hospital, adult training centres and Gateway Clubs are becoming interested in camping under canvas (see the Sheffield scheme and Outward Bound, pp 152 and 156). Scouts, Guides and the Camping Club of Great Britain have considerable expertise in camping, and may be willing to help train nurses and instructors in camp-craft.

For a few residents, camping can be arranged within the hospital grounds if a suitable site is found preferably out of sight of hospital buildings (Fig 15.1).

Those responsible for camping with adults and children with a mental handicap should consider the following points:

make sure the camp site is sheltered from the prevailing wind; that it is level; never pitch a tent on a slope;

water should be within easy reach;

whatever type of toilet is used it must be suitable for the lowest ability person — some have found the commode chair most suitable for severely handicapped people provided it is on a firm base;

advice should be taken on the type of tents used: don't overcrowd them— it is necessary for each individual to be able to get out during the night without falling over and waking the rest;

mark the guy lines with flags or pieces of cloth. It is all too easy to trip over them;

both camp beds/sleeping bags need ground sheets underneath and make sure there is plenty of warm material underneath — a lilo air bed, old eiderdown or blankets; closed foam insulating mats are now in common use. Roll up sleeping bags and bedding during the day;

use wellingtons and trainers first thing in the morning because of wet grass;

battery night-lights will help in the strange environment.

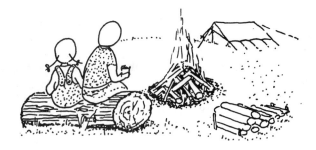

Figure 15.1 Camping within the hospital grounds can sometimes be arranged

Those leading the camp should be experienced to do so. Alternative indoor accommodation should be available in case of bad weather.

All equipment should be in good order and regularly inspected and repaired.

Safety regulations applying to all camping should also apply to camps for handicapped people.

A group from Aston Hall Hospital in the Trent Region camp every year, sometimes as far afield as Devon and the Lake District. Several physically handicapped residents and residents with a mental handicap, both children and adults, some in wheelchairs, enjoy the freedom of open air life — perhaps exploring the dried-up river bed or helping to feed the donkeys and chickens on a farm. Some help fetch water while others help with preparing food and washing up, and some make their own beds. Others may only be able to lie on the grass contentedly listening to their radio or picking the long grass.

What do they get out of living under canvas? The following are comments by the camp staff and campers:

'See their faces and listen to the things they have done - probably for the first time ever'.

'I saw a cow putting its milk in a pipe'.

' I saw a dog collecting sheep'.

'We saw a man on a rope on a mountain face'.

We went through a dark cave'.

and many more.

Some venture to the local pub, pushing wheelchairs and helping those who are unsteady on their feet.

Some hospitals play host to other handicapped groups, eg Gateway Clubs, who camp in the hospital grounds. This often proves to be a successful venture.

CANOEING

The British Canoe Union (BCU), which supports the promotion of canoeing for everyone, has appointed a coach whose responsibilities include canoeing for people with a mental handicap. It encourages members of its various disciplines, and particularly the Coaching Scheme, to contribute to this aim. Canoeists with disabilities are encouraged to take the Award Scheme Tests. The Union's policy is to avoid a separate system. Where a specific disability prevents a candidate from completing a particular part of a test the examiner may give the award with a suitable endorsement setting out the part of the test not completed (Fig 15.2).

One canoeing body for everyone is the aim, and members with a disability are encouraged to join existing canoe clubs and, wherever possible, use the same equipment. However, the formation of special groups and the development of specially adapted equipment is positively supported whenever this is necessary.

The BCU has a list of its Coaching Scheme members who are willing to support canoeing activities for disabled people. This list can be consulted to provide a specific response to any requests for help that may be received at the BCU office. In addition, the BCU has initiated a training programme for all categories of canoeists to make them aware of the needs of disabled people with particular reference to canoeing. This weekend course offers an endorsement to any canoe qualification held.

In January each year the BCU publishes a Coaching Programme for that year. Courses are available for all grades —from beginners to experienced coaches — and for all categories of canoeists.

The BCU can refer any queries or requests for help received at Weybridge through the Coaching Scheme to provide help in any of its regions.

Organisation

Geoff Smedley, a BCU Senior Instructor who works with disabled canoeists, describes the organisation of canoeing activities.

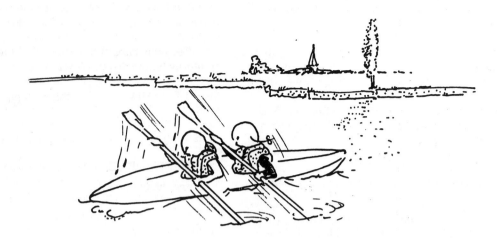

Figure 15.2 Canoeing — a buoyancy aid must always be worn in open water

'To introduce disabled people to the sport of canoeing a coach needs both teaching skills and an understanding of the effects of mental handicap on the potential canoeist. The latter often has implications for the former when seen through the eyes of the canoeing instructor. Perhaps more important, however, is the concern shown by parents, teachers and care staff regarding the effects, good or bad, that canoeing has on the disabled person.

'Liaison is the key to success. By fully utilising canoe sport and the education and care of disabled people, there is an increased possibility that a programme will be successful. Thus, the disabled canoeist will realise his or her full potential in the sport with the minimum of risk and the maximum pleasure and satisfaction.

'These notes are *not* for the inexperienced no matter how well intentioned. Canoeing is a sport that contains, perhaps more than most, an element of risk. The experienced canoe instructor has the expertise to minimise this risk to an acceptable level — this is paramount to the success of the sport and particularly to the involvement of disabled persons.

'Canoeing can be enjoyed at a diversity of levels and expertise. Some individuals will gain tremendous satisfaction from the white water kayak trip, but equally there will be those who gain the same thrill from sitting, perhaps as a passenger, in a canoe on a quiet backwater. This observation is not intended to be patronising or sentimental, but is based on the views experienced by a number of disabled canoeists who have expressed that feeling of achievement that comes from participating for the first time in a new and exciting venture'.

Getting started

The process of developing a suitable programme requires three basic stages:

1. environment, 2. equipment, and 3. education.

Environment

The best place to start would be in a heated indoor swimming pool. If this is not possible, then the situation should be sheltered, safe and comfortable, the weather should be fine and the water clean and calm with enough depth to allow the canoes to float but the canoeist and instructors to be able to stand up comfortably. There should be adequate support facilities (ie places to observe

from, places to leave canoeists and equipment safely, and a changing room—this is particularly important so that wet canoeists do not have to 'hang around' getting cold and uncomfortable).

Equipment

Clothes. All the participants should be clothed to stay warm if they get wet. This means wearing either woollen or fibre pile clothing with waterproofs over. Helmets are optional according to conditions, such as the composition of the bank (some reservoirs have gravel or concrete edges). Some form of footwear is advisable even in the swimming pool since the inside of a canoe can be less than smooth.

Buoyancy. A buoyancy aid of an approved type (BS 3595) must always be worn on open water, and it is also a good idea to wear one in the swimming pool since this gives confidence and familiarity. Bear in mind that a life jacket is only guaranteed to turn the person wearing it onto the back if it is fully inflated. The standard non-inflatable buoyancy aid may, therefore, be preferable for all but the most 'at risk' canoeist since it is a more comfortable garment.

Canoes. The type of craft is very important. Beginners can generally be introduced to the concept of being on the water by using an open Canadian Canoe with an experienced instructor. From here they can progress to a 'sit-on' type of kayak such as the Rob Roy (from Pyrana). A capsize in this type of kayak results in the canoeist falling off rather than going under and having to escape. From this the canoeist can move to a Caranoe (from Valley Canoe Products) which has a very large cockpit and, if capsized, the canoeist can escape easily and safely without having to go under the water. Going solo in one of these craft need have none of the trauma associated with closed cockpit kayaks; they are very stable and by no means as 'tippy'. In fact the Caranoe is one of the few kayaks in which people can stand up confidently. A progression to different craft can continue gradually up to full specialist specification canoes and kayaks, if appropriate. There is a tremendous feeling of achievement for any canoeist who paddles solo and these craft allow the person with a mental handicap to do this with success and in safety.

Paddles. There are also a number of ways in which the canoe or kayak can be propelled. Beginners can simply use their hands. From here they can progress to small paddles which they hold one in each hand, then to 'un-feathered' paddles and finally, if appropriate, to the 'feathered' paddle.

Education

Swimming. Water confidence is more important for the canoeist with a mental handicap than the ability to swim. People who fall into the water and float there confidently and without panic are less of a liability to themselves and the instructor than those who struggle and panic because their clothes, the buoyancy aid and the splashing of the water prohibit them from adopting their usual 'head-out-of-the-water' breast-stroke position. Swimmers are not necessarily water confident! Ideally, an assessment of a person's ability to demonstrate water confidence is in the swimming pool before a canoeing session. The canoeist should if possible be encouraged to learn how to put on the buoyancy aid and helmet, but not as a pre-requisite to being allowed to canoe.

Most of the early stages of the BCU Award Scheme tests can be achieved by canoeists with a mental handicap; if they are to pursue targets, it should be these.

Safety. Risk is a variable factor for everyone but is often exaggerated by disability. For some, the element of risk is the adventurous edge to the sport that gives the participant the sense of satisfaction and raises his self esteem. The element of risk must be determined according to the needs of the individual but careful planning will ensure that there is no undue risk.

Enjoyment. Canoeing is perhaps the only water sport in which initial success and independence can be achieved by canoeists with a mental handicap in a solo situation within an hour or so of getting into a canoe or kayak for the first time.

For further details contact: British Canoe Union, Flexel House, 45/47 High Street, Addlestone, Weybridge KT15 1JV (tel: 0932 841341). The BCU contact for canoeing for disabled people is: Geoff Smedley, 11 High Beech, Allesley, Coventry CV5 7QD (tel: (home) 0203 405395; (work) 0203 303776).

RAMBLING

Rambling is a simple and informal activity which can be enjoyed by all except the most severely handicapped people.

The equipment needed obviously depends on the type of walk planned. The main items are a rucksack, a pair of stout boots and some waterproof clothing, none of which need be very expensive (Fig 15.3).

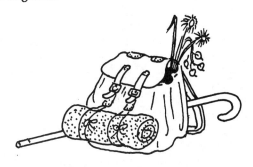

Figure 15.3 Rambling equipment

People with a mental handicap are invariably welcome to take part in walks organised by the many local clubs and groups,

as long as it is appreciated that the people leading the walks will not necessarily have any special expertise in looking after people with a mental handicap. People living in London, for example, can take advantage of the public rambles organised by the Ramblers' Association. Low-priced transport by coach and train is provided to different parts of the attractive countryside around London, the walks being conducted by experienced leaders. Information about these excursions can also be obtained from the Association, which provides fact sheets giving basic information about walking in the country and equipment for ramblers.

Many groups of the Ramblers' Association have prepared slide talks which can be adapted, if necessary, for presentation to groups of people with a mental handicap. There is usually no charge for this service.

ROUTE LEARNING

Route finding is necessary for some types of physical recreation, such as rambling, orienteering or even finding the way to a sports centre field or park. The following account of a study carried out by the Deputy Manager of Redditch Adult Training Centre, Worcestershire, may help some trainees and hospital residents to use photographs as clues to finding their way about.

Anyone using a route which he has used before looks for certain 'cues' along that route. The object of the Redditch study was to see whether people with a mental handicap could be taught to find their own way over a set route by looking at photographs of cue points.

The route

The chosen route — a mixture of roads, lanes and field footpaths — had a number of junctions giving a choice of direction and suitable cue points at each junction.

A number of factors had to be taken into consideration in choosing the route:

1. it had to be sufficiently far away from the trainees' home for them not to be already familiar with it;

2. although the ultimate aim was for the trainees to be able to traverse the route alone, the leader was still responsible for their safety and well-being while the study was in progress so that the route had to be in a fairly traffic-free area;

3. people with a mental handicap generally do not have the same chance to get out into the wider environment as able-bodied people, so any opportunity to get away from built-up areas should be taken.

Photographs

The route was photographed, suitable cues at every corner, and when the road was too long between these corners to see the next junction, or there was a bend in between, reinforcers such as a 'no waiting' sign, a lamp post within a garden, or some distinctive railings or piece of brick wall were photographed.

Prints were developed and printed, and extraneous areas of sky and foreground trimmed off. They were then mounted on uniform size cards in a ring folder (Fig 15.4).

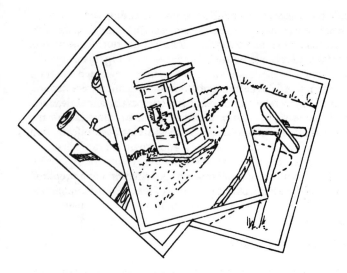

Figure 15.4 Route learning — photographs mounted on cards

Selection of trainees

Three trainees, of varying degrees of intelligence, were selected. An elementary form of assessment was necessary to attempt to get an idea of the functional level of the trainees involved. In selecting the three people for the experiment two factors were taken into account:

1. that the trainees must be able to walk at a reasonable pace for a distance of $2^1/2$ to $3^1/4$ Kms ($1^1/2$ to 2 miles), some of it over rough paths;

2. that, because of the mileage involved in travelling between the centre and the route, all three had to be taken together, two being left in the car while the other one was taken round the route.

Alan, the brightest of the three trainees selected, could read fairly well by ATC standards, and would probably have been working had he not had other problems. Brian suffered from Down's Syndrome, as did Charles, although he was less able than Brian. Charles was only able to do simple repetition work at the centre and could seldom repeat three digits accurately.

The first trip

On the first trip round the circuit the three trainees were driven to the car park at the beginning of the course and, after ascertaining that the other two would be all right sitting in the car together, the manager got out with Alan, showed him the first photograph, and asked him what it was.

'A telephone box', Alan replied.

'Can you see one anywhere round here?'

'Yes over there', said Alan, pointing to a telephone box about hundred yards away.

'Let's go down to it then'.

The box stood at a junction, with the main road bearing slightly to the right and a narrow lane branching off to the left. When they arrived at it the manager showed Alan the second photograph, taken from the telephone box, which depicted the main road going straight ahead and also the broken white lines across the junction with the minor road, as well as some cars on a car park further away. Alan quickly got hold of the idea and had no difficulty in finding his way round the course, taking forty-one minutes.

Brian had found it more difficult than Alan and needed a few prompts. His biggest fault was his tendency to make up his mind before reaching the next cue point and before seeing the photograph relating to the following cue point.

Charles, the least able of the three, was a rather slow walker, and sometimes had difficulty balancing on uneven ground, though he negotiated the stiles without any help. The sixty minutes he took for his first trip — half as much again as each of the other two — was, however, due more to the time he spent at all the major cue points than to his slow physical progress. At a cross roads, where the correct route to the right was denoted by a fence of white palings, Charles could not make up his mind which way to go, so the manager pointed to each road in turn and asked him if he could see any white railings as in the photograph. In each case he answered 'yes' and when asked which way he thought he ought to go, he indicated the road straight ahead.

Cueing points

It soon became obvious that what the manager had considered good cueing points were not necessarily so to the trainees. At one stage he had taken a photograph to include a 'slow' sign for traffic, but when asked what they could see, both on the photograph and along the route, each of the trainees remarked on a brick wall, some tall trees and a house, but none noticed the 'slow' sign until it was pointed out to them. It had not occurred to the manager that, being unable to read and not being drivers, the sign would have no meaning for them.

Second and third trips

The manager went round with the trainees three times altogether, on the second and third journeys letting them carry the book of photographs while he walked a yard or two behind.

Alan managed very well, not having to refer to the book at all. Brian thought he could do without it on the second journey, but had to be helped occasionally. Charles got in a complete muddle, not because he did not know the route, but because he could never find the photograph relating to the point he was already at.

Solo trips

Finally, each did a solo run. They all made it successfully, and then another boy, Dennis, who had walked twice with the manager round the course without seeing the photographs 'had a go'. He almost confounded the manager's theories and nearly ruined his study by going round without any help and with no mistakes!

Conclusions

As the manager commented, this was a preliminary study and by no means a scientific investigation. A lot more needs to be done before any decisions can be made as to whether photograph can play a useful part in teaching social competence to people with a mental handicap.

Because Alan, Brian and Charles used photographs on their initial journeys this is not to say that they would have found it any harder to have learnt the route without them. Dennis appears to have managed just as well with the photographs, memorising the course without being expected to.

If this method of teaching route learning was continued with a particular group of people, would they eventually build up a strategy of movement whereby they look for cues on all journeys?

The four trainees derived a great deal of pleasure from taking part in the experiment Most people with a mental handicap seem to enjoy open-air activities, and these four were no exception. They would have liked the experiment to have continued for a much longer period. The satisfaction which they obviously obtained would of itself have made the whole project worthwhile.

Since 1981, orienteering (see below) has developed as a sport for people with a mental handicap and could now replace other methods, such as route learning. However, if any member of staff is a keen photographer, further experiments could be carried out on the scheme outlined above.

ORIENTEERING

Sue Eccles, a Lecturer in Recreation and Leisure Studies, Co-ordinator for Recreation and Leisure Courses, Airedale and Wharfedale College, Leeds, and a member of the West Yorkshire Orienteering Development Association, writes: 'If a group of people with a mental handicap enjoy being out of doors and responding to a challenge, then orienteering may be the sport for them. It involves finding a way around a course by reading a map and making decisions about which way to go.

'One aim of orienteering is to provide an educational experience which will enable those who have participated in it to carry out a wide range of "life skills" with increased effectiveness. It can also foster the continuing development of physical and mental skills, encourage the individuals' personal development, as well as helping to broaden experience and introducing new environments.

'Ultimately, it can provide the basis for a programme which builds up self confidence, self reliance and self awareness, as well as being, above all, **tremendous fun.**

'A heightening of personal skills/awareness and an increased level of achievement in literacy, numeracy, and graphical skills, were the result of individual orienteering programmes tackled by several groups from adult training centres in the Leeds area. Overall, participants enjoyed an increased sense of well-being.

'The sport of orienteering affords participants the chance to integrate with people from a wide range of backgrounds at both local community level and further afield at national events.'

Further details of local clubs and events and a list of videos and permanent courses can be obtained from: the British Orienteering Federation, Dale North Road, Darley Dale, Matlock, Derbyshire DE4 2HX (tel: 0629 734042).

The United Kingdom Sports Association for People with Mental Handicap (see page 188) offer courses for 'Training the trainer' in orienteering skills.

SAILING

Sailing is now considered to be a very constructive and positive learning tool for people with a mental handicap. The progress

made has proved to be intellectually stimulating, socially valuable and emotionally satisfying, and also an enjoyable way for the participants to exceed society's expectations and to formulate ideas and beliefs of their own.

Several ATCs and Gateway Clubs now sail both on sea and on inland waters, making use of the co-operation and training facilities offered by fully qualified sailing instructors. There are also increasing numbers of recognised outdoor providers.

Experience at Blantyre ATC Centre in Cornwall suggests that anyone planning a sailing programme for people with a mental handicap should bear in mind the following guidelines.

Precautions and safety

1. Prepare yourself, your craft and your crew, and get to know local conditions.

2. Wear correct clothing and footwear.

3. Practise survival techniques in water.

4. Take life jackets to the local swimming pool and use them in shallow, warm water. Instruct the correct method of wearing and fastening them and how to remove them.

5. Discuss capsize and man overboard drills and, when the trainees are confident, practise these skills.

6. Read and use the Department of Trade and Industry Seaway Code and/or use the various British Waterways pamphlets.

7. Acquire a good stable tender, and never overload. It is better to make three safe journeys than one wet one.

8. Check weather conditions.

9. Carry appropriate safety equipment — flares, fire extinguisher (not appropriate for dinghies), life jackets, anchor — and know how to use them.

10. Understand the use and storage of toxic materials, and carry emergency spares for boat and marine engine(s).

11. Leave details of where you are going and how long you expect to be away with a responsible person.

Suggested plan

1. Carry out a feasibility study.

2. Discuss it with those in authority.

3. Look at the area of risk (see Chapter 20, 'Insurance').

4. Acquire the necessary skills and expertise before attempting to instruct.

6. Discuss the programme fully with all interested parties — management, parents, guardians, colleagues.

7. Acquire necessary safety equipment before acquiring the necessary craft It is all too tempting to use a boat without the necessary safety equipment and an initial programme can be made using safety equipment only.

8. When all equipment has been secured, choose a pilot group of people to work with, set short term goals for long term plans.

Resources

Allied Forces establishments

Boatyards

British Waterways Board

Chandlers

HM Coastguard Department of Trade

Ocean Youth Club

Outward Bound centres

Royal National Lifeboat Institution

Royal Yachting Association

Sailing clubs

Sea cadets

Sea scouts

Technical colleges

Youth service

(also many local charities and organisations).

WATER SKIING

In 1986 and 1987, the National Federation of Gateway Clubs set up a couple of taster days in water skiing, in conjunction with the British Disabled Water Ski Association (BDWSA), using the BDWSA facilities at the Tony Edge Centre, Heron Lake, Wraysbury, near Staines. The initial link was established by Dave Hurst, a volunteer at Stockport '66 Gateway Club, in Manchester. Among his many sporting interests, which include judo and mountain climbing, Dave numbers water skiing and ski-jumping in which he takes part at international level. As a blind water-skier, Dave is a member of the BDWSA, and was keen to introduce people with a mental handicap to the sport — initially with a small group to ascertain what difficulties might arise and what aspects should be given special attention.

The BDWSA readily agreed to set up a first taster day in 1986 — the first time they had specifically organised a beginners' day for people with a mental handicap. A small group of participants was assembled from Stonebridge ATC and Strathcona Social Education Centre (SEC) in Brent. They began by using 'Root 5 surf-skis' (rather like a large-hulled surf board with moulded top surface for seat, feet and legs). Each person was seated on a surf-ski and then tipped off to make sure that they were happy in cold water and could right themselves from a face down position. Once they had passed this test, they were towed behind the powerboat on a surf-ski, with a BDWSA instructor (depending on their level of physical co-ordination) either accompanying them on the same ski or seated alongside on another surf-ski. The final stage for the most able was using the 'Edge Triple Bar'. This is a specially designed tow bar which allows a skier to be towed with an instructor on each side. The instructors are able to detach their ends of the bar to allow the learner to ski solo. The other obvious advantage is that this device allows learners to overcome any difficulties of a water-start, as the accompanying instructors can help to lift the individual out of the water at the start of the tour.

The taster day at Heron Lake was repeated in 1987, when the same core group were joined by individuals from Acton Lodge ATC, Brentwood. Obviously, this initiative will have only limited potential on a yearly basis, and it is hoped that the local ATCs will eventually be able to use the BDWSA facilities on a more

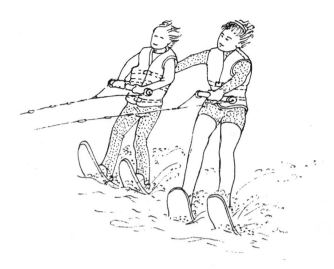

Figure 15.5 Water skiing

regular basis. As with most minority sports, however, and in this case one needing specialist equipment and instruction, problems lie in both voluntary staff time and the costs involved (although the BDWSA is able to provide skiing at a relatively low price). The sport requires a high degree of co-ordination between brain, arms, legs and torso; but given sufficient time and practice there is no reason why people with a mental handicap cannot become proficient (Fig 15.5).

People with a mental handicap have taken part in an annual two-day taster event at Sale Water-Ski Club, organised by the North West Branch of BDWSA. The Committee intend to increase the number of such days in the future, and to try to foster a process of integration, by using the facilities of other water-ski clubs in the region.

It is interesting to note that two members of the French team, which took part in the first World Water-Ski Trophy for the Disabled, held at Heron Lake in July 1987, were people with a mental handicap. See also Chapter 18.

YHA welcomes people with a mental handicap. For details see page 189.

WALKING

A well planned purposeful walk whether taken in a large city, town, country area or by the sea proves many opportunities for learning.

Here are some ideas for walks and ways in which they can be planned: a nature walk; a farm visit; a route finding walk leading to orienteering; a shopping expedition; a discovery walk; a hide -and- seek walk.

A nature walk

1.   Draw attention to some natural objects — a catkin, a stone, a flower, leaf. See how many of these can be brought back.

2.   Find a dark green leaf, a light green leaf and a yellow leaf. Gradually learn the tree names — later those of the different flowers and fruits.

3.   Identify some of the common birds. Show pictures first, eg robin, magpie, chicken, tit, thrush, blackbird, duck, swan.

4. Collect coloured pebbles from the beach.

5. Collect anything of interest in the neighbourhood.

A farm visit

Many farmers are willing for small groups to visit their farms — to see the animals, a tractor, a plough, farm buildings, dogs and cats, chickens.

A route finding walk (see p. 147).

This method has many possibilities.

A shopping expedition

This expedition needs careful planning and can only be undertaken with those who are learning about money.

A discovery walk

1. Plan a walk to find out the different types of buildings existing in the immediate environment, eg church, hotel, pub, post office, ambulance and fire stations, swimming baths, sports centres, adventure playground.

2. Take walks with different themes: how many different kinds of transport were seen on the walk?

   'Uniform' walks — how many different uniforms were seen, eg police, nurses, firemen, soldiers, bus drivers and conductors etc.

   'Work' walks — visits to factories, building sites, stores, to see people and their different kinds of work.

Hide and seek walk

This type of walk is particularly appropriate in places where there are low bushes or shrubs, logs, benches. Instruct the walkers that, at the whistle signal, they should all try to get off the ground or get out of sight; when two whistles are given, all should get to base.

Note: Suitable for hospital grounds. It is necessary to fix the route precisely and know the members of the group well.

Picnic walks

Walk to a picnic area with a good view, perhaps a lake or the beach. Take a picnic with you and sometimes cook outside.

Quiet walks

1. *Sounds* — how many sounds can you hear? What makes the sound — a bird, an animal, a bus or a train?

2. *Smell* — what do you smell? Is it the exhaust from a car, a flower, a factory?

3. *Look* — take a magnifying glass with you, study leaves, flowers and trees — what can you see?

4. *Feel* — what does the bark of a tree, pine needles, a stone, the water in a stream, feel like?

Note: To speed up walking, follow 12 to 20 walks by 12 to 20 runs (this also helps counting). Gradually lengthen the period of time allocated and encourage long strides.

2. GUIDELINES TO PLANNING AN OUTDOOR ACTIVITIES COURSE OR HOLIDAY

During the 1980s there has been an increasing awareness of the value of outdoor activities for people with a mental handicap. Many new outdoor pursuits/adventure/holiday centres have opened. These are maintained and run by local authorities, voluntary organisations, charitable trust and the private sector.

When planning an outdoor activities course it is prudent to:

● make plans well in advance;

● consider carefully with your clients/members what kind of activities they are interested in and want to experience for themselves;

● send for information/brochures from centres which seem to offer what you are looking for; study them carefully;

● contact the centre(s) of your choice and *visit it when it is operating*, before making a booking. This visit could make all the difference to the planning of the course and the value of its result and follow up.

When visiting a centre take note of:

● the environment — is it right for your members, including access to all amenities?

● are the activities well taught and supervised?

● are the safety regulations, including fire precautions, completely adequate and adhered to?

● is the atmosphere of the centre right? exactly how is a typical day's programme planned?

● what equipment is provided by the centre — how well is it cared for?

● where a ropes course, canoes, sailing boats, wet suits or climbing gear are used, are they well maintained and stored?

● what equipment has to be provided by your group, including any special personal clothing?

● what medical forms or other are required prior to, or at the time of, arrival at the centre?

● what, if anything, is required from members of staff/helpers you may take with you, both in the activities themselves and/or domestically? It is important to know what is expected of accompanying staff/helpers and where the responsibilities lie.

All this information is important when briefing your members, staff and parents.

It could be worthwhile to find out if any group near you has used the centre of your choice — personal recommendation can be very valuable.

Follow-up

What opportunities exist in your own area for putting into practice experiences and skills learned while on the course, eg canoeing, orienteering?

What specialist help can be obtained through national, regional and County Coaching Schemes?

Many ATCs, Gateway Clubs, hospitals and hostels are taking advantage of the help given by the Governing Bodies of Sport both regionally and locally with beneficial results.

3. SCHEMES OF TRAINING COMBINING SEVERAL ACTIVITIES

One well established scheme is described in detail — the Sheffield Adult Training Centres' Outdoor Pursuits Scheme.

Two other schemes — one involving the use of the Churchtown Farm Field Studies Centre in Cornwall by a Surrey adult training centre, and the other of Outward Bound Wales by groups from Hampshire — are described in some detail. Other groups attend the centres at the same time, so that the trainees have the opportunity not only to participate in the outdoor activities, but also to meet other students, to work together and learn to understand each other.

Some details are also included of other well known training centres for outdoor pursuits for people with a mental handicap — the Calvert Trust Adventure Centre in the Lake District and the Katharine Elliot Cottage Project in Scotland.

SHEFFIELD TRAINING CENTRES

Ways and means

The adult training centres in Sheffield are successfully answering the question as to how the natural desire of people with a mental handicap for adventure can be directed into exciting yet safe channels, and at the same time arouse a worthwhile interest that will survive in later years and be of use in their future training, giving them new motivation and means of communication.

About ten years ago a few of the more able trainees with a mental handicap were taken on country rambles and fishing trips. One of the instructors was a leader with the Edale Mountain Rescue team and, with the help of other team members, was eventually able to introduce rock climbing (Figure 15.6), fell walking, bivouacing, caving and mountain hut weekends.

Field studies are a part of all expeditions: the trainees observe local flora and fauna and items of geological interest. Collections can be made and mounted during the 'back at Centre' study sessions, but only of items which do not deplete the natural resources of the area. Other means such as sketches, plaster casts and rubbings are used for these. In some areas there are museum services which loan out collections and specimens.

Drawing and painting are often used as means of recording experiences and discoveries. This is helpful to those who cannot read or write, and can take the place of a log book. A group mural can also record the activities. The instructor comments, 'From experience over the years, the young men and women trainees so far involved have, without doubt, benefitted physically, socially and as individuals'.

Co-operation

What is it that makes a specialised team of instructors' objectives work? The co-operation of not only a few but of all the centres involved, and the parents of the trainees taking part; the staff who are not outdoor pursuit minded but willing to have extra

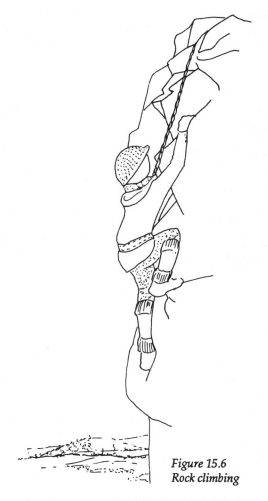

Figure 15.6
Rock climbing

group numbers in order to benefit the few; the kitchen staff who not only provide food for expeditions but also help to supervise the trainees in such tasks as sandwich making; also the other specialists such as the senior instructor engineer who has spent many hours canabalising obsolete wheelchairs in order to make one to our specifications, based on the principles of mountain rescue equipment. Sheffield now has a prototype chair with not only wheels but also sledge runners and anchorage points for stabilising ropes to be tied. This project is now in the hands of Sheffield University who hope to produce a new chair of maximum strength for maximum lightness, incorporating modifications found necessary on test runs.

Many of the Edale team members became interested in this rewarding work; they could see, from weekend to weekend, an improvement in the trainees' self-confidence and self-reliance and, in some cases, a marked improvement in gross motor co-ordination and balance. These outings also helped the trainees to become aware of the needs of others, and to be less self-centred. These activities were considered voluntary and, because they took place at weekends, the adult training centres were not officially involved. The work continued and a few far-sighted managers began to accept the importance of the venture. After a successful managers' meeting the activities were incorporated into the Centre's timetable, ie one day per month and the Friday afternoon prior to a weekend expedition. The use of the Centre's transport was granted and some time was allocated to the administration and paperwork involved.

The Outdoor Pursuits scheme is now accepted as part of the day-to-day training and assessment programme. Independence in curriculum and organisation is maintained and use is still made of voluntary help at weekends as well as centre staff. In this way contact is kept with other interested agencies, the Special Schools and the Royal Society for Mental Handicapped Children and Adults for instance, as well as the many individual experts who sometimes offer assistance.

Leaders' training

Before the more adventurous outdoor activities can be envisaged, the problem of training staff must be realised. Their extra voluntary training should be of a standard acceptable not only to the parents of trainees, but also to the authority. In Sheffield, staff are selected and trained not necessarily for their academic qualifications but, in the first instance, for their experience and suitability as mountaineers, cavers and rock climbers. Not only do they have to possess expert knowledge in any one subject, they must have an active interest in many others. They should also be able to work individually and yet be self-disciplined and able to work as a team. The staff as a whole must be prepared to work with enthusiasm. A harmonious staff relationship is 'Utopia' in any situation but this must be achieved if the aims of adventure training are to succeed.

A field team

A field team consists of an adviser, who takes full responsibility for safety and staff training; an organiser, who is responsible for equipment, bookings of huts and hostels and also acts as treasurer; four senior staff — all experts in their own field; and over 30 instructors who have completed an annual in-service training course. The organisation of the team mentioned above now includes several women which makes possible such events as female bivouacs.

Outdoor Pursuits development in the Sheffield training centres is not a full-time occupation for the staff, but one to which they give some time voluntarily, and with the exception of mid-week outings, carry on their normal teaching duties within the centres. The instructor training programme is a yearly event designed to include a great deal of navigation both night and day. Mountain safety and rescue techniques are covered with emphasis on First Aid and medical knowledge. Any medical condition, heart disease or tendency to chest infections more serious than is accepted as normal with trainees suffering from Down's Syndrome, must be known to the instructors, so that the programme can be modified to suit each group. In most Outdoor Pursuits centres the courses are aimed at the limits of strength and endurance of the individual, but a different approach must be adopted with handicapped people to allow a good margin of reserve strength and energy. Experience is vital; the instructor must know when to get off the hill or, more importantly, when not to be on the hill in the first place. Potential instructors are also given the opportunity to visit unfamiliar mountain countryside and to spend a night out in bivouac conditions, usually in winter.

A year's programme

A programme in booklet form is published each year and given to any interested trainee. The activities undertaken are fairly comprehensive and are aimed at all levels of intelligence: they vary from simple nature trails, including those for wheelchair cases, to mountain expeditions to over 900m (3000'). Many are mid-week day expediitions; a few take place at weekends.

Selection of those to take part

Individuals from adult training centres, Gateway Clubs and hospitals are selected and invited to join whichever expeditions coincide with their own particular level of training and ability and to join those which may expand their potential.

Planning the expedition

The types of expeditions, walks or scrambles undertaken and the length and strenuousness of the routes will depend on the individual trainee. However, walks of all grades can be found in any mountainous area and each course starts with the less strenuous and builds up to an expedition of suitable length and duration, including a camp under canvas, or, if the weather is poor, in a youth hostel. If the physical prowess of those taking part is such that they are not capable of carrying the tents, sleeping bags, and cooking equipment, the route can be so planned that equipment for camping is taken by transport and dropped off at a prearranged camp site, and collected later. If by using a shorter route the trainees could be self-supporting, however, they would benefit from the feeling of being self-dependent.

Obviously each walk or expedition requires a great deal of thought and planning, taking into consideration such factors as the medical condition of each individual, the time of year and, above all, the weather. Although orienteering is perhaps beyond the capabilities of most trainees, simple map reading can be interesting; for instance, north, south, east and west without the complication of degrees, and map references up to four figures, can be within their scope. The use of simple conventional signs can help to teach observation, while looking for churches, woods and streams marked on the map can add interest.

Rock climbing

Rock climbing, an exciting activity, well within the powers of most trainees, undoubtedly helps to build self-confidence, and provides the novice with a great sense of personal achievement.

Climbs of many hundreds of feet can be tackled with selected trainees if the safety rules are strictly observed, but the outcrop type of climbing reaching a height of not more than about 24m (80') provides trainees with sufficient scope and a spice of danger, while making an accident almost impossible.

The Peak District National Park is by far the best area for outcrop climbing. Gritstone Edges now boast many hundreds of climbs all named and graded according to severity. For instance, 'easy' — with large footholds suitable for beginners; 'moderate', — not much more difficult, but having one or two places that are a bit 'sticky'; 'difficult' — usually steeper and more exposed than the first two grades, but with adequate footholds and handholds, which there may not be in a climb that is rated 'very difficult' or 'severe'. The climbs get progressively harder and are graded 'very severe', 'extremely severe' and so on. People with a mental handicap should not undertake climbs any harder than 'difficult', as the harder climbs (although no more dangerous on a top rope) do demand an extremely good sense of balance and coordination. To tackle climbs graded higher than 'difficult' a much higher intellectual ability is required than can generally be found among people with a mental handicap. No doubt a trainee could be 'dragged' up harder climbs, but not only would this have no practical value, it would kill his enthusiasm.

Rock climbing would probably be number one on any list of dangerous pastimes. In fact this is not true; if certain rules are obeyed (ie if there is a ratio of two expert climbing instructors to one trainee actually climbing, and if equipment such as harnesses and crash helmets is used) the likelihood of a trainee falling more than a few inches would be slight, especially if the climbers were using an outcrop where the total height is not more than a rope's length. Rock climbing is also a suitable activity for the lest robust; it is a test of balance and co-ordination rather than of pure strength.

Caving

Caving is an activity which can be graded in severity from the easy, open-to-the public commercial caves, to the complex systems of the famous and often notorious potholers' caves. It rarely depends on the weather except after very heavy rain. Caving can usually be undertaken when rock climbing cannot. A wet day on the rocks can be a chilling experience and far less agreeable than a day spent in the constant temperature of the caves. This too is a sport involving little danger if treated with respect.

A pot-hole is a cave that has been formed or eroded so that it is vertical, or nearly so. Exploring a horizontal cave is usually quite exciting and quite difficult. A pot-hole can only be safely negotiated by a team of experienced people with ropes, ladders, wet suits and inflatable dinghies as well as many other items of equipment. This would be quite beyond the resources of even selected trainees. The commercial caves open to the public and several other famous caves can be used by small parties of trainees, but even then only after individual trials, since psychological factors could well be involved, ie, some trainees may suffer from claustrophobia or be afraid of the dark.

Water sports

Activities such as swimming, canoeing, and fishing can all be practised with success. Both swimming and fishing have been carried out in the Sheffield area for many years.

Pony trekking and horse riding are other possible activities — in Sheffield they are organised on a contract basis with a local riding stable.

CHURCHTOWN FARM FIELD STUDIES CENTRE

Churchtown Farm Field Studies Centre, which operates under the auspices of the Spastics Society, provides field studies and linked educational and adventure holiday courses for all types of handicapped children and adults. It has well equipped laboratories, classrooms with a range of audio-visual aids, a library and a photographic dark room. The dining hall and common room are in an old converted and modernised barn and an exciting feature of the development is an indoor pool. The Centre can accommodate 24 to 30 students plus the necessary visiting staff. Accommodation has been specifically designed for the handicapped with particular emphasis on the toilet/shower areas.

Selection

In 1977 the Colebrook Day Centre in Redhill decided to investigate the possibility of offering holidays involving more active pursuits than those provided by the usual seaside holiday. The Centre contacted numerous organisations including the Ramblers Association, Holiday Fellowship, Youth Hostel Association and National Students Travel, all of whom were willing to consider people with a mental handicap with certain reservations regarding their handicap. Finally, the Churchtown Farm Field Studies Centre, Bodmin, Cornwall, was selected because of the varied facilities it offered and the Centre's willingness to accept people with a mental handicap.

Staff

The Centre has its own team of fully qualified, experienced instructors and is admirably situated close to the coast, rivers and Bodmin Moor. It has its own nature reserve and trails. It was believed that clients would derive considerable benefit from physical pursuits and the staff of Churchtown Farm submitted the following programme:

coastal footpath walks; rambles on the moor; horse riding; sailing; rock climbing.

Preparation

With this range of activities in mind, plans were made to formulate a preparation programme, having first invited applications from clients. It was decided that a group of between 9 and 12 should be chosen at random, since the Centre did not know what response to expect and because it was difficult to select clients. A group of 10 women and 4 men with varying mental and physical abilities was chosen, in addition to 2 staff from Colebrook and a voluntary worker.

As walking would be the main activity on the holiday, part of the preparation consisted of a series of hikes which not only prepared the group physically but also gave them the opportunity of participating together as a team. Details about Bodmin and its environs given in the classroom proved valuable as some of the clients had little experience outside their own locality or had never been away from home or the family before.

The justification for preparation soon became apparent as many of the clients had little walking experience and some had never even encountered a stile. The group were taken out on three separate day hikes over different terrains, each hike being longer and more difficult than the previous one. It was evident after the first that adequate footwear and waterproof clothing were essential. This preparatory programme enabled clients to adjust far more readily to new situations and experiences during the holiday itself.

Aims and objectives

While primarily a holiday, this venture was also intended to provide the participants and those with whom they come into daily contact, considerable additional benefits. A major aim was to instil confidence through experiencing many new and challenging situations; to achieve this, each individual was extended to his maximum potential so that he should understand his capabilities. It was hoped that the holiday would also help to develop:

understanding and mastery of fear; awareness of safety factors; language; acceptance of criticism; ability to listen and comply with simple unaccustomed instructions; stamina; body awareness; confidence and trust in others; ability to make choices and make decisions; self-help and hygiene; understanding that different activities require different skills, perseverance, speed, patience etc, with changing emphasis; anticipation and recollection.

In addition, it was hoped to:

integrate academic education with constant reference to

basic concepts;

enhance the client's standing in the family, as their experience on the holiday may well have exceeded those of their brothers and sisters;

reinforce socially acceptable standards in a different environment;

improve staff's understanding of individual members of the group;

provide parents with opportunities during the absence of their son or daughter to have a vacation themselves without the normal pressures inherent within a family with a handicapped member;

make it clear to various authorities and fund-raising organisations that, given the opportunity, handicapped people can participate in a wide variety of pursuits and that learning through participating in outdoor activities can very often prove to be more profitable than learning in the classroom setting.

Activities undertaken on the holidays

Walking

These walks, which included walks along coastal footpaths and over rough moorland, were graded — the most difficult, the moorland walk, being undertaken towards the end of the holiday.

During the initial walk when obstacles were encountered, some people needed help and encouragement to overcome the awkward section. As their confidence increased they became more self-reliant and encouraged each other rather than awaiting staff assistance. The slower walkers raised their speed and on occasions a handicapped client, rather than a member of staff, led the party. The group also became more aware of their surroundings through looking for flora and fauna, some of which they collected for later use in the production of log books. The need to observe the environment was made apparent because of the different types of conditions underfoot. For example, anyone who did not walk carefully over rocks and boulders was liable to bruise and graze his hands, knees and shins, while the unobservant got wet when walking through marshland.

Stepping stones provided an excellent opportunity to improve confidence and co-ordination — at first several members negotiating them were unable to balance on the stones and received a bootful of water. This did not seem to upset them unduly, but on the second attempt fewer feet became wet.

Horse riding

This took the form of a one-hour ride, the horses being led by experienced riders on foot. At first clients were anxious at the prospect of mounting such large animals but, eventually, all but two did so and one of those was too large for the horses available. One girl remarked that 'she felt like a queen as she looked on everything'. By the end of the ride all the riders were far more relaxed, they conversed not only with the helpers but also with the horses, and were sufficiently confident to stroke the horses' manes.

Swimming and sailing

The Centre has its own fine swimming pool available each evening. During swimming sessions it was found that none of the clients were unduly frightened of the water even though a number were non-swimmers. This was important when considering sailing, as the boats were taken not only up river but also out to sea. Boating was an exciting exercise as the water was not calm and all learnt a certain amount about the sea and wind. Furthermore, a number of clients were given the opportunity to take the tiller for a short time.

Rock climbing

Individual clients climbed a small rock face and, on hearing that they were to climb and seeing the equipment, one comment was: 'people like us aren't supposed to do things like this', and the general feeling was one of considerable apprehension. This was no doubt due to the fact that no preparation had been given for rock climbing due to lack of facilities and lack of experience on the part of the organisers. To help them overcome their fears, the most able and active client was selected to make the first ascent. Having seen that one of their peers was able to negotiate the climb, most of the other members were prepared to attempt the face. They all appreciated the importance of listening to the instructions carefully and of complying with them. During the second holiday, all clients were prepared to climb the face and showed far less apprehension.

The climb had been extremely well prepared by the staff from Churchtown Farm who had anticipated that some would find the climb very difficult, they were, however, not prepared to let any members of the group fail, although this meant that several clients needed a great deal of encouragement and some assistance. Each client experienced the exhilaration of having achieved what seemed to him at the outset an impossibility. The thrill was further enhanced by the knowledge that he had possibly achieved something which was unique within his own family. How many brothers or sisters had climbed a rock face?

Waterfall — climbing the rapids (second holiday only)

This unexpected and therefore unprepared venture was more readily accepted than on the first holiday — no doubt prior experience helped many of the clients. The group were taken to the rapids of a fast running river — first three clients, and later the others, slid into the water fully clothed and were immediately engulfed in extremely cold, foaming, white water, varying in depth from 30.5 to 137 cm (1' to about $4^1/2$'). All were afraid but were able to control their fear and negotiated the river, crossing with some difficulty because they were unable to find secure footing since the numerous rocks beneath the surface were of different sizes. In addition, the strong current retarded their progress and the noise of the rushing water made the instructions of the staff virtually inaudible; although staff were in the river and in close attendance, the clients were very much on their own, in that they had to rely on their own initiative to make headway across the river, where they then had to climb up through the rapids. All the group were exhilarated by this adventure and proof of its popularity was the request of some clients that they be allowed to make a second crossing, which they did if time allowed. (Only one client did not take part in this activity because it was felt that the unpredictability of the individual might endanger her safety and that of others.) This physical and tactile experience obviously fired the clients' imagination and it proved to be the outstanding feature of a very successful second holiday.

Safety

The Churchtown Farm staff, who stressed the need for safety throughout the holiday, provided all the necessary specialised equipment and explained the various safety procedures to the

Centre staff accompanying the group. All activities were undertaken by clients voluntarily, persuasion rather than compulsion being employed. In fact, little persuasion was needed as the excitement generated by the activities themselves created sufficient stimuli.

Follow-up activities

Memories are precious to everyone, and since people with a mental handicap have great difficulty in recalling events, it was decided to follow up the holiday with a series of sessions designed to help them remember and retain as much about their holiday as possible. Clients were encouraged to express their thoughts and feelings on the events of the day into a cassette recorder and this was used later at Colebrook to aid memory. Sessions were devoted to compiling individual log books, dictating a transcript, painting pictures and discussing photographs and films taken during the holiday.

Films were made of both holidays to create and foster interest among parents and other people who may have little knowledge of the capabilities of handicapped people. In this way the Centre is able to provide visual proof of the ability of the participants.

Developments since 1981

Since 1981 the farm has been completely rebuilt with a new all weather facility enabling students to study rural life under cover. The new horticulture complex has also been developed; included in this is a horticultural teaching area and the Centre has plans to rebuild the greenhouse into another all weather teaching site.

Outdoor pursuits continue to develop and an approach has been adopted which is summarised in the term 'challenge education'. This is an existing concept which matches the 'abilities' of the students to the level of activity from which they can develop. For example, the student may start the week at a relatively low level of challenge, such as involvement in new games, and move through the sequence to finish his/her week at a high level of challenge such as rock climbing.

Short term camping expeditions are now featured in the weekly programmes. This leads to involvement in longer term international expeditions. Currently, one member of staff is co-leading a Canadian Canoe expedition on the lakes of Canada. The Principal has travelled extensively in the United States, gathering material and information which is now incorporated in Churchtown's programmes. Students attend the centre from many different countries which adds to the social atmosphere.

Finally, in an effort to promote the idea that ability rather than disability is important, in-service courses for professionals are run on a regular basis at Churchtown.

OUTWARD BOUND

Outward Bound has schools at Eskdale and Ullswater (England), Lochiel (Scotland), and at Aberdovey and Rhowniar (Tywyn) (Wales). All these schools run courses for people with disabilities.

The Centres have comfortable dormitories, living and dining rooms, assembly halls for drama, music and movement, and

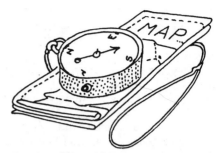

Figure 15.7 Outward bound

good facilities for laundering and drying clothes.

Courses

'Each course strikes a balance between physical and mental challenges. The adventures and risks are real, so is the satisfaction of achievement. The classroom of Outward Bound are the mountains, the sea and the storms; the elements become the examiners of young people brought up in the urban industrial environment created by man'. (Duke of Edinburgh, Patron of Outward Bound).

First course for residents with a mental handicap

Six 'higher' grade residents (3 men and 3 women) with 3 members of the nursing staff from Chelmsley Hospital, Birmingham, were the first people with a mental handicap to attend a course at Outward Bound Wales. This venture happened as a result of one member of staff hearing a BBC programme featuring Outward Bound courses.

Preparation

To prepare for the course the residents and hospital staff walked and pursued other activities at weekends (Fig 15.7).

First course for adult training centre trainees

The first adult training centre to take trainees on an Outward Bound course was the Bournemouth Adult Training Centre. A group of 12 men and 2 training centre staff arrived in the second week of a standard junior course, age range 14 to 20 years.

Concurrent Outward Bound courses

The groups arrived in the second week of a three week course. Each group of Outward Bound students worked with the group with a mental handicap for 1 day in a one-to-one ratio. The handicapped group seemed to adapt very easily to the different faces and were not confused by having different students with them each day. They also enjoyed relating the day's events to students they had worked with earlier in the week.

Course aims

1. To give the students a challenging and enjoyable 'holiday' experience;

2. to give the students on the Outward Bound course the opportunity to mix with handicapped people and vice versa.

Programmes

Since the Outward Bound staff had little previous knowledge of the handicapped individual's abilities, the programme had to be somewhat flexible — but all took part in the following activities:

> camping, canoeing, canoe building, cleaning camping gear, climbing practice and rock climbing, map and compass course (competition in pairs with one student), disco, exploring the shore, games, life line, picnics on beach, rope course (see Fig 15.8), shopping, swimming, trampoline, walking, watching badgers.

Meals

Both groups shared tables in the dining room with the students on the Outward Bound course who were working with them on that day. This arrangement seemed to help the students to mix and communicate with one another.

Comments

From the Voluntary Service Department: 'The first year, "higher" grade patients took part in the second week of a normal three week course so that usual course members, especially those working for their Duke of Edinburgh's Gold Award, became involved with our patients and their activities. During the first venture the patients were able to make their own small canoe, which was brought back to the hospital, where it is used quite often in our hospital swimming pool.

'The following year six of the more dependent patients were selected to attend a one week course. Unfortunately, there was no involvement with other course members, as there were no three week courses on at that time. However, this venture was still very successful and our patients very obviously benefitted from the experience.

'It was generally agreed that in future we would endeavour to take part in the usual three week course, as experiencing these activities with other young people was beneficial to everyone'.

From the Senior Nursing Officer's report: 'The instructor had obviously given a great deal of thought to our activities programme. In fact, all the instructors had prepared the ground with each group of students who assimilated our group into their group activities. They all showed a great deal of interest, kindness and understanding for our residents.

'I am sure that many people would be surprised to know that those suffering from Down's Syndrome and epileptics can climb and swim in the sea quite safely provided due precautions are taken. Swimming in the pool and surf were greatly enjoyed. All patients wore life jackets'.

'I never thought that building our own canoe would stimulate so much interest, but thanks to the instructor who organised this activity it turned out to be a very interesting venture. He gave us all a task to do, some had to polish the mould, some had to cut the fibre glass mat, some had to stir the resin and we all had a hand in stapling and rolling on the resin. The canoe was taken back to the hospital'.

From Outward Bound instructors: 'For Outward Bound students and staff it was interesting to work with six such different people and to learn to adapt to each. Judy was always happy, whereas Elaine lacked confidence and needed a lot of encouragement. Martin would remain interested in what he was doing until the task was completed whereas Kevin wandered from one thing to another. Michael had a good sense of humour, always wanted to know "why", and could reason things out for himself. Barbara

loved to use the tambourine to the record player and had a marvellous sense of rhythm. She seemed to live in a world of her own but would give a big affectionate hug when something pleased her. . . .

'Our two walks were quite short but we found that they got pleasure from simple things like shouting to get an echo. They each managed a roped scramble during the rock climbing day, and the boys and Barbara went on to do a second route'.

From the Bournemouth ATC report: 'The week which trainees from Dorset spent at the Outward Bound school was a time they will never forget. Ten out of the group of twelve men have already asked "when can we go again"'?

A sense of achievement and, most important of all, an increase in their self respect may be brought about by attempting activities which some of their families and friends had not tried'.

From parents: 'We feel that, in the final analysis, all must be on the credit side. I was certainly prepared for our son to find things too much for him, but, to your credit, he didn't, and we knew that the basic idea and aim of your course was a good one'.

'Christopher particularly liked the rock climbing, rope swinging, trampolining and his first experience of sleeping under canvas. This has been a big step forward . . . I am sure this venture has helped him to gain more confidence in doing things for himself and another big factor is the chance for him to mix and converse with complete strangers. It has also given me a "break" from normal routine'.

'Although Stephen has always enjoyed outside activities and has usually been ready to have a go at any new challenge, as parents we were a little apprehensive about this venture, not knowing to what extent Stephen would be able to participate. At the same time having a chance to be able to get involved with so many different activities where normally because of the handicap he might not have ever had such an opportunity, was a challenge not to miss . . . Also, mixing with a group of girls (other than those he meets every day at the Centre) would possibly help to develop a more social understanding between the normal and handicapped person'.

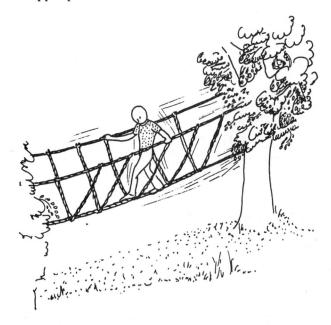

Figure 15.8 Rope walking

From Outward Bound student who worked with the Bournemouth ATC: 'On Wednesday while I was helping to make breakfast in the barn, Stephen came over to me and said that this holiday was the best he had ever had and he would like the staff and girls to know how grateful he was. Nobody had told him to say this. . .

'I must admit that as time went on I found it a lot easier to talk to them and the atmosphere became more relaxed. They told me about their lives, and what they do at the Centre where they work, I think it was of great value for these young men and an experience they will enjoy for the rest of their lives.'

From a social worker who spent the entire week with the second group of trainees from the Bournemouth ATC : 'This week had proved to be one of the most wonderful I have spent in my career in social work. I saw these twelve people become caring, capable individuals whose ability to make their mark on all they came into contact which will never be forgotten. They probably touched some hundred people during their week at Rhowniar and the impression they made would make anyone proud to have known them. The development in self esteem and physical and co-ordinating skills was truly remarkable. They became sharing and caring people both as individuals and as a group. I could never express my gratitude to them for allowing me to have been associated with them and I shall never forget our week at Rhowniar. I don't believe that any other type of experience could have made the impact that this did, and it must be the beginning of a continuing process of providing opportunities for people with a mental handicap to show what they are capable of.'

A recent course for people from ATCs

During the last few years Outward Bound has attracted groups of people with a mental handicap to its courses. One such course at Rhowniar is described by the then manager of Alton ATC, Graham Hiscock.

'The motto of Outward Bound is "to serve, to strive and not to yield" and is very much more than outdoor pursuits, adventure skills, group living experience or physical or practical survival. It provides all these things but much more in a facility that has a reputation second to none for commitment, learning and safety (the experience is actually "apparent danger but hidden total safety"). Participants do not just turn up in the mornings at Outward Bound — they are the course. As can be seen from the activities carried out, the skill learning is there and all the benefits are apparent from them but such is the skill of the staff and the way the schools are organised that those taking part get much more than that. They become more complete people, more aware of themselves and others, more aware of the environment and how they relate to it and more confident of their position in relation to the rest of society. This does not just happen, it is the Outward Bound philosophy that does it — it is part and parcel of Outward Bound not just incidental as it is in most other activity centres.

'As Kurt Hahn said: "It is wrong to coerce people into opinions, but it is a duty to impel them into experience". Outward Bound is an impelling and compelling experience'.

The course programme

1. *Group living/tasks/discussion.* The group completed its shared tasks around the house and dormitories with good spirit and efficiency. As far as the tasks went a lot of emphasis was placed on inter-dependance and responsibility. The group's self-advocacy was always brought to the fore in planning and in debriefing sessions. The only real hiccup came when the group, having spent two hours in the mine collecting items for lunch, then spent the next two hours waiting to be told it was lunchtime — they were not, so we did not eat. However, as the result of discussion, this was not repeated — people ate when they wanted to, now, not when it suited the management.

   'Picture orienteering and the beech walk confirmed the group's ability to get on together, and certain individuals' awareness of their abilities or disabilities in the assembly/meeting was marvellous.

2. *The Wharf.* 'A lot of wharf activities depend on the weather. They are always well received — experience of the water is often limited — regardless of the extent to which the group manages itself.

   'Bosun's chair was an excellent exercise and all the water work was fun as well as educational. . . . Again, many of the nautical terms don't bear repeating.

3. *Local activities.* '"Ropes 1", with its low, less spectacular climbing bars, swinging tyres and cargo nets is a good activity to settle in with, as is "kitting out". Getting all the group equipment together is an excellent familiarisation exercise, especially as the next two days tend to be spent looking for all the places that the kit may have been left (staff only, of course).

   'The "small zip wire" as a prelude to more daring activities is excellent — especially if undertaken at night. The person descending the wire, locked-in to the helicopter strop, is certainly given a taste of things to come. "Ropes 3" is full of more difficult, close-to-the-ground activities with balance beams, ladders and so on — but it does let everyone know where they start the "big zip wire". "Big zip wire" — the high climb, the safety measures, the swaying platform high in the trees, the speed of long descent towards the sea after pondering for 30m minutes on whether or not to jump and trust the safety measures — was brilliant.

   'The work in the climbing store was first class, from trampolining to the training walls, The indoor climbing walls were a good preparation for the real thing. On "night line" the organisers suspected that the group had been pre-warned about what to expect by previous groups. They seemed to know they were being followed as they picked their way through the woods, blindfolded, hanging on to the rope line. They certainly expected to be left in the wood, to find their own back at the end — and knew they were being trailed! But this might be too unjust on the group's obviously burgeoning skills.

4. *Birdrock.* 'The walk was another good introduction for the expedition to come. It is spectacular and achievable, as are most of the activities if carefully planned.

5. *Swimming/Canoeing.* 'The pool session at Aberdovy is useful as a known experience, leading to the Canadian canoeing or singles on Broadwater. Both were fun and valuable experience in lots of ways. This session on the first course led to the Centre taking up canoeing in a major way — we now have fifteen boats and many ace members.

6. *Climbing.* 'We climbed at Tonfannau with the "trainers" course. The details — safety gear etc was as usual an integral part of the activity — appreciated by the group during a full

day. The wide range of abilities was well catered for from abseil to climb.

7. *Expedition and mines.* The expedition was another success. Everyone had new experiences in the cottage, tents and activities. The mine exercise was terrific — quote: "Is this dangerous" — Answer: "No, not for someone as tall as you!"

8. *Conclusions.* This report serves mainly as an aide memoir for planning future courses. We don't feel that we should be too self critical at all, whilst reflecting on things that could be done differently. This course was an unqualified success and our Outward Bounders are easily seen around our centres.

'We shall always return to Rhowniar, as long as they will have us. We wear our sweatshirts proudly and there is an unseen bond between all ex-Rhowniar people — the thing that only going there can give you.'

FIELDFARE TRUST, SHEFFIELD

The British Telecom Kielder Challenge is an adventure project for mixed teams of able-bodied and disabled children organised by the Fieldfare Trust, which promotes access to the countryside and environmental education for people with disabilities.

The Challenge started in 1985 to try to get youngsters into the countryside and, by introducing them to problem solving situations, to encourage them to work as a team. A team is made up of eight youngsters, four able-bodied and four disabled. The physically handicapped members are, typically, one ambulent, one who uses a self propelled wheelchair and two people who use electric wheelchairs.

The Trust sees the integration of able-bodied and disabled children not as a one-off event, but as a continuing process and the Kielder Challenge as a link in the chain. The two most difficult problems in achieving the aims of the Kielder Challenge are: is it possible to introduce activities that involve all the team members whatever their ability, and is it possible to stimulate the process of integration beyond the actual competition?

To answer the first question it is necessary to explain how the project is judged. Although competition is an integral part of the Kielder Challenge, bonus points are introduced for initiative, communication and teamwork. The tasks are designed so that all the team members can play a significant part in the competition and those that look to involve everyone are most likely to be successful in terms of winning the competition, as well as learning and benefiting from the experience. A simple, water moving exercise, for example, can be adapted and made more fun (as well as fitting the criteria for involving everyone) by simply attaching everyone, by means of short ropes, to an octagonal plywood board on which they have to transport 'highly volatile chemicals' that, if split, will kill all the flora and fauna in the immediate vicinity.

The BT Kielder Challenge is now a national competition. It is hoped that the teams that take part will, when they return home, spread the message that it is possible to involve mixed groups of able-bodied and disabled children in exciting and stimulating activities. These need not involve high adventure but simply aim to progress the process of integration.

Some of the lessons learned from the Challenge recently enabled the Trust to work with a group of unemployed people and young people from an adult training centre for people with a mental handicap to organise a Canadian canoe expedition down Scotland's Caledonian Canal. Obviously, back-up support for such an arduous expedition is essential if the process of integration is to occur, but also the participants were encouraged from the outset to view the project as their own. They had to raise much of the funding before the expedition could take place as well as committing themselves to a taxing training programme.

The event proved to be successful in that the participants completed all 60 miles of the Caledonian Canal and thoroughly enjoyed the experience. The process of integration occurred, however, just as much when the group practised capsize drills in a swimming pool and when they organised a sponsored walk and overnight camp in a bunk barn, as it did when they crossed Loch Ness.

The aim of the BT Kielder Challenge and the Caledonian Canal Expedition is not simply to give the opportunity for mixed groups of people with and without handicaps to participate in adventurous activities, it is also to provide a catalyst that will encourage other integrated projects.

For further details contact: Ian Newman, Director, Fieldfare Trust, 67A The Wicker, Sheffield S3 8HT.

THE CALVERT TRUST ADVENTURE CENTRE, KESWICK

The aim of this Centre is to provide the facilities for disabled people to enjoy the Lake District National Park as far as possible in the same way as able-bodied people.

The Centre is built in traditional Cumbrian style and is set in two acres of grounds overlooking Bassenthwaite Lake. It commands a beautiful panoramic view of the nearby fells.

The Centre is open from mid-January to December for sailing, canoeing, fishing, bird-watching, archery, riding (own stables), hill-walking, nature trails, orienteering, swimming (own heated indoor pool).

The accommodation is suitable for both sexes, in mixed groups, and is specially designed for wheelchair use. Up to 38 people can be accommodated in pleasant two-, three- and four-bedded rooms.

A self-catering unit for up to 12 people can be hired for a small charge during certain times of the year.

A similar Centre has been established at Kielder Water on the Kielder Reservoir. It caters mainly for families with one or more handicapped people in them.

KATHERINE ELLIOT COTTAGE PROJECT, HAWICK

The Elliott Centre, having decided to develop an outdoor pursuits programme, discovered a likely base for their project in a cottage on an estate in the Border country; they contacted the Factor and the Hawick Rover Scouts, and the Scouts, the owners, decided to give the Centre the use of the cottage and donated a gas cooker and light fittings.

The cottage roof was repaired and a new window added; the guttering was renewed and the walls repaired for decorating. A fireplace with surround was built and flooring apoxy resin was laid. A local Women's Guild donated two calor gas fires and several pieces of furniture were forthcoming from other sources. A path was laid and rock and stone embedded in the cart track to 'firm up' the ground. All this was accomplished through the hard work of staff and trainees. Curtains and bed covers were made from offcuts of material donated by local mills.

Angling and canoeing

The Centre investigated the possibility of using a local loch for angling (Fig 15.8) and canoeing. This was not possible, but did lead to discussion with the Border's Education Outdoor Activities Staff and the Roxburgh District Council, who offered 'Williestruther Loch', providing certain guarantees were given to angling clubs, shooting clubs and other bodies.

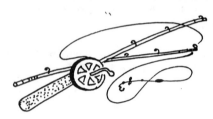

Figure 15.9 Angling equipment

A suitable seasonal timetable was evolved. A shingle beach is ideal for canoeing and dam stonework offers a suitable dinghy wharf. The 'Spetch', part of the River Teviot, running through the Hawick Park, also offers ideal canoeing on grade 1 water for training canoeists.

The Hawick Angling Club allows members from the Centre complimentary passes to use any of their waters.

Equipment

A two-seat kayak was built from a Moonraker kit and has proved an ideal trainer stability craft on loch and river.

The three/four seat dinghy was built from plans and base materials and given rubber section safety grabs by the Centre; over 50% of the Centre members use this. It can be, and is, used:

1. as a basic paddle craft — Canadian paddles;
2. as a basic rowing boat;
3. with an outward motor as a recovery and motor vessel.

A Water Bat KW7 and KW4 are the property of the Katharine Elliot Centre and small Water Bats — Panthers and Snipes — are available via Selkirk High School Canoe Club.

Integration (Border's 'Snap In' Club)

The Manager of the Katharine Elliot Centre joined the Teacher's Train-Ins organised by the Education Outdoor Activities. As a result of this the following year Selkirk High School staff and Canoe Club members, with Selkirk baths staff, developed facilities for evening 'integration session clubs' with Selkirk High School Canoe Club, Friday evening 'Snap-In' Club, Joint Week-

end Slaloms (river races, camps and youth hostel tours), Thursday lunch time Katharine Elliot Centre swim/canoe preparatory sessions in which the Selkirk High School teachers and baths staff work together with Centre staff.

WING-WAY OUT

A disabled voluntary organisation in Gateshead — WING-Way Out — that provides outdoor activities for thousands of youngsters is proving a great success. WING-Way Out started in 1984 and now provides a programme featuring canoeing, rock climbing, abseiling and skiing in Scotland and the Lake District.

Thousands of youngsters from all backgrounds including unemployed, disabled people and people with a mental handicap have benefited.

The Sports Council has provided a grant for activities, help with leadership training and, with Gateshead Education Department, pays the salary of a development worker/instructor.

Kevin Pearson of WING says: 'The Sports Council enabled us to do the activities that proved we were needed and effective. Thanks to that we have now got funding over four years from the Inner Area Partnership Fund and that will enable us to take on two more instructors'.

WING can be contacted at: Whinney House, Durham Road, Low Fell, Gateshead, NE9 5AR (tel: 091-487 9356).

LEE VALLEY PARK

The Lee Valley Park, which stretches 37 km (23 miles) from Bow in East London, along the borders of the River Lea to Ware in Hertfordshire, offers variety of indoor and outdoor sports, and leisure facilities, swimming pools and parks, all of which can be visited by people with a mental handicap.

Further details can be obtained from the park's Marketing Department (tel: 0992 717711 ext 226). The park also organises many specific events for disabled people throughout the year; for details contact Terry Phillips at the Picketts Lock Centre (tel: 01 803 4756).

4. HOLIDAYS PROVIDING AN INTRODUCTION TO OUTDOOR PURSUITS

The holiday schemes described serve primarily as an introduction to one or more of the foregoing activities or just to 'the out-of-doors'. Such is the popularity of some of these schemes that facilities, clubs, qualified instruction and help are searched for locally, so that some of these pursuits become a part of the hospital's or ATC's general programme.

More and more hospitals and ATCs are looking for holidays for residents and trainees where new activities can be tried and new ideas born. An activity enjoyed on holiday can easily become part of the everyday programme.

Some examples of such holidays are given in this chapter. Many more exist, organised either by local authorities or voluntary organisations. It is a case of 'shopping around' to find the best package, not only from the financial aspect but also the standpoint of instruction and safety.

See also 'Guidelines to planning an outdoor activities course or holiday, pages 151-152.

BRIGHOUSE ATC

Brighouse Adult Training Centre in West Yorkshire took nineteen adults to Low Mill Askrigg (a centre set up by the village trust). From this village in the dales the trainees took part in a wide range of activities which included, for the more active — climbing, walking, canoeing and potholing — and for the less active — country walks with visits to a cheese factory, a 96-year-old fairground organ, a farm and a pottery.

PETER LE MARCHANT TRUST, COLSTON BASSETT

The Peter Le Marchant Trust, based in Nottinghamshire, arranges day and weekend boat trips for handicapped people of all ages and with all types of disability. Those with severe mental or physical handicaps can and do enjoy the exhilerating experience of travelling through some of Britain's loveliest countryside. 'A day of brightness' was the way one visitor summed up his experience.

In 1976, only one 12m (40') narrow boat was in use, now there are more, including a 70-footer.

The Trust will accept bookings from all sources, voluntary organisations, social services departments and families with a handicapped child.

AVON ATC

An Avon Adult Training Centre staged a pilot scheme in 1977 which has now been extended.

The Manager of the Blackhorse Adult Training Centre suggested that, rather than take a large group of trainees to a holiday camp, it would be far better to take small groups throughout the summer, on a variety of holidays according to the apparent individual need. It seemed likely that many trainees would benefit from living in small groups rather than in the more overpowering environment of a large holiday camp. It was therefore agreed that, as a pilot scheme, two separate groups of twelve trainees would spend five days in an area of wild country to assess the suitability of some adventure activities for adults with a mental handicap.

It was found that the Fedw Adventure Centre owned by the Methodist Association of Youth Clubs would be a suitable place for the initial trials. The hostel, high on Llangattock Hillside above Crickhowel in the Brecon Beacons National Park, is an old converted farmhouse.

During the first week the most exacting activity was the climb by the three trainees from Llangenny to the summit of the Sugar Loaf—594m (1950'). However, during the second week six trainees from a similar group to the first, climbed the Sugar Loaf and three later in the week climbed Pen-y-Fan—886m (2907').

From two groups of 12 in 1977, four ATCs visited the Fedw Centre in 1978 with 90 trainees. The choice of activities has widened to include pony trekking, boating on a nearby canal and visits to caves and castles in the district. Fedw is not staffed by qualified outdoor pursuits instructors, but the Avon Authority feels that this is no deterrent. 'For the present, an unstaffed Centre such as Fedw would appear to offer the greatest potential. It allows our staff to structure their programme to suit their group, without the constraint of fitting it to a standard day common to most staffed centres.

'If it found that there are small groups with a particular interest, such as pony trekking, climbing, canoeing etc, consideration might be given, in the future, to mixing trainees from more than one centre a for a specialised week, with an accent on that activity.

'Should specialised groups be formed, then the use of a staffed centre with expertise in that activity should be considered. Numerous centres of this kind would tailor a course to cater for groups of disabled people'.

EIGHT YEARS ON

It is now some eight years since the first edition of this book was published. At that time, a few pockets of excellence, working in isolation, provided outdoor opportunities for people with a mental handicap; these pockets have now expanded beyond all expectations.

At that time only a few countryside managers were aware of the needs of handicapped people and only a few outdoor pursuits centres had thought of offering them a service. Now, day centres and community based projects, as well as social education units, include countryside recreation and environmental learning in their activities.

What has brought about this change?

Graham Hiscock (see p 158) suggests that the following are the main influence that have been at work.

1. *The Community Sports Leaders Award*, with particular reference to the South Yorkshire initiative and its provision of basic taster courses in outdoor pursuits, with its focus on safety and awareness of one's own limitations.

2. *The Initiatives of the United Kingdom Sports Association for People with Mental Handicap (UKSAPMH) Training Committee.* The publication of the booklet *Outdoor opportunities* (for people with mental handicap) was followed by several national courses in outdoor pursuits aimed at instructors and nursing staffs within the mental handicap services. The first course was held at the Knowsley Trust Parson House Farm, near Sheffield, and was directed by Mike Devlin. This has been followed by many others, the most recent has been organised by the Yorkshire and Humberside region of the UKSAPMH and again held in the Peak District. The course tutors, Judith Russell and Martin Shaw, have already received requests for further courses.

3. *Outward Bound* held one of the most inventive courses — aimed at senior staff with responsibilities for providing outdoor activities within their own authorities. The course was not about teaching the rudiments but designed to use the environment to develop management skills. The course

was hosted by Outward Bound Wales at the Rhowniar Centre, Tywyn, and tutored by Steve Gough (see p 158).

4. *The Fieldfare Trust* has helped many individuals and agencies to achieve their objectives. The Fieldfare approach, whether running an adventure weekend for able bodied and disabled youngsters, or advising on the design of an informal interpretive facility in a country park, is to work with handicapped people to meet their special needs in the countryside. This means involving disabled people directly in the work of the Trust, asking what they want and listening to what they say. Public authorities, private firms and voluntary bodies can benefit from the consultancy service the Trust operates in North of England from the Peak District to the Scottish border. In fact, ATCs, social education centres and hospitals are making increasing use of field centres as alternative holidays.

As camping, canoeing, climbing, caving, horse riding, sailing, and skiing now seem to be very much a part of everyday activities and part of the curriculum of day centres, it would seem that these high risk sports, once introduced with trepidation, are now accepted as normal.

FURTHER READING

General

Cotton, M. *Outdoor adventures with handicapped people.* London, Souvenir Press, 1983.

Cotton, M. *Out of doors with handicapped people.* London, Souvenir Press, 1981.

Croucher, N. *Outdoor pursuits for disabled people,* rev ed. Cambridge, Woodhead Faulkner, 1981.

Croucher, N. *Adventures of their own.* Cambridge, Woodhead Faulkner (in press).

Department of Education and Science. *Safety in outdoor pursuits.* London, HMSO, 1972.

Girl Guides Association. *Guiding for the handicapped,* rev ed. London, Girl Guides Association, 1988.

Price, B. *Coaching disabled people.* Leeds, National Coaching Foundation, 1985.

Scout Association. *Extension activities handbook: guide to scouting activities with the handicapped.* London, Scout Association, 1972.

Smith, R. *Outdoor directory.* Edinburgh, Holmes McDougall, 1979.

Sports Council, Advisory Panel on Water Sports for the Disabled. *Water sports for the disabled.* Woking, Royal Yachting Association Seamanship Foundation, 1978.

United Kingdom Sports Association for People with Mental Handicap. *Outdoor opportunities.* UKSAPMH, First Floor, Unit 9, Longlands Industrial Estate, Minler Way, Ossett, WF5 9JN.

Water sports for the disabled. Wakefield, EP Publishing, 1983.

Angling

Beaver Book of Fishing. London, Arrow Books, 1983.

Know the Game Series. *Coarse Fishing; Game Fishing; Float Fishing; Sea Angling.* London, A & C Black.

National Anglers' Council. *Guide to fishing facilties for disabled anglers.* National Anglers' Council, 1977.

Wrangles, A. *A line on sea fishing tackle, rigging and bait.* Havant, Kenneth Mason, 1979.

Wrangles, A. *Daily Express Guide To Fishing,* London, Star Books, 1982.

Camping

Know the Game Series. *Camping.* London, A & C Black.

Scout Association. *Enjoy camping.* London, SA, 1973.

Canoeing

British Canoe Union. *No 1. Choosing a canoe and its equipment; No 2. Canoe handling and management; No 7a Canoe building (soft skin moulded veneer); No 7b Canoe building (glass fibre).* Weybridge, BCU.

British Canoe Union. *Canoeing handbook.* Weybridge, British Canoe Union, 1981.

British Canoe Union. *Disabled update in Canoe Focus,* 1983, Spring.

Know the Game Series. *Canoe games.* London, A & C Black.

Smedley, G. *A guide to canoeing with disabled persons.* Weybridge, British Canoe Union, 1986.

Caving and Potholing

Know the Game Series. *Potholing and caving.* London, A & C Black.

Mountaineering

Blackshaw, A. *Mountaineering.* Manchester, British Mountaineering Council, 1970.

British Mountaineering Council. *Booklet on safety; leaflets on helmets, ropes and hypothermia.* Manchester, BMC.

Langmuir, E. *Mountaincraft and leadership.* Manchester, British Mountaineering Council, 1984.

Orienteering

Disley, J. *Orienteering.* London, Faber, 1978.

Harris, N. *Orienteering.* Tadworth, World's Work, 1978.

Know the Game Series. *Orienteering.* London, A & C Black.

Rambling

Sharp, D. *Walking in the countryside.* Newton Abbot, David and Charles, 1978.

Spurbook of map and compass, 2nd ed. Bourne End, Spurbooks, 1980.

Sailing

Bond, B. *Handbook of sailing.* London, Pelham Books, 1985.

Know the Game Series. *Sailing.* London, A & C Black.

Royal Yachting Association. *Learn to sail* (a guide to RYA recognised teaching establishments). Woking, RYA.

Royal Yachting Association Seamanship Foundation. *Water sports for the disabled.* Woking, RYA.

Water Safety

Royal Society for the Prevention of Accidents (several publications on specific sports including water safety). London, RoSPA.

Chapter 16

Riding and Driving

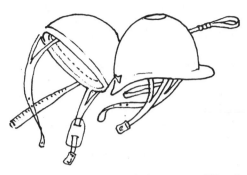

Riding and driving are exceptionally popular with people with a mental handicap and an increasing number of facilities now exist.

The Riding for the Disabled Association (RDA) should be contacted for help and advice by any establishment or club thinking of encouraging its members to ride.

During the 25 years of its existence the RDA has been one of the fastest growing recreational charities concerned with disabled people. Through riding and driving most people with a mental handicap can attain levels of physical and mental performance that are seldom possible in any other way.

The Association has over 600 groups in the United Kingdom divided into 18 regions. Working closely with the medical, paramedical, educational and equestrian professions, local education authorities, the National Health Service, Adult Training Centres and many voluntary bodies, the RDA organisation can provide therapeutic and recreational activities to suit the specific needs of people with a mental handicap.

More and more purpose-built riding centres are being set up, but people with a mental handicap are sometimes better catered for at a regular riding school, riding the same horses as anyone else. A horse considered too frisky by other riders can sometimes be ridden successfully by a handicapped rider, because the rider is unconcerned with the horse's reputation, is calm and relaxed, uses a long rain and has a calming influence on the horse which then behaves beautifully. At one time, the Association catered mainly for physically handicapped people needing a lot of support, but now an increasing number of people with a mental handicap are benefiting from riding. Obviously, the degree of handicap will dictate the amount of assistance needed; those with less ability may always need physical support from a helper, while the more able are capable of riding independently, given the opportunity.

RIDING GROUPS

Official RDA riding or driving groups meet regularly each week at approved establishments where suitable ponies are available and there are experienced helpers.

Group programmes are devised with reference to the individual's disabilities. Every session is 'fun' although an equally important objective is to develop the physical and mental potential of each member through riding.

EQUIPMENT

All riders and/or drivers must wear either jodhpurs or long trousers and suitable footwear with heels.

The RDA insists that crash-helmet-type riding hats as approved by the British Horse Society must be worn.

It says that while its riders, with few exceptions, are riding in a safe, controlled situation and that their requirements are not the same as those of able-bodied riders, it is desirable for member groups to take account of what is currently recommended by the Society as good practice and that, when new hats are bought, they should be at least of BSI 6473 Standard or the Jockey Scull Cap Riding Helmet BSI 4472. Where riders are not able to wear hats conforming to the above standards, advice should be sought on alternatives. If there are any problems, write to RDA headquarters. In addition, the new style Jofa Riding Helmet (from Jofa UK, P O Box 8, Petworth, Sussex) has been given BSI approval (BSI 4472). S Patey (London) Ltd 15b Amelia street, Wellworth Road, London SE17, will make extra large and small hats.

Jackets, when worn should be fastened — a flapping anorak can startle a horse and cause it to bolt.

Driving groups are particularly careful to ensure that the carts used ensure maximum safety. The specially designed cart for disabled drivers approved by the RDA has shown itself to be highly successful. Carts with tailboard ramps and arrangements for securing wheelchairs on board have made it possible for non-ambulant people to drive. Riders are encouraged to become involved in pony care through such activities as grooming, feeding and stable management.

COST

No one is excluded from riding or driving with RDA groups because of lack of finance. All groups endeavour to be self-supporting, although help for major projects and advice may be sought from RDA headquarters. Special arrangements are made with riding establishments and private owners to provide horses and ponies, and operating funds may be 'topped up' by grants from local authorities, donations from charitable organisations, money raised by the groups themselves and, where possible, contributions from those responsible for the riders themselves.

Anyone wishing to join a group must produce a doctor's certificate, and, in the case of riders under 18, parental consent is also required.

SAFETY

Every precaution is taken to avoid accidents. Special attention is given to the correct technique for helping participants to mount (whether by lifting from ground level, from a trench or a mounting block), supporting the rider in the saddle or cart and leading the pony in such a way as to maintain complete control. Most people with a mental handicap are able to learn how to mount correctly. The basic technique involves a helper on the opposite side of the horse from the rider stabilising the saddle by bringing weight to bear on the stirrup leather so that unnecessary slipping of the saddle is prevented while the less agile rider gains the correct position on the pony.

Helpers should not be over-protective; if they are, they may prevent a rider becoming more proficient. If too many allowances are made for a handicapped person, lack of success may be attributed to the extent of their handicap, when it may be due to lack of experience. Having due regard to safety precautions, handicapped people should have the opportunity to take the same risks as anyone else if they have the necessary ability.

RDA GROUP ACTIVITIES

Although most RDA groups are based on a riding establishment with the use of a manage or paddock and sometimes an indoor riding school, where possible they take disabled members out on hacks or drives in the countryside. Some riders progress to vaulting while others compete in local RDA competitions leading to a national championship. Residential RDA members become sufficiently proficient to be integrated into pony club groups and units of the riding clubs.

If a rider moves from one group to another it is the responsibility of the new group to ensure he is competent and safe before allowing him to ride independently, even if he holds proficiency tests of certain standards.

Strange ponies and new surroundings can often produce very different results.

One or two cases have come to light where a rider has passed a proficiency test, moved to another group or to a riding school, and has been allowed to ride alone, with unfortunate results.

Group organisers should make it clear to parents that passing a test does not necessarily mean that a rider can ride any pony anywhere, and that adequate supervision must be given to all disabled riders in a new group or at a commercial riding school.

THE DIAMOND CENTRE FOR HANDICAPPED RIDERS

The Diamond Centre in Surrey was first opened in 1968 to give handicapped children the opportunity to experience the joy of riding a real pony. Since then the group has expanded. Today it has 28 ponies with their own stables and a large indoor riding area and a smaller covered school where 400 people ride every week. Many of these young riders are now adults because no one had the heart to say they could not come any more as they grew older. The following account is based on the experience of Helen Henn, a physiotherapist who has worked at the Centre since it began.

Riders

Many of those who come for lessons at the Diamond Centre are people with a mental handicap. They come from adult training centres (ATCs), special schools and hospitals around south London. Pupils from the schools go on to the ATCs and, having ridden while at school, are proud to show their colleagues at the centre what they have achieved, be it the rising trot or just mounting successfully from the floor. Sometimes they have a

sympathy and rapport with the pony which makes their hour at the centre the only time in the whole week when they can demonstrate to themselves and others their skill in managing to make a pony go where they want.

Rides usually end with a game of some kind: this is the moment when the rider becomes sufficiently excited to use his legs strongly enough on the pony's side to win. If the same rider is likely to be the champion every time, the helper leading the pony can hobble the best and let the slowest have a chance of the accolade.

Organisation

A full ride consists of eight people. Some ATCs have so many who wish to ride that they take 16 people each week, eight watching for half an hour while the first eight ride. However, this half hour can be instructive and fun. The waiting trainees can go down to the stables and see the ponies in their boxes and perhaps help to 'tack up' or watch the ponies being groomed. After the ride is over the riders learn to run up the stirrup irons and, if the ponies are not wanted again immediately, they assist their leaders to put them away in the stables.

Helen Henn says: 'Perhaps one of the many good things that develop from riding is when a clumsy hyper-active person slows down and is gentle and kind to that warm soft creature waiting so patiently to allow them to mount. Often the pony is a better teacher than we are.'

Preparation

Training courses are organised for instructors, therapists and for helpers to help them appreciate all the problems involved.

Before any group starts riding, those in charge, be it head teacher or manager, should visit the centre to see for themselves what riding involves. There is more to riding than sitting up and staying on, and a careful assessment must be made of which trainees gain most from it. To appreciate this to the full, the instructors/teachers are asked to ride if they have never done so before; often they are surprised to find that it is not as easy as it looks. Riding requires balance, co-ordination and concentration, and those who are slow to begin with and need a lesson to be repeated many times often become better riders in the end.

Ponies and weight limit

The ponies at the Centre are mostly native breeds — small and stocky — but even these ponies will suffer back trouble before long if ridden by someone over 11 stone sitting like a sack of potatoes. The fact that riders cannot weigh more than 12 stone is often an incentive to some who are overweight to slim.

Cost

Unfortunately, riding is an expensive sport and always will be. Ponies must be fed and buildings maintained, so it is essential that every minute of riding time is used to the full and to the maximum benefit of the rider. Riders pay something towards the cost of their ride but the charity supports about two-thirds of the actual cost.

Anyone who has balance problems in learning to walk or run will find riding a great stimulant and an incentive to hold himself upright and maintain a better posture. Trotting, cantering or going over small jumps are some of the goals, but everything achieved can be a real morale booster, especially to those who score very few goals during their lives. Meeting their voluntary helpers is a two-way event, rewarding for both helpers and riders who are so often isolated in their institution or home. Realising how much they rely on their helpers as well as the pony for an enjoyable ride can make them less self-centred, and remembering to thank both helper and pony at the end of the session with a handshake or a pat can mean a great deal.

Physiotherapists and instructors

Considerable responsibility is put on the shoulders of the riding instructor and this is shared by the physiotherapists who provide the necessary link between the medical and horse riding worlds. Physiotherapists often attend during rides and will advise on the best ways of helping the people with different disabilities. The riding instructor is not only responsible for the safety of the ride but needs to have eyes at the back of her head to keep eight ponies and riders working hard, but not on top of each other, and to see that those who are impatient learn to wait their turn. Everyone is encouraged to have a kind and considerate feeling for the pony they are riding.

A good instructor will incorporate many things into the lesson which will not only teach the trainee to ride but help him in his day-to-day living. Trotting over poles can be exciting, a lesson in good rhythm, and the rider can count out loud — an exercise which can help those with communication problems. 'At the Diamond Centre a non-communicating person has been heard to shout out a whole sentence in the excitement of a game', says Helen Henn. Those who succeed in mastering the rising trot have achieved a real feeling for the movement of the pony and have learnt to move in rhythm with him. All good movement is rhythmic. Learning which is 'left' and 'right' can be a problem, but anyone whose pony goes the opposite way from everyone else's when the instructor asks for a right turn, soon understands the difference between the right and left rein.

Liaison

Good liaison is essential between the ATC, school or hospital and the Riding Centre. Also, before riding lessons commence the instructor must be told as much as possible about the trainees, in particular about any aspect of their condition which might affect their attitude to riding, especially if any of them have a fear of animals or of heights.

Trainees should have their doctor's consent.

Helpers

Good leaders should build up personal relationships with the riders so that they know them as individuals and anticipate the moments when they are most likely to need help during the lesson: Johnny may ride quite safely on the straight, but a sharp turn during a game may unseat him; Jane can reach and put a ring on a pole quite easily, but Mary requires her pony to stand quite still before she will stretch out very far, and even then the helper may have to offer a little assistance (Fig 16.1).

Clothing and equipment

Riders must have a good riding hat, lace-up shoes with a heel or boots, and trousers; these things are necessary for safety and

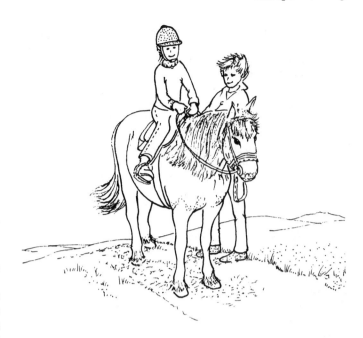

Figure 16.1 Building up a personal relationship with a rider

comfort. Shoes that are likely to catch in the stirrup must not be worn. The bridle and girth must be checked for each rider if he is unable to do so himself; the bridle and saddle and the health of the pony are the responsibility of the riding school.

Insurance

A riding centre which is a Member Group of the Riding for the Disabled Association is fully insured for public liability. The Diamond Centre is a Member Group of the RDA and is also approved by the British Horse Society.

Safety

Mounting must be taught carefully and those who have no spring will need some assistance, either a helper's strong arm, a stool or a mounting block, so that the saddle is not damaged or the pony's back hurt.

Riding holidays and other events

Sometimes 'hacks out' are arranged from the Centre during the summer months. The RDA organises very successful riding holidays. Sponsored rides, horse shows and gymkhanas all add interest to the sport; even the slowest pony and rider can win a rosette in the fancy dress parade.

HAVERING GROUP RDA

The Havering RDA group started in 1979 with just eight riders taking lessons in preparation for a pony trekking holiday in Wales. Both the holiday and the lessons were so successful that the group now organises two riding holidays every year. The pony trekking holiday is for the more adventurous handicapped riders who, like any other guests at the trekking centres, ride unled over the Welsh mountains. For the less able who need more assistance in a more structured environment, the Havering Group organises riding holidays.

Since the number of riders with a wide range of ability has grown to 36, the four weekly lessons are graded — one for beginners and low achievers, two lessons for intermediate riders, and one for the 'stars' who include jumping in their activities as a prelude to competing in the dressage and show jumping section of the Mini Olympics (see below and p 188). All the riders take part in some competition during the year, whether in the group's own One Day Event, the best rider classes in the riding school's annual horse show, or in the regional competitions. Almost without exception, all the riders in the Havering Group are keen to be involved in the RDA proficiency tests and, in 1987, four achieved Grade One, eight Grade Two, ten Grade Three, ten Grade Four and four Grade Five. The group is completely integrated with the riding school at which it is based, and the only concessions for handicapped people are the few helpers and a mounting block for those who are handicapped. Riding takes place mainly in the indoor school so that riders can ride all the year round and progress with a minimum of risk. Separate lessons on the theory of horsemastership and stable management are arranged; however, these tend to take place only when tests are imminent.

MINI OLYMPICS

These started in 1979 to provide a week's competitive sport at national level for adults with a mental handicap and, in 1980, it was decided that equestrian events should be included. Each member of the Co-ordinating Committee of the Mini Olympics takes responsibility for organising a different sport.

It is the philosophy of the organisers that people with a mental handicap should be consciously accorded the same rights and expectations as anyone else. Hence, normal competition rules are applied to their events which, in the case of horse riding, means no leaders. The dressage tests and the show-jumping courses are simple, straightforward, and are geared to independent success for the rider. Entries for the dressage competition outweigh those for jumping by three to one, probably not because those with a mental handicap cannot take part in show jumping, but because those in authority, influenced by people who think (wrongly) these riders cannot manage the jumps, do not give them the opportunity to try. People who have ridden with the Havering Group RDA gained the first four places in the show jumping section of the 1986 Mini Olympics, and the organiser looks forward to the day when riders from other groups will share the honours.

RDA RIDING TESTS

For the majority of people with a mental handicap the degree of competence needed to be successful in the RDA's tests is beyond their ability, but the few minutes they spend on horseback every week can represent an achievement and be of a therapeutic value quite disproportionate to the time involved. It is with this kind of 'riding' that the Society's fund is especially concerned.

Evidence suggests that a handicapped child can gain in confidence from the knowledge that even he, for a change, is in control of, and responsible for, a creature who is dependent on his whims and wishes — he who is usually so heavily dependent on the support of parents and friends. Difficult children learn to relax, non-communicating children to adopt a more responsive attitude.

In addition, some people with a mental handicap, for example those at Lufton Manor, MENCAP's rural training unit for horticulture and farming, have the opportunity to learn stable maintenance.

RIDING WITH A DIFFERENCE

To overcome the difficulty that very severely handicapped people cannot sit astride or even side saddle on a horse, one riding school found a trap, refurbished it and trained a pony to draw it. It was then possible to lift people into the trap so that they too could experience 'riding'. It is worth inquiring locally to see whether a local farmer has a forgotten pony trap hidden in the corner of a barn.

DONKEY RIDING

At a donkey sanctuary at Slade House Farm, Salcombe Regis, Devon, the first indoor donkey riding centre for disabled people is nearly complete. Donkeys are placid and very suitable for the young to ride.

The founder of the Slade Centre, a qualified teacher, assesses the value of donkeys on trial visits — 'The results are shattering: autistic children begin to relate, the hyperactive quieten while riding, and even spastic and severely handicapped children make movements previously thought impossible by doctors, therapists and teachers' (*Therapy*, Dec 7, 1978).

The intention is that the Centre will be used by schools during the week and that on Saturdays it will welcome parents with disabled children.

FURTHER READING

Peacock, G and Saywell, S. *Introduction to riding for the disabled*. Riding for the Disabled Association.

Riding for the Disabled Association, *RDA Handbook* (articles on riding for people with a mental handicap). Riding for the Disabled Association, 1978.

Riding for the Disabled Association, *RDA News*. National Agricultural Centre, Avenue 'R', Kenilworth, Warwicks CV6 2LY.

Sayer, K.K. *Look at this! Signs for the deaf and non-communicating riders*. The Diamond Riding Centre for the Handicapped, Carshalton, Surrey, 1979.

FILMS/VIDEOS

Riding towards freedom; The right to choose; Twenty one years on. Available from: Landscape Film & Television Productions Ltd, Thames Wharf Studios, Rainville Road, Hammersmith, London W6 9HA (tel: 01 385 3344).

Chapter 17

Adventure Playgrounds

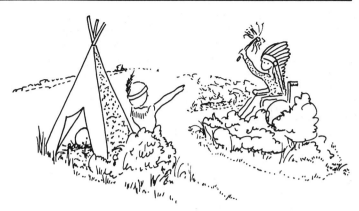

The object of an adventure playground is to stimulate the mental and physical development of a child or adult by the use of imaginative, adventurous play.

A number of hospitals have built an adventure playground within their grounds. Without doubt, these playgrounds afford excellent opportunities for residents to explore, to be 'active' in, or to be quiet.

The late Drummond Abernethy who was Consultant to the NPFA (National Playing Fields Association) said:

'In this country we realise the urgent and imperative necessity for children and young people to be able to play in the manner which nature predestined. In other words, the process is so diverse that it includes physical and mental growth, learning, fun, experiment, social conduct and many other skills. Because of the extraordinary conditions in which we live in this (so-called civilised) modern society, this whole growing up process is now quite impossible in its original and natural form. Twenty years' experience of ordinary adventure playgrounds has taught us this: as soon as children identify with the scheme and with the adult and teenage workers and helpers one is constantly staggered by the initiatives and liveliness which stem from what at first sight had seemed the most unpromising child and teenage material. The same goes for the parents and adults who begin to move into these schemes. Over and above all this, one also releases a torrent of help from able bodied young and old'.

The Handicapped Adventure Playground Association and the National Playing Fields Association work together to find ways and means of establishing more adventure playgrounds for handicapped children, and will advise anyone considering setting up any facilities for children or adults with a mental and/or physical handicap on lay-out, equipment, building, organisation and leadership, and can arrange for them to visit a handicapped adventure playground scheme in progress. Owing to the complexity of an adventure playground and the wildly varying ideas as to what constitutes such a playground, it is essential to discuss all plans for development with one or other of the two organisations mentioned.

PLANNING AN ADVENTURE PLAYGROUND

The success of an adventure playground depends on the initial planning and the skill and imagination of the play leader and many experienced leaders feel that the following ideas should be taken into account when planning a playground.

Layout

See the section on informal play areas in Chapter 6 (see p. 20) and consult the National Playing Fields Association and/or the Handicapped Adventure Playground Association (see p. 189).

Equipment

Everyday removeable equipment, which can be replaced or interchanged, should be the basis for a good adventure playground and trainees should be taught to handle and care for these items. Equipment which can provide the concepts of 'up', 'down', 'height' and 'through' 'round', etc, to provide stimulation should be emphasised. Natural mounds or cuttings help to provide such stimulation.

Swings, see-saws, slides and roundabouts are expensive pieces of equipment both to buy and to maintain but could become a more economic proposition if a group of parents, ATCs and hospitals co-operated in purchasing and using the equipment (Fig 17.1).

Types of playground

For those who are only slightly handicapped, the playgrounds outlined in *Adventure playgrounds for handicapped children* (see Further Reading, p. 170) can be suitably adapted, although some of the equipment could be expensive. For the more severely handicapped the playground need not be sophisticated. Simple equipment, such as wooden boxes, wooden planks on bricks (so that the height can be adjusted quite easily), old car tyres and everyday functional items not normally seen in the hospital (such as suitably placed old tree trunks, immobilised old cars from which all projections and wheels have been removed, old road rollers etc) can be easily used to provide obstacle courses. It is a good idea to keep a store of such objects for creative play.

Climbing ropes should be trailed down natural or artificially made banks rather than, or in addition to, being hung from trees. People can pull themselves up such banks and are not likely to injure themselves should they fall.

Artificial sand dunes rather than sand pits, or sand in small holes to allow people to dig easily, should be provided. Trees and shrubs and the whole of the natural terrain of the area can be utilised for exploration leading to adventure play. It is, however, essential that the equipment provided for this group is readily adjustable to meet their needs.

Profoundly physically handicapped people and people with a mental handicap can also benefit from the use of adventure playgrounds — their handicaps are no bar to some form of physical play. Water pools at ground level for water play and gardens with sand dunes in which to dig can be particularly enjoyed by this group.

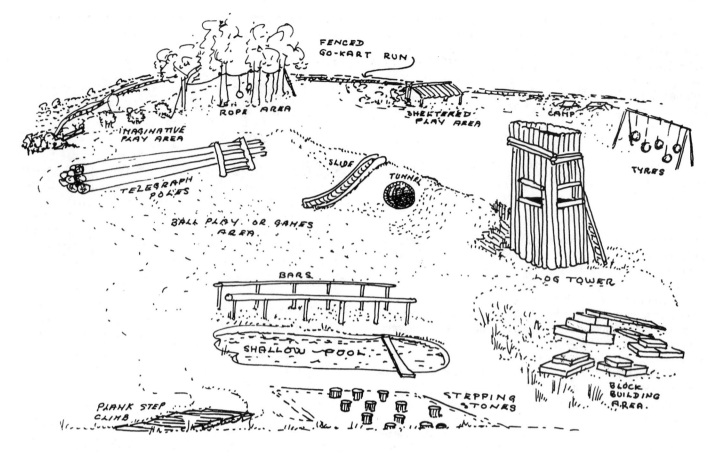

Figure 17.1 Examples of adventure playground equipment

The various types of adventure playgrounds suggested for different types of patients are not separated functionally. In many hospitals with large numbers of people with various handicaps it may be necessary to provide a full range of adventure play. In small hospitals with perhaps only a small number of children, most with a profound mental handicap, the type of playground required will have to be adjusted in relation to the abilities of the users.

Adventure playgrounds need not be limited to outside areas: the use of wards as indoor play areas should be considered. Everyday, cheap equipment coming into the hospital and used on the ward, such as cardboard boxes, packing cases, tins, string, can be adapted for play in these areas. Ropes, hoops, coloured ribbons, large blocks of wood, can all be used in imaginative play on the wards.

Storage equipment

It is desirable, whatever the type of adventure playground, that suitable storage space for material and equipment is provided adjacent to the playground itself.

Staffing

To get the best out of either outdoor or indoor adventure play areas, trained play leaders should be employed. These play leaders, together with help from volunteers, staff and interested parents and friends, can make an adventure playground work.

A description of the planning, building, development and running of the adventure playground at St Lawrence's Hospital, Caterham, Surrey, illustrates the variety of resources that can be utilised, and how a playground can be equipped and managed.

PLAYGROUND AT ST LAWRENCE'S HOSPITAL

At the beginning of 1974 the League of Friends considered whether some of the old farm buildings in the hospital grounds could be used as a centre for the League's first major project — a new adventure playground. The Regional Board's Surveyor reported that the old buildings could be repaired.

An ambitious fund raising campaign was launched and contact made with various local youth organisations. The National Playing Fields Association immediately gave encouraging advice and a promise of financial help; local volunteers also offered assistance.

Boys from a local school started to clear the site after which a mechanical digger excavated a huge sandpit, the earth being used to form a landscaped range of hills. The pit was lined with concrete and surrounded with an 2.4m (8') wide patio.

Materials — including wide concrete pipes, railway sleepers, telegraph poles, timber and polystyrene cylinders — were very generously provided by a local firm. The band of the First Battalion the Irish Guards worked for a week moving a line of fencing to extend the area of the playground, levelling and grassing part of the site, building a drainage sump, two concrete jumping pits, an area of stepping stones and constructing a balance walk and a barbecue.

The derelict old three bedroomed farmhouse was repaired with the first instalment of the NPFA grant and voluntary labour. The outside was painted by a group of International Volunteers and the interior reconstructed and decorated to professional standards over a period of a year by members of a local organisation — the materials used being supplied by the organisation.

In late 1974, the first play leader was appointed and, although much of the playground and buildings were still under construction, she withstood cold, wind and rain and organised order from chaos. At this stage, the support of the NPFA was invaluable and in 1975 they organised a Study Day on 'Play in Sub-normality Hospitals' at St Lawrence's. Speakers included Alfred Morris, MP, then Parliamentary Under-Secretary of State for the Disabled, and Lady Allen of Hurtwood, Chairman of the Handicapped Adventure Playground Association.

By this time a new toilet block and washroom had been build, a Go-Kart track constructed and also a fountain, waterfall, stream, paddling pool and a castle moat. Local school children gave great support.

In the summer of 1975 regular users of the playground included the children of St Lawrence's, many adult residents (who particularly enjoyed paddling during the hot weather), members of the hospital staff children's club and several groups of handicapped children. With the help of donations and grants from trusts, charities, business interests, private individuals groups of children as well as the Croydon Area Health Committee, two old barns have been re-roofed, re-floored, made stormproof, decorated and equipped with gas-fired warm air central heating and fluorescent lighting. Additional play features provided in 1975 included a fibre-glass 'igloo', an aviary with budgerigars and a look-out tower, built as a leavers' project by pupils from a local school.

On the first Open Day held in October 1975 the playground's specially designed flag — made and given by a local firm — was hoisted. It depicts a bluebird of happiness and a yellow background symbolising the role of the playground as a place where the handicapped children and adults can emerge from the hospital ward and spread their wings in the sunshine.

The playground was well used during the winter by residents and staff, children and parties of handicapped children from the community. By the beginning of 1976 the project was so well established and successful that Croydon Area Health Authority sanctioned the appointment of an Assistant Playleader. The large barn was used as a Play Hall for games and play, singsongs and concerts and the occasional film show, and the small barn was ready for fitting out as a 'Soft Play' Gymnasium with specially designed equipment for blind and severely handicapped children and adults. Extra features added include a rabbit hutch (with rabbits), a guinea pig hutch, an embankment slide, swings, a climbing-tower and a cyclodrome.

The hours of opening have gradually been extended to enable more of the older residents to use the facilities. Time is divided between play sessions on the wards and others on the playground. Many more departments are now using the facilities and the older residents enjoy erecting tents, building Go-Karts and mask making.

The headquarters now consists of playrooms, storerooms, office, kitchen, washroom and toilets, connected to the barns and soft play area. Outside the adventure playground has a great variety of unconventional and challenging equipment. Adjoining is a camping ground of one acre.

Extensive and increasing use is being made of the playground by handicapped children from the community. The reputation of the playground has spread and several teams of medical and administrative staff from other hospitals, anxious to provide similar facilities, have visited St Lawrence's.

The playleader

The author talked to many playleaders and feels that the points made by the St Lawrence's Hospital Playleader are general applicable.

Seeking co-operation

Armed with little but enthusiasm the playleader at the hospital began to develop the playground. During the mornings, when she visited every ward and department in the hospital she found out the sisters' problems and observed those under their care who would eventually use the playground. The afternoons were devoted to building equipment, cleaning the paddling pool and painting floors, and in the evenings many of the adults who worked during the day helped to build pedal go-carts or helped the local kids and volunteers doing their Duke of Edinburgh Award paint pictures on all the walls. The art therapy department provided paints, paper and sticky paper, and the two small rooms in the house were used for general crafts. After a Baby Belling cooker was installed, cookery was included.

Equipment

Rather than expensive equipment, most playleaders favour sturdily made improvised equipment which can be easily replaced when worn out, hence the need for skilled volunteers. Equipment in the large barn includes an eight-seater rocker-box made out of two table tops and two bed frames; a circular bicycle on a track with two wheelchairs, two seats and four seats with pedals; a trampoline 305cm (1') high made out of a bed frame covered with a plaited and woven nylon wool, and a boat to climb in and out of, given to the hospital. Some of the most used objects are balls made out of foam bits stuffed into a nylon stocking, and plastic hoops. A milk float, virtually given by a dairy for transport, was adapted by volunteers.

Using the playground

The playground was eventually used by patients from most of the departments and from as many of the wards as the playleader and her two assistants could collect. Most of the groups begin by pushing, rolling and swinging in the soft play room which not only gave the adults more freedom of movement but made them more independent. After this they began to explore and make up their own activities, and could soon get themselves on to the swings, down the slides and up rough grass.

Camping

During the summer the residents with behaviour problems were taken camping. At the end of their camping holiday, the young men looked content, well fed, and had developed the initiative to take themselves to bed at night. A similar scheme was successfully tried with female residents (Fig 17.2).

Voluntary help and integration

The playground has grown from empty buildings to a community centre. As the playleader says: 'Local mums with their own handicapped children come. Adult training centre trainees 'drop in' for an afternoon. Help is given by six local schools doing term-time community service. It is nice having one to one ratio for our severely disabled groups, and cups of tea at four sort out any

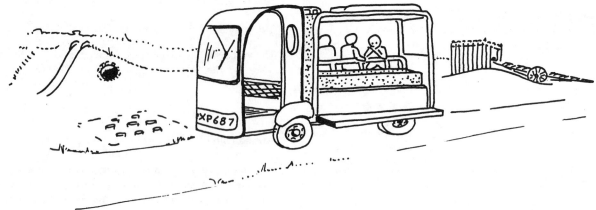

Figure 17.2 Transport to adventure

problems. These young adults often lend a hand on Saturdays and during school holidays as well. Adults residents now help with children in a very understanding and caring way. Sunny days can be used spontaneously by four or five wards as well as organised groups. Nurses from different wards then find time to chat when everyone is occupied. Sometimes even the hospital workmen drop in for a chat and a repair. One could say that the playground now belongs both to the hospital and the local community. It is easy meeting a stranger when both are involved in an activity, the job now is facilitating the right activity.'

Safety

Playleaders find that if heavy equipment is placed where it is not easily moved, and light equipment put where it will not injure anyone if it is thrown, there is little chance of accident. Broken toys are always repaired quickly or thrown out if they are irreparable. Every new piece of equipment is tested by the playleader and by volunteers.

FURTHER READING

Handicapped Adventure Playgrounds Association, *Adventure playgrounds for handicapped children.* HAPA, Fulham Palace, Bishop's Park, London SW6 6EA.

HAPA, *Handicapped Adventure Playground Association.* HAPA, 1987.

Soames, Paul, *Adventure play with handicapped children.* Souvenir Press, 1984.

Chapter 18

Gateway Clubs

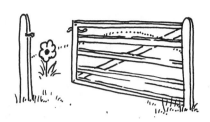

In 1966 the National Society for Mentally Handicapped Children and Adults, recognising the need to co-ordinate and develop the many clubs for handicapped children which were springing up as result of the initiative of parents, promoted the National Federation of Gateway Clubs as a national voluntary youth organisation with the needs of people with a mental handicap particularly in mind. Since that time the Federation has been particularly concerned to secure the recognition of these needs in the field of leisure and recreation by both central government and local authorities with the result that Gateway Clubs are now recognised throughout England, Wales and Northern Ireland as an integral part of the Youth and Community Service, many of them receiving assistance from their local authorities in a variety of ways, including payment of leaders, provision of premises, assistance with transport and equipment and allocation of teaching resources. In these activities sport and physical recreation have played a prominent part, stimulated by the organisation of competition at regional and national levels and, as yet to a lesser degree, by the physical activities sections within the Gateway Award Scheme.

Gateway Clubs exist to provide for people with a mental handicap in the community what the rest of the community enjoys as of right in a mixture of youth clubs, community centres, sports centre and evening institutes. The integration of people with a mental handicap into existing organisations is not necessary in their best interests. Needs, pace and performance are too disparate to enable them to obtain full value from services shared with the rest of the community. Gateway Clubs attempt to achieve a degree of integration through the services of helpers and friends and through access to the resources at the disposal of the local authorities, though at present only a few clubs make use of facilities for informal further education in the form of teachers taking responsibility for games coaching or special activities such as dance, drama and cookery.

THE MEMBERS

In broad terms the membership of Gateway Clubs is drawn from two categories: the people with a severe mental handicap of whom there are some 124,000 in England. Wales and Northern Ireland, with about 77,000 in the age-group 15-64, and those who, while less severely handicapped, are nevertheless at a considerable social and cultural disadvantage to the extent that they are unlikely to integrate successfully in normal youth clubs and organisations of a similar nature. So far as the latter category is concerned it is possible only to guess at a figure, but it is unlikely to be less than 100,000 and could be considerably greater.[1] With nearly 700 clubs and a membership of about 40,000 and with a potential membership in excess of 200,000, the National Federation can be said to be only touching the fringe of the problem.

It should not be concluded that Gateway Clubs are intended

more particularly for, and are largely the preserve of, the less severely handicapped members of the community, through which they can enjoy participating in sporting activities. Gateway Clubs, quite rightly, are seen as places in which their members can enjoy their leisure time in relaxation. It is, however, not always fully appreciated that relaxation may take an active form and call for more stimulating interests and experiences than being entertained or 'occupied'. This applies particularly to the more severely handicapped members of the community, especially those with multiple handicaps, for whom simple movement exercises, with or without music, and even simpler dance-drama can provide new and pleasurable experiences.

THE CLUBS

As part of the preparation for this publication information was obtained from nearly 453 clubs representing approximately 70% of the total number of clubs affiliated to the National Federation at the time (1986). Of particular interest were the type and size of clubs, the nature and quality of the accommodation in use and the sporting and physical activities engaged in.

Type and size

Over 70% were 'open' clubs of which two thirds were for members over the age of 16, one quarter catered for members of all ages and the remander were junior clubs. Of all the clubs included in the survey 16% were based on schools, 13% on training centres and 6% on hospitals.

The majority of Gateway Clubs, nearly 60%, had a membership of between 20 and 50, with a further 30% in the bracket 50 to 100. School clubs tended to follow this pattern whereas, perhaps understandably, hospital clubs tended to be larger. 44% of the membership fall into the age range of 7 to 25, while 55% were aged 25 and over.

Accommodation

The most popular meeting places appeared to be schools, the premises of local societies for children with a mental handicap, local authority youth centres, church halls and adult training centres. 60% of the accommodation in use at the time of the survey was considered adequate for club purposes, 30.3% was excellent and 9.3% was classified as unsatisfactory. The clubs were fairly evenly distributed between those having the use of only one space, those having two spaces, and those having three or more spaces within which to operate. In most clubs indoor facilities for sport and physical activities other than dancing were limited. Nor was there any indication that this deficiency was compensated for by access to outdoor facilities, other than grassed areas and public parks.

Sports and physical activities

The range of interests and the range of abilities require that Gateway Clubs should offer a wide programme of activities covering the whole spectrum of interests associated with youth clubs, community centres and adult education of an informal nature. So far as sport and physical recreation is concerned almost any activity, with appropriate modifications to the rules, is likely to be found in a Gateway Club. However, closer examination of the actual number of clubs engaging in the more imaginative and adventurous pursuits reveals how comparatively few of the members have the opportunity of participating in them. For this, a major share of responsibility must fall upon the shortcomings of the accommodation available and the absence of qualified instructors and helpers. Few Gateway Clubs have regular access to such specialist facilities as gymnasia, sports halls and swimming pools, even in urban areas. Even the use of playgrounds and all-weather surfaces does not feature prominently in reports of activities undertaken by clubs.

The results are predictable: the activities receiving the most frequent mention are dancing, especially jiving, darts and table-tennis. The various forms of football, five-a-side, six-a-side and eleven-a-side, came well down the list after swimming, rounders and country dancing. Gymnastics, movement and music, net-ball, keep fit classes and athletics come even lower, emphasising the deficiencies noted above. Yet the members of some clubs can enjoy riding, camping, relaxation classes, tennis, cricket, and trampolining and individual clubs have experimented with roller skating, squash, ten pin bowling, volley ball, canoeing and sailing. Gateway and similar clubs need greater resources to develop interest in activities which promote self-confidence as well as pleasure, such as sailing, canoeing, trampolining, riding, climbing and especially swimming. One of the conclusions of an International Symposia on the Leisure Time Needs of the Retarded[2] was that: 'The forms of leisure activities for the retarded need to be even more varied than those for the rest of the community.'

Competitions

Features of the Gateway year are the national competitions for five-and six-a-side football, rounders; indoor games (darts, table tennis), swimming galas, international eleven-a-side football, athletics. Most of these events feature adapted activities suitable for the more severely handicapped person. Behind these events are the regional competitions which attract widespread support and which in turn are based upon inter-club competitions at a local level. Most regions also organise athletics meetings which arouse considerable enthusiasm among the comparatively few clubs which participate and which effectively demonstrate the value of athletics as a Gateway activity. Both track and field events produce good standards of performance and the rules and track disciplines are well understood by the majority of competitors.

JUNIOR GATEWAY CLUBS

The demand for, and the provision of, leisure-time interests and activities for children of school age have been a feature of youth work for as long as voluntary organisations have been active in this field. Young people with a mental handicap are no exception; indeed it can be argued with some justification that their need for participation in stimulating activities and experiences outside the home is greater than that of normal children. From the point of view of parents and siblings the opportunity for a handicapped child to belong to a club, if only for one evening a week, comes as a welcome break from the tasks of constant attention and constant amusing out of school hours. Junior Gateway Clubs have therefore featured in the work of the National Federation of Gateway Clubs from the easiest days of its existence and there is now a growing number of such clubs operating either in their own right or as a special evening (or Saturday) of Gateway Clubs which cover the full age-range.

Activities centre around games, music and movement, simple crafts and art. A high ratio of helpers to members is required, with leaders who have at their command special knowledge and experience of handling children whose need of physical expression is quite inconsistent with their comparatively low mental ages. Collaboration between club and school and the incentives offered by the Gateway Award Schemes at the upper end of the age-range can do much to supplement the work of the schools and the resources of the home.

GATEWAY CLUBS IN HOSPITALS

As a result of past policies many severely multiply handicapped people can still be found in sub-normality hospitals, together with still large population of active people with a mental handicap who by now are so thoroughly 'institutionalised' that life outside the walls can offer little prospect of security and happiness.

For the residents of the hospitals themselves the organisations of Friends and Visitors almost invariably offer a lively programme of activities and entertainments covering most evenings in the week. A growing number of hospitals, however, are beginning to appreciate the value of Gateway Clubs as being something in which the residents cannot only be actively involved as members in their own right but also where they can share the activities with helpers from outside. In this respect a Gateway Club can be a valuable adjunct to a programme of preparation for transfer from hospital to living in the community, while encouraging discharge residents to retain their contacts with Gateway Clubs in the area.

One hospital club has found that, because of a lack of helpers, the members have had to learn for themselves how to be self-sufficient and to be concerned for their less able fellow members. Not only has there been a noticeable improvement in social behaviour but members have also learned to participate in club policy-making, in entertainments, in running a tea-bar and in the collection of subscriptions.

The same hospital encountered a problem of how to provide physical recreation for a group of high-spirited abolescent girls. The boys, with football and cricket on a competitive basis, were already catered for. The result was the formation of a keep-fit class team which, with coaching and practice, became so successful that it now gives public displays. Special features of the displays are rhythmic exercises to music, sword and country dancing, mat-work, Indian club swinging and solo gymnastics.

GATEWAY CLUBS IN SCHOOLS AND TRAINING CENTRES

Comparatively few Gateway Clubs are based on a school or adult training centre although there are signs of growing interest, especially arising from a desire to participate in the Gateway Award Scheme. There are two inhibiting factors: in the first place there is a feeling that leisure time is more profitably spent in an atmosphere and surroundings which are quite distinct from work programmes in terms of time as well as of place. Also, it must be accepted that however generous the response to transport needs, it is often impracticable for children to go home after school and return for club activities in the evening, especially when they are likely to be drawn from a very wide area. The same can be said of the adult training centres which serve mainly rural areas, with the added disadvantage that there are often few opportunities for activities outside the centre and the home in these circumstances.

Staffs in both establishments might examine ways in which either the daily programme can be extended into the 'twilight' hours to enable the people or trainees to enjoy leisure activities, especially those of an informal nature, or ways in which links can be established with existing Gateway Clubs or new clubs formed as the need requires.'For many people with a mental handicap their visit to, for example, the Gateway Club is the high spot of the week. SEC (Social Education Centre)/ATC staff should maintain contact with their local Gateway organisers to explore areas in which they might usefully co-operate.'[2]

GATEWAYS NATIONAL FIELD TEAM

Considerable development of the full-time support offered to Gateway Clubs took place during 1985/86. In June 1985 a National Sports and Outdoor Pursuits Officer was appointed to develop initiatives for both participation in, and training for, sport/recreation among Gateway members and volunteers, as well as to develop links with sports-based and disability-based organisations.

Gateway's work throughout England is guided by five full-time Divisional Advisers. In addition there are development Officers in Wales and Northern Ireland, and Regional Development Officers in the West Midlands and Yorkshire and Humberside Regions (1986). The entire field team operates to support and encourage regional developments in sport and recreation, alongside Gateway's other interest in the field of leisure. County groups have been established in many ares, some being supported by part time Gateway County Officers.

The establishment of a full-time field staff has had a considerable impact, and greater links have been forged with sports organisations and governing bodies of sports both regionally and nationally.

EXAMPLES OF GATEWAY CLUB PROGRAMMES

Halesowen and Stourbridge Gateway Club

Leader: Mrs Janet Ingram

Sports scheme

Many of the club's sports schemes have amalgamated with the local Special Olympics Group so that they work together as one body for people with a mental handicap in the area.

1. *Monday* — Gateway Swimming Class - held at local swimming pool

7.45pm — 8.15pm Main pool (swimmers only)

7.30pm — 8.30pm Learner pool

The club runs its own Learner Pool Awards Scheme to help develop the members' water confidence.

Stage 1: award 1

a) Walk around the pool holding the side, not aided (shallow end of big pool, from one side to the other).
b) Wash face in the water.
c) Get in and out unaided — using steps.
d) Holding someone's hands, kick legs from behind.
e) Support from behind, kick legs in front.

Stage 2: award 2

a) Walk around not holding sides.
b) Put head in water.
c) Get in and out not using steps unaided.
d) Use float on front and back, then go half width (help can be given).

Stage 3: award 3

a) Blow bubbles.
b) Kick legs for 15 seconds holding bar.
c) Using floats, swim half width.
d) Swim with helper using one hand and two legs (as little assistance as possible).

In the main pool novice swimmers follow the STA awards whilst the more advanced swimmers have moved on to some lifesaving awards.

Members are being trained for the Aquapark awards and some of the more able members should cope with the Lifesaving 1 award. The outside, fully qualified examiners who test members have been very impressed with their ability and the skills gained and this does not just apply to the most able members. Members also enjoy the opportunity to take part in many swimming galas.

2. *Tuesday* — Football Practice — held at Ridge Hill Hospital. This is operated in conjunction with Dudley Special Olympics.

3. *Friday* — Dudley Special Olympics run the Athletics evening at the Stourbridge ATC.

4. *Saturday* — The club runs horse riding sessions at Hagley Hall riding stables once a month. This involves rides over the Clent Hills, and, when the weather is bad, indoor instruction is given, eg learning how to mount and dismount, guide the horse, team races.

5. Other sports offered by the Club include: ladies rounders, netball and indoor games.

Once a year annual indoor games are held at the Automobile Association Social Rooms at Halesowen. Everyone participates in the three main sports of darts, table tennis and dominoes.

There are different competitions for women and men.

Those who do not qualify for the next round have their own uni-shuffle, skittles and quoits competitions; these are all geared to less able and elderly people, but the trophies for winning are just the same. Those who the Club classes are 'very able' have their own 'Superstar' competition in which they take part in all the sports on offer and are awarded points for each event. The whole emphasis of the competition is to give the ordinary member and elderly members a chance of winning a sports trophy which they keep for one year.

Tiverton Gateway Club

Leader: Mrs Pauline Bayliss

1. *Monday evening*

Green bowling at Tiverton Bowling Club

The club tries to use as many of the established sports and social clubs within Tiverton and the surrounding area as possible. Firstly, it enables the club to give its members a taste of a much wider variety of sports than would otherwise be possible. Second, it is hoped that once the club has escorted members to a particular club, they may find it easier to continue with a chosen sport and might even become members of that club. Third, it would appear that the greatest obstruction to the integration of people with a mental handicap into their rightful place in the community is not, as was initially assumed by many, to be the fears of Club members but ignorance of society in general about how to interact with people with mental handicap. Quite often, when negotiating with different clubs and organisations, any hesitancy in agreeing to a visit from the club is caused by some misconception that people with a mental handicap have to be treated differently from the rest of society. After an initial visit to a club, Gateway members are always invited back. The same can be said of the club's use of local pubs for activities such as darts, pool and skittles.

2. *Thursday evening*

Archery Club

Again some members expressed a wish to have the opportunity to take part in the sport of archery. Having advertised on local radio for volunteers experienced in teaching archery, the club was surprised when the Archery Association offered its services for six weeks. East Devon College offered the club the use of its equipment and a weekly venue. The only cost to the club was travelling expenses. Two volunteers underwent training to enable the club to continue after the initial six weeks.

The Tiverton Gateway Club also takes advantage of some of the Gateway national and regional events such as five-a-side football, six-a-side football, rounders, land yachting, sports taster days, and adventure holidays. It is also used as a contact point to pass on information about sports and activities available within the area.

Newtownards Gateway Club, County Down, Northern Ireland

The Keep Fit leader of this club suggests points to remember when preparing a keep fit lesson for people with a mental handicap.

Class members have a very different ability levels; they like to be treated as individuals and to be called by their names.

They may have difficulty in hearing and have speach problems.

Movement itself, co-ordination, posture, balance and rythm, all need special training.

Useful exercises, dance and methods of teaching can be found in Chapters 3, 4, 10 and 11.

See also Gainsborough Gateway, page 173.

Further information about Gateway Clubs, their management and administration, leadership and training can be obtained from: the National Federation of Gateway Clubs, 117 Golden Lane, London EC1Y 0RT.

References

1. Stuart, Francis. *Leisure services for the mentally handicapped. The role of Gateway Clubs.* Mencap, 1976.

2. National Development Group for the Mentally Handicapped. *Day services for mentally handicapped adults.* Pamphlet No 5, London, HMSO, 1977.

Chapter 19

Facilities, Equipment and Toy Libraries

FACILITIES

Apart from the facilities available at the hospital or ATC, it may be possible to use other community and private facilities if the right approach is made to those in charge of them.

Before making the initial approach, find out to whom the first enquiry should be made, either to:

1. United Kingdom Sports Association for People with Mental Handicap (UKSAPMH);

2. British Sports Association for the Disabled;

3. National and Regional Sports Councils;

4. local authority recreation and leisure departments.

SOME SUGGESTIONS

1. Park facilities — contact the local parks department which is usually based at the town hall (the number will be in the local telephone directory).

2. Sport/leisure centres — contact the director/manager.

3. Swimming baths — contact the baths manager.

4. School halls for use during holidays, evenings, weekends — contact the education office at the local town or county hall.

5. Public schools — contact the headmaster/headmistress.

6. Church halls — contact the vicar, priest or minister in charge.

7. Colleges of further education — contact the principal.

8. Polytechnics — contact the principal.

9. Universities — contact the registrar.

10. Hospitals, eg use of swimming pool, outdoor facilities, contact the hospital administrator.

11. Club premises — contact the leader.

12. Industrial sports grounds and indoor facilities for large events — contact the personnel officer.

13. Sports club grounds for large events — contact the secretary.

14. Hotels for use of swimming pool or other facilities — contact the manager.

15. Riding schools — contact the owner/secretary.

16. Halls belonging to other organisations — village halls, dance halls, scout and guide halls and camp sites — contact the secretary.

17. Private facilities — swimming pools, tennis courts, paddocks etc — contact the owner.

EQUIPMENT

People with a mental handicap need the same sports wear as anyone else. It is important that it is suitable for physical activity in general; shorts, slacks, skirts, T-shirts and track suits are the most common. When a specialised game or sport is practised and a trainee or resident joins a club, sports wear for that sport is essential — he/she must 'look the part' and feel comfortable.

Sports equipment of all kinds is expensive; sports manufacturers produce a great variety of goods. When considering the purchase of equipment it is important to:

select what is good value for money;

select equipment which can be used by the maximum number of people.

CHOICE

Before purchasing, investigate what is offered (cheap may not be durable). Seek expert advice from:

(i) UKSAPMH;

(ii) British Sports Association for the Disabled (BSAD);

(iii) the Sports Council or local governing body of sport;

(iv) advisers of physical education or physical education teachers;

(v) catalogues of well-known sports manufactures *of repute*.

CARE OF EQUIPMENT

When buying equipment, ask for guidance on its care and maintenance and stick to the directions. Durability and safety depend on constant overhaul and repair.

Store equipment carefully when not in use — careful storage can lengthen its life, eg balls should hang in nets. A well organised, **tidy** equipment store with clearly labelled shelves saves time and is an excellent way to help trainees and residents to be tidy. It is wise to have a rota of equipment helpers from class members.

OTHER SOURCES OF EQUIPMENT

Used badminton or tennis racquets, golf clubs, fishing tackle, tournament balls, shuttlecocks, may be available either by direct approach to the secretary of the appropriate sports club or through advertisement in the local press. When introducing a new sport it is well worth trying it out with secondhand or loaned equipment before laying out money on equipment which may or may not have any future use. Equipment may also be available on loan from local sports centres, through social services or recreation/leisure departments of the local authority.

If the staff of ATCs, hospitals and clubs in an area want a demonstration of a sport or game and its equipment, some sports manufacturers will send a representative and/or demonstrator either to a joint conference or to make individual visits in an area, eg Unihoc.

Coaches and instructors from county or local sports organisations will help to introduce their game or sport by demonstration and group coaching 'taster days' (trainees or residents can have a go!).

In some cases it is possible to make special equipment for a person with both mental and/or physical handicaps. Advice can be obtained from: PLAY MATTERS (see below)

IMPROVISED EQUIPMENT

Improvised equipment can be used in simple team games and races — and, in the early stages of learning skills, bricks, tins, old tyres can be found, and skittles, bats, stumps, targets, bean bags and soft balls can be made in a workshop. Usually it is possible to find a friend or someone in a hospital (or ATC) who has the 'knack' of making or adapting simple games and play equipment, often from unusual materials and unusual sources.

HAND APPARATUS

Some hand apparatus is used in movement training — balls, hoops, clubs and scarves can be bought or, in some cases, made.

EQUIPMENT FOR ADVENTURE PLAYGROUNDS

This equipment — fixed, moveable or improvised — should be bought or made to suit the needs of those who will use the adventure playground. Advice is readily available (see p 167).

PERSONAL SPORTSWEAR

Where possible each individual should have his or her own personal sports gear, particularly sports shoes. It should be regularly laundered and kept in good repair. Shoes should be cleaned. A number of ATCs and hospitals make some of the personal sportswear, often with the co-operation of parents, and funds seem to be raised for more expensive items such as track suits. If there is space for lockers for sportswear, these should be kept tidy.

Where the teachers, coaches and instructors are themselves immaculately 'turned out', this example sets a standard, usually followed by the class members.

TOY LIBRARIES

WHAT IS A TOY LIBRARY?

A toy library is a centre for lending the best — and sometimes specially adapted — toys to all children, including those with special needs or those who are socially deprived. The majority of toy libraries in the United Kingdom are organised by voluntary groups and run by volunteers; many of these have professional advisers. A growing number of toy libraries are run by professionals in connection with their work — as social workers, teachers or therapists. Toy libraries are found in village halls,

community and family centres, clinics, special schools and 'mainstream' schools, hospitals, including residential units, and in assessment centres.

It is widely recognised that the early years of life are vital to the future development of the child; how much more this is true of the child whose potential has been limited by disability. Children with special needs may have a short span of concentration; those with a mental handicap have an extended childhood — sometimes for life — and handicapped children generally may lack the stimulus that other children receive through exploring their surroundings. They live in a limited world. But the right play material can do a lot to make up for this. These children and adults therefore need more toys and leisure equipment which is carefully chosen to develop their fullest potential by encouraging their imagination, teaching them skills and helping them to become involved socially with other people. Toy libraries fill this need. Their aim, however, is to provide friendship as well as toys. They constitute what is often the only really local meeting place for parents and children.

Toy libraries are open to all children, no matter how young they are. The sessions are happy occasions with all the toys on display for their parents and children to choose from. Returned toys are cleaned before being returned to stock. Most toy libraries will have a helper with a special knowledge of handicap — an occupational therapist, physiotherapist, speech therapist or nurse — who will advise the parents on request on the choice of toys for their children. Tea, coffee and juice are usually on offer. and many friendships are formed in the informal atmosphere of the toy library.

PLAY MATTERS/NATIONAL TOY LIBRARIES ASSOCIATION

The work of the Association includes:

- providing information and advice for people who want to start a toy library or an 'active' group and for those who are running one;

- holding training courses and conferences for people involved in toy libraries and 'active' groups;

- publishing booklets about play and toys, especially for children with special needs;

- publishing *Ark*, the magazine for members;

- jointly publishing *What Toy*, a magazine for parents and other people interested in toys and play (this is sold through newsagents);

- talking to toy manufacturers and people who sell toys about toys best suited to children at each stage of development and about the importance of good quality toys;

- working with other organisations which are concerned with children's play and with disabled people.

For further information or details of publications please contact:

PLAY MATTERS/National Toy Libraries Association, 68 Churchway, London NW1 1LT (tel: 01 387-9592).

FURTHER READING

Play matters. Toy Libraries Association (see above).

Chapter 20

Insurance

Those responsible for sports or recreation projects for people with a mental handicap should consider carefully which insurance they need to cover any liability which might arise as a result of the activities and also the property used.

LIABILITY INSURANCE

Employers

Public liability insurance

This insurance provides the protection an organisation needs against legal liability claims for injury to people other than employees and for damages to their property. Such a claim could, for instance, arise from an accident caused by the negligence of an employee or voluntary worker and, in view of the greater than normal duty of care which would be owed to people with a mental handicap taking part in sport or physical recreation, the correct arrangement of adequate Public Liability insurance will be essential. Since this cover is important, it is essential that the insurance company is made fully aware of the particular circumstances of the activities to be undertaken. There is always a limit to the amount payable for any one incident and any organisation would be unwise to think of insuring for less than £500,000, in view of the current level of court awards.

Employer's liability insurance

This type of insurance protects an organisation against legal liability claims of any amount for injury or disease brought by its employees and is made compulsory by the Employer's Liability (Compulsory Insurance) Act, 1969. It is important to remember that this insurance covers only any legal liability of the employer – it is not Personal Accident and Sickness Insurance described in the next paragraph.

Personal accident and sickness

If any organisation wishes its members or employees to receive a benefit in the event of accident or illness, irrespective of the question of legal liability, it can provide for this by means of a Personal Accident or Personal Accident and Sickness policy on either an individual or a group basis. Accident cover can be for a lump sum payable on death or loss of limbs or sight and a weekly benefit, usually payable for up to two years, while sickness insurance is for a weekly benefit normally payable for up to one year.

Motor insurance

If any motor vehicles are owned by the organisation, they must, by law, be insured against third party personal injury risks. A choice can be made between Third Party, Third Party Fire and Theft and Comprehensive cover. The main distinction between these three versions of motor insurance is that Third Party provides cover against legal liability claims for injury to other people or damage to their property. Fire, Theft and Comprehensive cover are dealt with under property risks below.

Perhaps it is more likely that employees or voluntary workers will use their own vehicle on the organisation's behalf. If so, it would be wise to consider a Contingency Liability policy, which would protect the organisation against claims resulting from an employee's or a voluntary worker's negligence in those circumstances, should there be no other insurance in force. Such a policy would give no protection to the employee or voluntary worker, who must have his own policy—it is really a case of 'belt and braces' by the organisation, just in case it incurs liability.

Should any motor vehicle be taken abroad the insurance company should be told as soon as possible, so that your normal level of cover may be maintained for the trip.

Employees and voluntary workers

Those employed by, or providing voluntary services to a body organising sports or recreation projects for people with a mental handicap should check with that body to see that insurance cover has been arranged to protect them and their charges, so that they know what insurance arrangements they themselves need to make.

An employee's or a voluntary worker's liability for injury to someone or damage to property should be provided for by the organisation's Employer's Liability or Public Liability insurance, as described above, but a voluntary worker may also have cover under a Personal Liability insurance, usually included in a Home Contents policy.

If the organisation does not provide personal accident or sickness cover, an employee or voluntary worker may wish to avoid any hardship, which may arise from being out of action, by taking out his own insurance. He/she could also consider a Permanent Health insurance.which, once granted , stays in force until a previously chosen age—provided the premiums are kept up. To anyone suffering a serious illness, the weekly benefit would be payable continually — until that chosen age if necessary.

Employees or voluntary workers using their own car on the organisation's behalf should tell the motor insurance company exactly what the car is used for and by whom, so that the cover may be extended, if necessary.

PROPERTY RISKS

A number of different types of insurance may be necessary.

Fire

Fire insurance is a very important and, at the same time, inexpensive form of cover for both the buildings and their contents. If the building is owned by the organisation using it, that organisation will want its own insurance; if it is leased or simply hired, check the lease or hiring agreement to see whether it requires the hirer or lessee to insure — it might not mention insurance, but simply make them responsible for damage to the building — so do read it carefully. Similar considerations apply to the insurance of the contents of the buildings, for example sports equipment.

Special perils

Special Perils insurance is normally an optional extra to a Fire policy and can cover both the building and its contents against explosion, riot, earthquake and impact by vehicles, animals and aircraft and, with the insured being responsible for the first few pounds of any claim.

Theft

Theft insurance is designed to cover loss of, or damage to, contents of the building following theft or attempted theft — resultant damage to the building itself will also usually be covered.

All risks

All Risks insurance effectively includes all of the above — and more — by covering against accidental loss or damage (whereas the policies described above cover only the perils they specify, eg fire and theft). The wide cover provided make this type of insurance more expensive and it is usually bought to cover office machines and similar expensive equipment vulnerable to accidental damage.

It is essential to choose very carefully the amount for which buildings and their contents are insured. For a building, it needs to be adequate to provide for full reinstatement or rebuilding, including clearing the site and architects' and surveyors fees. A reduction would need to be made from this figure for 'betterment', if the building were in poor condition, as it could well be impossible to repair it without improving its condition and the principle of indemnity requires that an insured person should not profit from a claim. However, the resulting figure needs to be increased to provide for the expected rise in building costs during the year of insurance and any subsequent period when reliability might be taking place. Contents cover should be for an amount adequate to replace the damaged goods with new, less an amount for wear and tear and, again rising prices must be borne in mind.

Motor insurance

Compulsory Third Party insurance is dealt with under liability insurance above. In addition, Third Party, Fire and Theft and Comprehensive cover are available. Third Party, Fire and Theft cover includes claims for loss of or damage to your car by fire or theft; comprehensive cover extends to claims for accidental damage to your own car.

Personal possessions taken to work

There is unlikely to be much, if any, cover for these unless you have your Home Contents insurance extended to provide Temporary Removal or All Risks cover for them. In this case, the insurance will protect you all the time, not just at work.

CONTENTS

Anyone discussing insurance with an insurance company or broker must ensure that he tells all there is to tell — if in doubt, 'tell': otherwise, the insurance could be rendered invalid when a claim arises. Anyone in doubt about what they should disclose, whether at the time of taking it out or when claiming, should seek the guidance of the insurance company or broker.

Further details about insurance problems can be obtained from the Central Council of Physical Recreation or from the British Sports Association for the Disabled (see Appendix 2).

Chapter 21

Parents' Views

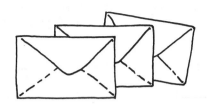

'If only parents would let their sons and daughters "have a go", then we could make many more activities available for them — activities which they could enjoy'. How often is this said.

When talking to parents who have encouraged their children to take part in physical recreation, sports and outdoor pursuits it became evident that they should 'speak for themselves' and so share their experiences with others. Comments from parents on particular projects appear throughout the text — the following accounts and letters are more general in character.

SPORT FOR ALL — TRY IT

A father relates how his 17-year-old son has been encouraged throughout his life to take part in various sporting activities with the rest of the family.

'Peter, who is now 17, has from his earliest days taken part in all family activities in which he was able to participate. From children's party games, hide-and-seek and putting, he has graduated via trampolining, swimming, table tennis and family football and hockey, to carpet bowls and badminton. Like all of us, he takes part because of the pleasure and sense of achievement which he gets and which are not necessarily — and certainly not always! — related to excellence in performance or winning. Like all of us too, as a bonus, he gets healthy exercise, improved co-ordination and companionship.

'Nothing unusual about the story so far — and there shouldn't be! But Peter has a mental handicap having Down's Syndrome and, unfortunately, many like him have been denied the opportunity to take part in any physical activity. For them, mental handicap has come, for some inexplicable reason, to be equated with complete physical disability. Parents, I regret to say, have often acquiesced in this view. To them I would say *"give your child the chance to enjoy physical recreation and add a new dimension to his or her life"*.

'How then was Peter encouraged to participate and develop his ability in specific sports, such as swimming and badminton? Truth to tell, there is no ingenious secret or deliberate plan. It has simply been a case of taking advantage of what opportunities and facilities exist.

'Thus, so far as swimming is concerned, we were fortunate to be able to make use in the early days of the facilities obtained by the swimming club organised by our local branch of the Scottish Society for the Mentally Handicapped. There Peter (and I might add two of his sisters!) learnt to swim in the usual way — playing in the water, swimming with supports and, eventually, (at about age 7) swimming unaided. Family outings to the local swimming pools are just part of our normal activities and, whilst none of us are dedicated swimming enthusiasts, all, including Peter, thoroughly enjoy them.

'Badminton is the latest sport in which Peter has been given the opportunity to take part. It is one of the activities provided at an evening class for people with a mental handicap run by the local Further Education College. He is still at the initial stage of hitting (or attempting to hit!) the shuttle back over the net, but he is enthusiastic and improving all the time. Provided his enthusiasm for his new love continues, there is no reason why he should not be able to go to the local Church Badminton Club and enjoy both the sport and the company there'.

RISK TAKING

A mother recounts the advantages of allowing her son to take calculated risks like other young people.

'I am the mother of an educationally sub-normal son of twenty-nine, called Christopher. My husband and I both have a genetic abnormality which has effected eight out of eleven pregnancies, three sons aged twenty to thirty-five are normal, two babies died two months after birth and the others were spontaneously aborted at three to four months.

'At two years Chris was blind, brain damaged, weighed ten pounds, had cirrhosis of the liver and kidney stones. He spent most of his first three years in the Hospital for Sick Children, Great Ormond Street, where he received wonderful treatment. Next came daily speech and physiotherapy, travelling daily from home to the hospital. After many eye operations he was registered eventually as partially sighted and learned to use a white cane.

'He started at the local Educationally Sub-Normal (M) School at six years and made good progress. He learned to read and cope with numbers and money, but his writing is still poor. He was promoted from the school bus to public transport at 14 — this was one of the early risks!

Living dangerously

'When Chris was eight-years-old I joined the local group of the national Society for Mentally Handicapped Children. I met a widow at the first meeting who said: 'Do your best to feel it is better that Chris might die young living dangerously, rather than wrap him in cotton wool until he's eighty'. This made a great impression on me and, while it is still difficult to let him take risks, I have tried very hard to put it into practice. I know that as a result Chris has gained in self-confidence and independence and developed as a person of whom the whole family are proud.

'He joined the handicapped swimmming club at 14, travelling alone, and very slowly learned to swim. Eventually he progressed to helping other learners, besides helping others to dress and pushing wheelchairs. He had the normal need to be needed and was invaluable on outings, while the physically handicapped members gave him immense support and stimulation. The risk in this case was often in finding him safely at 2 a.m. after a long day trip, perhaps to Liverpool, as a member of the swimming team. Chris started a Saturday job at the age of 15, filling shelves at a local store. This time we risked him being rejected by the other staff. He was, but he survived for 18 months.

'On leaving school at 16, he attended a three-month residential course for school leavers. He then worked his way through the three graded workshop/training establishments in Croydon, ending up in six years on a special assembly line for people with a mental handicap at a local factory. He has an hour's journey on two buses, and this work at present seems the limit of his capabilities because he can't cope with pressure or crises. He has done a typing course and tried clerical work, but not very successfully. Incidentally, his sight in one good eye gets him by.

Leaving home

'Three years ago he left home, after much heart searching, to live in a mixed hostel for 29 young people. Our local parents' group had help to raise the money for the hostel, and I preached to all and sundry as their Chairman how necessary it was for the residents to leave home while still young enough to be flexible. When the day came, and for week after, I was very tearful and felt I had thrown Chris out of the family. Chris came home to supper every night for about three weeks, unable to talk but obviously unhappy. It was very hard to send him off to the hostel every night when his old bedroom was still upstairs, but by the end of the month he had settled down and began to drop in only sporadically. Looking back and talking to Chris we know that this experience has matured him and he has enjoyed his independence as his brothers do. He acts as an elder brother to the other less able residents, helps with their money, teaches bus travel, how to order a meal in a restaurant, etc.

'He has also enjoyed being a volunteer at the old people's home on Sundays. He comes home weekly , but does not ever want to live at home again. We are now looking forward once again with mixed feelings, to Chris leaving the hostel with four friends to live in a house independantly, but we hope with some support from the hostel staff. I accept intellectually that this is the next logical step towards a flat of his own evenually, but I still worry emotionally about how they will cope in a emergency. Unless we give them the opportunity to cope with crises, they will never learn.

'I think back to all the emergencies and risks that have arisen—going to Cub and Scout camps and mixing his own synthetic milk; being lost on Victoria Station three times before he learned to travel safely to London and back; the day he took six hours and seven buses to reach Guildford just as the MCC stopped play for the day, and the excitement on his return last year from caving and riding adventure holiday on Dartmoor. We used to worry, ten years ago, about marriage and children and wanted to have him sterilised. He's now decided he doesn't want to marry, but enjoys his brothers' children.

Important things learned

The most important things I have learned in these 30 years are firstly, that I shall never accept the fact that I gave birth to Chris,

but I have learned to live with all that mental handicap means and hopefully am a better person for that knowledge. Secondly, other people are much better at risk-taking with Chris than I can ever be, because they are not emotionally involved. I can quite happily encourage risk-taking with other people's children or adults in my work as the Co-ordinator of Voluntary Services in a very large sub-normality hospital. I find too that my reactions as a parent can be both helpful and constructive when talking to other professionals in this field'.

OUTWARD BOUND COURSES

A former Manager of Alton Adult Training Centre, felt that parents'/carers' views were most important in every aspect of the day service curriculum. He therefore gathered together a few examples of their views on sport and physical recreation and what it means to them, their children and their families:

'Pauline's involvement in recreational activities has opened up a whole new world for her. She now has common interests with her brothers, whilst we are too old to compete now of course. She has made many new friends and met many more people now that she can take part in fitness sessions'.

'We thought that Rose was too old for anything as energetic as Outward Bound activities. Having listened to her and having seen the photographs, we know that she has a lot of potential as yet untapped. We were also amazed at how her confidence and self esteem grew in such a short time'.

'Maisie has always played a big part in Robert's life and I suppose that dance and movement is a progression from that. Other people might not think so, but I am sure he is expressing himself in a way that is very real to him'.

CARRICKFERGUS (NORTHERN IRELAND) ATC's PROJECT

The Centre's manager, describes a scheme to increase parent involvement in the provision of leisure time pursuits.

'As Manager of Carrickfergus Adult Centre I invited the parents/guardians of the trainees to a meeting at the Centre to discuss the setting up of a Parents' Group and a Tuesday evening Social Club.

'After a lengthy discussion parents were very keen on the idea. A committee of six was elected with the responsiblity for:

    raising funds'
    organising transport to and from the Centre
    organising and supervising trainees.

Senior staff from the Centre are always in attendance to guide and assist.

'Every Tuesday evening (7-9.30pm) approximately 30 trainees and 12 parents (on rota) are involved with other groups invited from the community (adult centres, schools, police cadets, etc.).

'Our Club closes for summer recess in June and re-opens in September.

Encourage parents' participation

'It is most important that parents should be encouraged to participate and are given responsibilities so that they become part of everything, thus giving them self-satisfaction and a feeling of achievement.

'Many managers do not encourage parents to attend clubs or social evenings because some parents tend to be overprotective in the presence of their son or daughter, and managers feel that more adventurous activities can be attempted if parents are not present. I believe that despite this valid point, parents have much to offer in the formation of a family atmosphere. First, parents provide the much needed transport, not only to bring their son or daughter to the club, but also friends who live near them. Second, many adults with a mental handicap learn by example — it is hoped that the mature behaviour of the parents will be copied.

'The growing number of parents and friends at meetings illustrates how parents are interested in helping in a practical way, not only with their own children but with other families as well.

'Parents know much about the background of their children and it is wise to listen to constructive suggestions and criticism.

'Trainees enjoy every Tuesday evening in the Centre, but not all wish to take part in vigorous activities. Provision should be made for this group to sit in a quiet room playing card games or discussing topics with parents.

'Parents perform a much needed service in helping with the provision and preparation of refreshments at club meetings.

'The many activities include: disco, table tennis, billiards, darts, bowls, drama, yoga, choir, music, discussion etc.

'It is essential that trainees embark on activities that are adult in outlook, purposeful, and as far as possible on terms similar to normal people.

'Our club is a tremendous success — it helps to make parents more aware of the activities of the Centre, creates better relations with the staff, thus ensuring that many benefits are gained by the people who matter, our trainees'.

TEN-PIN BOWLING

An appreciation by a mother of a community bowling scheme.

'In opening the doors of the ABC Ten-Pin Bowling Alley (free of charge) to the trainees of the Senior Occupation Centres in Aberdeen, the managers, Mr and Mrs Ron Parry, have opened the doors to a wider and more fulfilling life for our handicapped people.

'This weekly, lively activity is stimulating our sons and daughters to realise an undreamed of potential and quality of life. It encourages effort, team spirit, and healthy friendly rivalry with ordinary people, on equal terms.

'The bowling T-shirts, donated by BP Oil, are proudly worn and matches are played against teams from Grampian ITV, the local newspaper *The Press and Journal* and the local BBC.

'Working in the centres, bowling, swimming and dancing at their club discos, means a better deal for people with a mental handicap with the co-operation of, and integration within, the community. In the field of sport, the horizon for our trainees has no limits.

'What Mr and Mrs Parry have done is just the beginning'.

FINAL COMMENT

As a Gateway Club helper and mother of a severely hyper-active boy says: 'In the early days of learning to cope with the everyday problems of a child with a mental handicap one feels so very much alone, even within one's own family circle. It is as though yours was the only family with a handicapped child. But there are many of us, one in every hundred so statistics tell us. Most are very willing to pass on the benefit of their experience to new parents and that is generally done through membership of a Society formed to help the people with a mental handicap and their families'.

Chapter 22

Co-operation within the Community

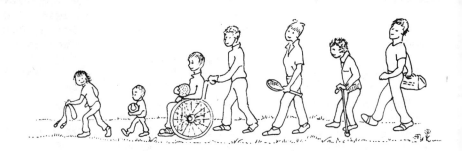

In the past people with a mental handicap were treated as a group unto themselves; they were seldom seen and their abilities were sadly under-estimated. This section contains examples of the ways in which hospitals (Brockhall and Offerton House Hospitals), adult training centres (Woodfold, Oakbank, Brighouse, Marlborough ,and Alton ATCs) and clubs (the Keep Fit Association and Children's Leisure Club, Sheffield) have co-operated and integrated with the local community to the benefit of all concerned.

BROCKHALL HOSPITAL, OLD LANGHO, BLACKBURN

In 1959, Dr. Bland, the Headmaster of the School at Brockhall Hospital, started an Evening Centre as a club for residents. In spite of initial difficulties the club has grown over the past 30 years. It is part of Lancashire Education Authority which provides further education services under the terms of the 1959 Mental Health Act.

Dr Bland retired as Headmaster in 1982, and a year later as Principal of the Evening Centre. J H Geddes became Headmaster of the school until its closure in 1986; he also became Head of the Evening Centre.

In January 1983, anticipating the school's closure, a 'Tutor-in-Charge' — N J Duckworth — was appointed to co-ordinate the work of the Evening Centre and to initiate day-time adult educational provision within the hospital.

Classes were started during the daytime to complement the initiatives of the hospital's training areas. The provision has grown steadily and five full-time tutors and over 60 part-time tutors are now involved in the work. Classes cater for all ages and degree of disability, from the most profoundly handicapped to those poised for discharge.

In 1988 Calderstones Hospital was also included under the responsibility of the 'Tutor-in-Charge' and some 190 two-hour classes now take place each week over five days and three evenings on both Brockhall and Calderstones sites.

New Initiatives

In addition to the music and movement, physical education and dancing classes, which were already in existence, successful new initiatives include survival cookery, basic education, current affairs, communication skills, outdoor pursuits, combined crafts and oral history.

In accordance with the recent drive towards more community orientation classes, a variety of venues in the local community are used, including Whalley Adult Centre, Youth Clubs, YMCA and public swimming pool.

A new collaborative venture is planned with the Health Authority — a 'computer assisted' learning project with equipment financed by the Health Authority and a tutor provided by the Education Authority.

Co-operation

Good co-operation exists at all levels between the Health and Education Authorities. The Education Authority finances the tutors and their further training, while the Health Authority contributes towards the consumables budget, transport, provides refreshments and assists with accommodation. Nursing staff accompany residents to classes where possible and, where required, classes are held on the wards to enable non-ambulant residents to attend. No fees are charged to students.

Evening activities

Trefoil Guild

This is an active group which has survived from the 1930s when every hospital had their own scout and guide movement. The Guild meets every Tuesday and is closely associated with other Guilds in the community.

'62 Club

Belonging to the National Association of '62 Clubs, this Club is for physically disabled people; it enables its members to compete at regional and national events on an equal basis without help and assistance from more able bodied people. This Club meets on a weekly basis for social activities.

Gateway Club

Affiliated to the National Association of Gateway Clubs, this Club meets every Friday evening and enables residents to participate in all activities at regional and national level. Brockhall was represented at the 1979 Special Olympics in America.

Cinema

Every Thursday evening a cinema performance is held within the Recreations Hall, showing the latest films on the circuit.

Inter Hospital Sports and Social Activities

As members of the North West Inter Hospital Sports and Social Association, residents compete in all activities from football, rounders, quizzes, 'It's a Knockout' and 'Miss Personality' contests.

Recreational activities do not stop here, for, in addition to the Christmas programme of pantomimes and carol services, there are the usual bonfire night fire-work displays, Valentine's Dance, arts and craft show, visiting superstars and performers. This ensures that a well balanced and extensive programme is provided.

Assistants

In spring 1988, to cater for the needs of the ageing residents and declining level of handicap, three care assistants to the Further Education Unit were appointed to assist both during the day and evening. The appointment of the care assistants has averted an imminent crisis, but voluntary help is still much appreciated

MARLBOROUGH ATC: SIXTH FORM INVOLVEMENT IN PHYSICAL ACTIVITIES

Marlborough Adult Training Centre works in the reverse way from the Brighouse ATC (see p.185) — sixth formers from St. John's Comprehensive School help with physical activities on one afternoon each week under the supervision of their physical education teacher.

First contact

The manager of the Centre contacted the physical education adviser in 1975 to ask for the use of a school swimming pool. The possibility of sixth formers from the adjacent St John's Comprehensive School giving some help with the swimming was explored at the same time. This proved impractical due to the travelling time involved. Swimming for the trainees went ahead nevertheless, and other ways in which the sixth formers could help at the Centre were found, including some extension of the physical activities programme on Wednesday afternoons, a plan readily agreed to by the headmistress.

Co-operation

A lecturer in physical education and dance at King Alfred's College, Winchester, started movement training which proved helpful to a group of shy young women trainees. A teacher at the Adult Training Centre has continued this movement work and netball is now played as well as the traditional football, with rounders, cricket and athletics in the summer. Sixth form girls work with the trainees in movement training, netball and rounders.

Matches

Inter-centre matches have provided an undoubted stimulus in widening the range of physical and social activities. The manager is concerned that the value of physical work and its contribution to the personal and social development shall be made available to as many people as possible. There has been an improvement in the way the young women move and hold themselves, and opportunities to increase language vocabulary and understanding have been created.

Daily activity

A daily activity session is now taken by a member of the ATC staff to develop body and spatial awareness and co-ordination

Organisation

No sixth form boys are involved in this particular project although they help with other projects in the county. Careful liaison between all the people concerned is essential because of the many interruptions in sixth form life — interviews, exams — and the need for continuity of help in the Centre. The sixth formers themselves agree that they have learned a lot about getting to know and understand people who at first talk and appear to communicate very little.

Future development

This project and others involving people from the community coming into the Centre is seen as a first step in helping men and women to go out from the Centre into the community in ways which are suitable for them.

Developments since 1981

The practice of using volunteers from the local comprehensive school to assist students in physical activities is one that is still valued by all concerned. There have been 'cosmetic' changes since 1981 in order to meet the changing demands of the students and curriculum changes at the school. Volunteers now come from the fourth and fifth year, as well as the sixth.

As well as being involved in sport and keep fit at the Centre, pupils from the school have been, and are, assisting students at sports halls, and with swimming, at both public sessions and in the hydrotherapy pool.

Negotiations are taking place to enable staff from the Education Service to run music and movement sessions at the school for both pupils and students from the Centre. Sixth form pupils from Marlborough College have helped students involved in field sports.

As a result of this co-operation, volunteers continue to come to the Centre in their holidays, and other opportunities such as using College facilities for developing films, have been explored.

The school's flexibility and co-operation makes it easier to meet the demands of students using community resources.

OAK BANK CENTRE, CHADDERTON, OLDHAM

Informal leisure activities play a major part in the free time after lunch when facilities are provided for those who wish to join in. These lunch time activities include bowls, carpet bowls, music, dancing and darts.

Oak Bank has a 'Fun Day Committee'. Attenders on the committee are able to choose and organise recreational and sports activities for themselves and other attenders.

Several people at Oak Bank have taken advantage of the Oldham Leisure Pass Scheme. This enables leisure pass holders to use facilities within the authority at a reduced rate. This is a fairly new project, but the Centre hopes that it will allow people with learning difficulties to take full advantage of local facilities.

Horse riding is a regular part of the timetable. Those attenders who are interested in riding are able to go on a regular basis to a local riding school.

Other recreational and sports activities at Oak Bank include hiking, boating, musical movement and dance.

WOODFOLD (SHEFFIELD) ATC'S WEEKLY PROGRAMME OF PHYSICAL ACTIVITIES

This centre is able, within its resources, to meet individual off-centre programmes, and, in order to offer a variety of opportunities, expeditions are repeated during the centre's weekly timetable.

Day	Activity	Comment
MONDAY	Outdoor pursuits	Groups of up to 13; trips into Derbyshire or Yorkshire Peak Districts for walking, rambling, socialising and field study.
	Shopping — and/or interest visits	These offer the opportunity to experience other cities' facilities and resources.
	Ten pin bowling	In local bowling alley.
TUESDAY	Swimming	Organised sessions when schools are open, public sessions at other times.
	Horse riding	This helps to boost confidence and offers new experiences.
	Interest visits	Using local amenities.
WEDNESDAY	Outdoor pursuits	(As Monday but a different group)
	Interest visits	
THURSDAY	Weight training	In local sports centre — mixed groups using public facilities.
	Badminton	In local sports centre as above.
FRIDAY	Indoor football	In local sports centre
	Horse riding	Repeat of Tuesday's programme with a different group.

The ATC is sometimes represented at sports meetings and also offers a 6-session introduction to canoeing using, initially, local swimming baths and progressing to a Country Park lake.

Home economics, adult education, literacy, numeracy, coping skills, music appreciation, DIY, physical development, communication, integration, and use of college and community resources are also provided in local education establishments.

Team entrants to Five-a-Side Football competitions involving handicapped and non-handicapped people are also supported by staff throughout the year.

PHYSICAL ACTIVITIES AT OFFERTON HOUSE HOSPITAL, STOCKPORT

This, a much smaller hospital than Brockhall, manages to maintain a well-balanced programme of recreational activities and sports in spite of the fact that it has lost its more able residents. Through the energetic efforts of the recreation officer, supported by other staff members, the hospital is well known in the community; this ensures a healthy supply of helpers to the hospital and opportunities for the residents to be absorbed into the community.

The number of residents at Offerton fell to below 90 in 1988, with a slight increase in day care places as care in the community in social service provision gathers pace.

The departments have been restructured to cope with the changes, and a programme that caters for the needs of residents leading up to discharge into the community provision is offered.

The recreational department has been reorganised into three units each with its own functions.

The Recreation Hall functions as a 'drop-in' centre and a place where people can congregate before moving to other activities. The atmosphere is robust and because of this a 'quiet room' for withdrawn people has been opened; the aim is to offer a stable social environment where interactions can begin and, it is hoped, progress to integration with a wider social spectrum.

An area for simple cookery and hobby skills — scalextric, model railways, model making and stamp collecting is also provided.

Links are maintained with local schools and colleges and the district voluntary service co-ordinator; through these links Offerton obtains a number of voluntary workers.

Since 1986, increasing use has been made of community facilities to accommodate the recreational and social needs of residents. Groups of no more than three take part in social training activities in the local community; a floor exercise/trampolining group uses the local sports centre; and local swimming pools are used. In addition, a group of men go out for weight training and for occasional horse riding sessions at a nearby riding school.

In 1988, with Stockport and EEC funding, a group of sports professionals was founded — Action for Sport — and the hospital has formed close links with this group. Offerton has experience of people with a mental handicap and the group has knowledge and access to a wide range of sporting activities. At present the hospital and the group are co-operating in weekly sports sessions.

A recent innovation is a package of outward bound activities with high dependency residents at venues outside the local area — Peak District, North Wales and West Pennines. So far residents have been canoeing, caving, climbing, sailing, fishing and skiing. Everyone has been surprised at the latent abilities demonstrated within this group and there are plans to extend these activities as far as is practical to all those who want to take part. Given the opportunity and the right level of staff commitment, the hospital has found that highly dependent people with a mental handicap can derive a great deal of pleasure and increase their confidence by taking part in all the activities outlined.

CO-OPERATION BETWEEN THE CITY OF SHEFFIELD EDUCATION DEPARTMENT, THE FAMILY AND COMMUNITY SERVICES AND THE KEEP FIT ASSOCIATION

The national movement and dance organisations are becoming more aware of the need for their activities for mentally handicapped adults. Some Keep Fit, League of Health and Beauty, Medau, Sesame and dance teachers are working in hospitals, adult training centres and clubs. One such scheme under the guidance of an adviser of physical education is described.

A percentage of people with a mental handicap are physically handicapped and/or elderly. The following account draws attention to the need to train keep fit teachers and other specialists to appreciate the special needs of those with a physical and mental handicap and the elderly.

A number of keep fit teachers and experienced class members in Sheffield have been interested for some time in helping special groups. These include physically handicapped people and those with a mental handicap in day and residential care.

This work began in a small way with just a few keep fit teachers who had a natural instinct for the quality and type of work needed when they entered any special field, who learnt quickly, and readily sought advice and help from those with expertise in the care of handicapped people. These teachers are in the minority and some form of training should be provided for those wishing to be involved in this kind or work.

The Education Authority, the Family and Community Services and Keep Fit Association have held meetings and introductory days for teachers to make them aware of the need for some form of training before working with handicapped people.

The 'extras' which these teachers need to know include some basic knowledge of physical and mental handicaps and of the ageing process; a simple knowledge of physiology and anatomy related to handicapped people; an understanding of the support services available, some simple knowledge of nursing, First Aid

and general care; practical sessions on suitable work to be undertaken with specific groups, opportunities for discussion, supervised teaching practice and opportunities to work with experienced teachers.

Teachers and experienced class members have responded well to courses and meetings. The result has been that an even greater demand for teachers has been received from other establishments. Most of the work is done on a voluntary basis, although some efforts to obtain funds through adult education have been successful but estimates do not always allow for this. Though talks have been held with various agencies, this aspect of finance is still unsatisfactory and the leaders are relied upon to give their help without financial reward.

Two leaders visited Conisborough Adult Training Centre and the special care unit, to work with the trainees and patients with a mental handicap.

Developments since 1981

A number of Keep Fit teachers and experienced class members who were involved originally still work with groups of physically handicapped people, those with a mental handicap and with the elderly in hospitals and in residential and day care centres.

A follow-up course has not yet been organised, but in some cases, and in particular in the case of the Conisborough Social Education Centre, staff have responded with enthusiasm, have attended courses in movement and dance, and have taken over the teaching themselves. People with a mental handicap in this Centre have enjoyed their involvement and great progress has been made.

It is hoped that another training course will be set up in the near future.

BRIGHOUSE 5-7 CLUB, WEST YORKSHIRE

The Brighouse 5-7 Club was established in 1976 to provide social activities for students attending the local ATC. Initially, the club established a relationship with a local secondary school which enabled ATC students and school pupils to work together on both classroom and outside sports and social activities.

In recent years the ATC has moved away from contract work and put greater emphasis on personal skills, social and recreational activities. In many respects the ATC has begun providing similar activities to those provided by the 5-7 Club. Consequently, the 5-7 Club has had to evolve, and the changes reflect the wishes of members. While still meeting between 5 and 7 pm, the Club no longer has a base. Instead, the members gather at the ATC and then usually go to a restaurant, burger bar, public house, cafe or sports centre. The accent is on socialising and winding down in a 'normal' setting after a day's work.

Volunteers and school children take part in Club activities, although six-formers are now preferred to the younger children who were involved in the earlier years.

Contact with local secondary schools has been maintained

and now takes the form of a group of sixth formers putting on an occasional 'evening' for the Club during which there is joint use of art, craft and cookery classrooms.

Affiliation

The 5-7 Club has affiliated to the Gateway Organisation to benefit from its insurance cover. It is also registered with Calderdale Council Youth and Community Service and there is a provision for a paid leader and ancillary worker. Club membership averages 30, many of whom have been members since the Club was founded. Club members decide the Club programme.

DEVELOPING COMMUNITY LINKS AFTER OUTWARD BOUND COURSES

The questions concerning 'integration' are complex. Without developing those issues too much, it is important to stress that the activities undertaken have the ultimate goal of integrating people with a mental handicap into sport and recreation. It must of course be tempered with realism, and take into consideration the wishes of the individuals concerned who may wish to remain within their peer groups.

However, this realism can lead to interaction within the whole world of leisure activities. If community resources are used then people with a mental handicap become familiar with all the issues involved and, if they wish, their participation can, and should, lead to membership of 'mainstream' clubs. Of course, it is essential that this goal is applied to high achievers, otherwise they will simply remain 'top of the tree' in a fairly restricted world.

As an illustration of this Alton ADC has been able to develop some of its sportsmen's and sportswomen's all round skills to such an extent that they have advanced outside the training centre circle. Regular use of local sports facilities has helped to move people into local clubs using those facilities. For example, two of the people taught by the local canoe club eventually joined the club and attend evening sessions in their own right, and several people from the groups coached by the local athletics club are now regular joggers. The same thing has happened with cricket, football and darts — with people competing as often and at a level that they feel is appropriate.

Perhaps the best example of interaction is the most successful — the continuing use of an Outward Bound Centre (see p ....) in Wales by a group of people from Alton and Aldershot Training Centres.

CHILDREN'S LEISURE CLUB, SHEFFIELD

A Leisure Club has been established in the City of Sheffield which offers structured activities for children with disabilities, aged between 7 and 14 years, in a variety of sport and leisure pursuits.

The Club is based at Notre Dame Roman Catholic School in Fulwood, which welcomes the opportunity to make its sports hall and grounds available for community use.

The main core of volunteer help is provided by the students on the full time Leisure and Recreation Management course at the Totley site of Sheffield City Polytechnic.

Specialist Training

Since the students have obvious sporting knowledge, but little knowledge of disability, specialist training in that area is provided by the Yorkshire and Humberside Sports Association for People with Mental Handicap who act as co-ordinators for the whole project.

Specialist coaching in the sporting field and some small items of equipment is provided by the Sheffield City Council's Community Recreation Department.

The benefits to the children as a result of this inter-agency co-operation are already evident in the obvious increase in sporting skills and confidence in social situations.

Appendix 1

Steering Group

STEERING GROUP (September 1976 - February 1988)

LADY HAMILTON CBE MA (Chairman) *   *Chairman, Disabled Living Foundation*

W D ABERNETHY OBE **   *Consultant for Handicapped Children and Play, National Playing Fields Association*

C ATKINSON MCSP   *Technical Officer, British Sports Association for the Disabled*

G BUCKLEY Dip TMH MISW *   *Manager, Brixton Adult Training Centre*

MISS B L BUSHELL TMAOT   *Retired Principal, Botleys Park School of Occupational Therapy, Chertsey, Surrey*

D CARTER   *Federation to Promote Horticulture for Disabled People*

MISS E DENDY DipPE *   *Senior Executive Officer, The Sports Council*

MISS M DICKS   *Senior Clinical Psychologist, Winchester Health Authority, Mental Handicap Services*

MISS K EVANS MBE MCSP DipPE *   *Project Officer, Disabled Living Foundation*

Dr R FIDLER MRCS LRCP DPH   *Assistant Controller Health, Non-Hospital Services, London Borough of Harrow*

T FRENCH JP SRN RNMS RNT   *Nursing Officer (Mental Health), Department of Health and Social Security*

F HEDDEL   *Director of Education Training and Employment, Social Security for Mentally Handicapped Children and Adults (MENCAP)*

C T HEDDITCH SEN   *Physical Recreation Officer, St Lawrence's Hospital, Caterham, Surrey*

G HISCOCK *   *British Sports Association for the Disabled*

MISS F HODGSON *   *Education, Training and Employment Adviser, Royal Society for Mentally Handicapped Children and Adults (MENCAP), Southern Division*

Dr H HUNTER MD DPM   *Medical Superintendent, Balderton Hospital, Newark*

MISS S H JOHNS *   *HMI, Department of Education and Science (Metropolitan)*

W LLOYD DMA OHA   *Project Training Officer, Trent Regional Health Authority (Regional Training Section)*

MISS B NORRICE DipPE *   *Former Senior Lecturer in Physical Education, Keswick Hall College of Education, Norwich Physical Education Association of Great Britain & Northern Ireland from January 1979*

MISS C PECK *   *Head Occupational Therapist, Chase Farm Hospital, Enfield, Middlesex*

K R PUGSLEY SRN *   *Department of Health*

A G ROGERS RNMS *   *Nurse Tutor, Lea Castle Hospital, Kidderminster*

MISS J RUSH SRN DipSoc   *The Kings Fund Centre*

M SOUTHAM *   *National Development Officer, UKSAPMH*

Dr V SIMMONS MRCS LRCP DCH   *Medical Officer, Department of Health and Social Security*

F A STUART MA   *UKSAPMH; National Officer, National Federation of Gateway Clubs*

R STUART BA DipPE   *Development Officer, Scottish Sports Association for the Disabled*

P THODAY MSc NDH MIBiol   *Lecturer in Amenity Horticulture, University of Bath, School of Biological Sciences*

DR T VANIER MB BChir MRCP   *Trustee, Disabled Living Foundation, Regional Co-ordinator, L'Arche Ltd*

MRS M WILLIAMS *   *Education Officer, English National Board for Nursing, Midwifery and Health Visiting*

J WYATT JP DPA   *General Secretary, Disabled Living Foundation (until June 1987)*

Observers

MRS E CAVE   *Department of Education and Science (until June 1979)*

J R FISH   *Department of Education and Science (from June 1979)*

MRS K LATTO (MASKELL) DipPE MCSP   Project Officer, Sport and Physical Recreation for People with a Mendatl Handicap, Disabled Living Foundation

MRS J DUVAl, MRS H WILSKER   *Secretaries to Project*

MRS E BATT   *Illustrator*

* Present members of the Steering Group (1989).
** Died in May 1988.

Appendix 2

Organisations concerned with Sport and Physical Recreation

The organisations listed under 1, 2, 3 & 4 can supply general information on events, visual aids and publications.

1. Organisations which promote sports and physical recreation (activities) for people with a mental handicap

Mini Olympics for the Mentally Handicapped Ltd, 23 Mansfields, Writtle, Chelmsford, Essex.

Northern Ireland Sports Association for People with a Mental Handicap, Secretary: Miss A E Moorhead, Sports Council for Northern Ireland, House of Sport, 2A Upper Malone Road, Belfast BT7 5LA.

Special Olympics UK, Management Office, Willesborough Industrial Park, Kennington Road, Willesborough, Ashford, Kent TN24 OTD.

United Kingdom Sports Association for People with Mental Handicap, National Development Officer: Mark Southam, 1st Floor, Unit 9, Longland Industrial Estate, Milner Way, Ossett, Wakefield WF5 9JN.

2. Organisations which promote sport and physical recreation for people with any form of handicap

British Sports Association for the Disabled, The Mary Glen Haig Suite, 34 Osnaburgh Street, London NW1 3ND.

Northern Ireland Committee on Sport for the Disabled, House of Sport, 2A Upper Malone Road, Belfast BT7 5LA. Secretary: F Kelly.

Scottish Sports Association for the Disabled, The Administrator: Miss Margaret MacPhee, Fife Institute, Viewfield Road, Glenrothes KJ6 2RA.

Welsh Sports Association for the Disabled, T Edwards, Brynn Erddig, Erddif Road, Wrexham, Clwyd.

3. Organisations concerned with the development of physical education and recreation

British Association of Advisers and Lecturers in Physical Education, G Edmondson, Nelson House, 3/6 The Beacon, Exmouth, Devon EX8 2AG.

Central Council of Physical Recreation, Francis House, Francis Street, London SW1P 1DE.

New Games UK, PO Box 542, London, NW2 3PQ.

Physical Education Association of Great Britain and Northern Ireland, Ling House, 162 Kings Cross Road, London WC1X 9DH.

Sports Councils (see Appendix 3).

4. Organisation concerned with the provision and landscaping of play areas and the training of play leaders

Handicapped Adventure Playground Association, Fulham Palace, Bishop's Park, London SW6 6EA.

National Playing Fields Association, 25 Ovington Square, London SW3 1LQ.

5. Organisations which support and encourage sport and physical activities as part of their programme

Association for Professions for Mentally Handicapped People, Greytree Lodge, Second Avenue, Ross-on-Wye, Herefordshire HR9 7EG.

British Association of Occupational Therapists, 20 Rede Place, London W2 4TU.

British Institute of Mental Handicap, Wolverhampton Road, Kidderminster DY10 3PP.

British Red Cross Society, 9 Grosvenor Crescent, London SW1X 7EJ

Chartered Society of Physiotherapists, 14 Bedford Row, London WC1R 4ED.

Disabled Living Foundation (Project: Physical Recreation and Sport for People with a Mental Handicap) Project Officer, 380-384 Harrow Road, London W9 2HU.

Duke of Edinburgh's Award Scheme, 5 Prince of Wales Terrace, London W8 5PG.

Girl Guides Association 17 Buckingham Palace Road, London SW1 WIPT.

Inland Waterways Association, 114 Regents Park Road, London NW1 8UG.

Institute of Baths and Recreation Management (IBRM), Giffard

House, 36-38 Sherrard Street, Melton Mowbray, Leicester-shire LE13 1XJ.

Institute of Leisure and Amenities Management (ILAM), Lower Basildon, Reading RG8 9NE.

Institute of Park and Recreation Administration (address as ILAM above).

King's Fund Centre, 126 Albert Street, London NW1 7NF.

Methodist Association of Youth Clubs (Methodist Church Division of Education and Youth), 2 Chester House, Pages Lane, Muswell Hill, London N10 1PR.

MENCAP Royal Society for Mentally Handicapped Children and Adults, 117-123 Golden Lane, London EC1 YORT.

MIND National Association for Mental Health, 22 Harley Street, London W1N 2ED.

Mobility International, 228 Borough High Street, London SE1 1JX.

National Association of Teachers of the Mentally Handicapped, Secretary: Eva Smith, Hillside Cottage, 2 Overhill, Wood Lane, Kingswear, Devon.

National Council for Special Education, 1 Wood Street, Stratford-upon-Avon, Warwickshire CV37 6JE.

National Federation of Gateway Clubs, 117-123 Golden Lane, London EC1 YORT.

National Youth Bureau, 17-23 Albion Street, Leicester LE1 6GD

Outward Bound Trust, Chestnut Field, Regent Place, Rugby.

RADAR Royal Association for Disability and Rehabilitation, 25 Mortimer Street, London W1N 8AB.

Royal Society for the Prevention of Accidents, Cannon House, Priory Queensway, Birmingham B4 6QS.

Scout Association, Baden Powell House, 65 Queen's Gate, London SW7 5JS.

Spastics Society, 12 Park Crescent, London W1N 4EQ.

Women's Royal Voluntary Service, 17 Old Park Lane, London W1Y.

Youth Hostels Association, Trevelyan House, 8 St Stephen's Hill, St Albans, Herts AL1 2DY.

Appendix 3

Sports Councils

The address of all the national governing bodies of sport, outdoor pursuits, movement and dance can be obtained from the Sports Councils, both at national, regional and county level.

The Sports Council, 16 Upper Woburn Place, London WC1H OQP.

Scottish Sports Council, Caledonia House, South Gyle, Edinburgh EH12 9DQ.

Sports Council for Northern Ireland, House of Sport, Upper Malone Road, Belfast, BT9 5LA.

Sports Council for Wales, National Sports Centre for Wales, Sophia Gardens, Cardiff CF1 9SW.

Regional Offices of Sports Council (England)

North (Northumberland, Cumbria, Durham, Cleveland, Tyne & Wear), Aykley Heads, Durham DH1 5UU.

North West (Lancashire, Cheshire, Greater Manchester & Merseyside), Astley House, Quay Street, Manchester M3 4AE.

Yorkshire and Humberside (West Yorkshire, South Yorkshire, North Yorkshire and Humberside), Coronet House, Queen Street, Leeds LS1 4PW.

East Midlands (Derbyshire, Nottinghamshire, Lincolnshire, Leicestershire, Northampton), Grove House, Bridgford Road, West Bridgford, Nottingham NG2 6AP.

West Midlands (Hereford-Worcester, Shropshire, Staffordshire, Warwickshire), Metropolitan House, 1 Hagley Road, Five Ways, Birmingham B16 8TT.

East (Norfolk, Cambridgeshire, Suffolk, Bedfordshire, Hertfordshire, Essex), 26/28 Bromham Road, Bedford MK40 2QP.

South (Hampshire, Isle of Wight, Berkshire, Buckinghamshire and Oxon), 51a Church Street, Caversham, Reading, Berkshire RG4 8ZX.

Greater London and South East (Greater London, Surrey, Kent, East and West Sussex), PO Box 480, Crystal Palace National Sports Centre, Ledrington Road, London SE19 2BQ.

South West (Avon, Cornwall, Devon, Dorset, Somerset, Wiltshire, Gloucestershire), Ashlands House, Ashlands, Crewkerne, Somerset TA18 7LQ.

Note: The address of the Regional Offices of the Scottish, Northern Irish and Welsh Sports Councils can be obtained from the national offices listed above.

Appendix 4

Atlanto-axial instability in people with Down's Syndrome

The following 'Dear Doctor' letter giving advice about atlanto-axial instability in people with Down's Syndrome, was issued by the Chief Medical Officer of the then DHSS in May 1986 (ref CMO (86) 9).

In recent years the quality of life of individuals with Down's Syndrome has improved considerably through opportunities to take part in sports and other physical activities. In the recent Olympic Games for the handicapped in Ireland, people with Down's Syndrome took part safely and successfully, the pleasure and opportunity for personal development clearly justifying the risk involved.

However, amongst the several problems which can affect a person with Down's Syndrome, one concerns the development of the bones in the neck. Perhaps 2 or 3% of people with Down's Syndrome will have instability between the atlas and the axis bones at the top of the neck, which can lead to pressure on the spinal cord and in exceptional circumstances to death. In some of these individuals, spinal cord compression develops slowly over a number of years, while in others, accident or injury produces immediate damage. The question arose therefore, whether, given this knowledge, the lives of people with Down's Syndrome were being put at unreasonable risk, and in what way the risk should be limited. The Standing Medical Advisory Committee were asked to advise the Secretary of State on this matter, and I am writing now to let you know their views.

The first thing to say that *at present only one case of injury to the neck and spinal cord during sporting activity has been reported in the world literature* and that occurred during unsupervised trampolining to a girl already known to have nerve damage. Deaths have occurred however in a variety of other circumstances including car accidents involving whiplash injury, to which these individuals are more vulnerable. It is possible to identify the instability by x-ray from the age of six onwards and one response has been to suggest radiological investigation for all people with Down's Syndrome. Although this might be appropriate if there was an effective treatment available current advice is that this is not so, and that it is not possible to stabilise the bones satisfactorily by surgery. The Standing Medical Advisory Committee therefore recommend the following compromise:

● that people with Down's Syndrome should continue to participate in a full range of daily activities including running, jumping and horse riding;

● where more vigorous sporting activity such as diving or trampolining, which involve acute flexion of the neck, or violent contact sports, such as karate, are envisaged, the individual should first be x-rayed;

● where an instability is demonstrated, the individual should be medically examined. In the event that compression of the nerv-ous system is demonstrated, consultant advice should be sought without delay. Where there is no evidence of compression, individuals should be encouraged to continue previous activities but be dissuaded from more vigorous activities such as diving or trampolining;

● care should be taken to support the body and head of a person with Down's Syndrome when travelling by use of seat belts and head rest;

● because pressure on the spinal cord occasionally develops without any accident or injury, examination of the central nervous system should form an integral part of the medical examination of all people with Down's Syndrome. On finding exaggerated knee jerks the doctor should arrange radiological investigation to exclude atlanto-axial instability;

● at the time of a general anaesthetic or following a road traffic accident, particular attention should be paid to people with Down's Syndrome because of the possibility of instability and its attendant complications.

Knowledge of this disorder has generated considerable anxiety which I trust this advice will allay, enabling people with Down's Syndrome to enjoy an active life at reasonable risk.

(signed) E D Acheson, DM FRCP FFCM FFOM, Chief Medical Officer

Appendix 5

Bibliography

GENERAL READING

Many books are published which could be of value to those working with people with a mental handicap. The following are a selection.

Books describing the lives of people with a mental handicap and those caring for them

Brosnan B, *Yoga for handicapped people*, Souvenir Press, 1982.

Brudenell P, *The other side of profound handicap*, Macmillan, 1986.

Council of Europe, *Measures to promote the social integration of mentally disabled people: partial agreement*, COE, Strasbourg, 1986.

Department of Health & Social Security, *Mental handicap - progress, problems and priorities*. HMSO, 1987. (A review of mental handicap services in England since the 1971 White Paper 'Better services for the mentally handicapped').

Jeffree D, McConkey R and Hewson S, *Let me play*, 2nd edition, Souvenir Press, 1985.

Moody P and Moody R, *Half left*, Dreyers Forlag, 1986 (Distributors: George Philip & Son Ltd.)

Moore P, *Dressing matters: a handbook to help people with learning difficulties to dress themselves*, Disabled Living Foundation, 1988.

Upton G, *Physical and creative activities for the mentally handicapped*, Cambridge University Press, 1979.

Willis P and Kiernan C, *A new way evaluated*, Mencap, 1984.

Young F, *Face to face, with assistance from Arthur, a boy with severe mental handicap*, Epworth Press, 1985.

MAGAZINES AND PERIODICALS

The following are a selection.

Assessment, Down's Syndrome Association, 12/13 Clapham Common Southside, London SW4 7AA.

British Journal of Special Education, National Council for Special Education, 1 Wood Street, Stratford-upon-Avon, Warwickshire CV37 6JE.

CP Leisure News, Sport and Recreation Department, The Spastics Society, 16 Fitzroy Square, London W1P 5HZ.

Camphill Village Trust News, Vivian Griffiths, Bolton Village, Danby, Whitby, Yorks YO21 2NJ.

Calvert Trust Newsletter, Calvert Trust, Little Crosthwaite, Under Skiddaw CA12 4OD.

Community Care, Business Press International, Oakfield House, Perrymount Road, Haywards Heath, West Sussex RH16 3DH.

Consumer Voice, National Consumer Council, 18 Queen Anne's Gate, London SW1H 9AA.

Contact, Royal Association for Disability and Rehabilitation, 25 Mortimer Street, London W1N 8AB.

Disability Now, The Spastics Society, 16 Fitzroy Square, London W1P 5HZ.

Gatepost, National Federation of Gateway Clubs, 117 Golden Lane, London EC1Y ORT.

HAPA Journal, Handicapped Adventure Playground Association, Fulham Palace, Bishop's Park, London SW6 6EA.

New Games Newsletter, PO Box 542, London NIN2 3PQ.

Parents Voice, Mencap National Centre, 123 Golden Lane, London EC1Y ORT.

RDA News, Riding for the Disabled Association, National Agricultural Centre, Avenue 'R', Kenilworth, Warwickshire CV8 2LY.

Special Children, 73 All Saints Road, Kings Heath, Birmingham B14 7LN.

LIBRARIES

Most public and college libraries acquire books partly in response to the demand they perceive from their readers. If the required titles are not in stock, librarians are able to borrow them on request for a reader, through the inter-library loan system.

Some non-public organisations have their own libraries to support the work of the staff. Outsiders may arrange to visit the following libraries for reference and research:

British Institute of Mental Handicap, Wolverhampton Road, Kidderminster, Worcs DY10 3PP (tel: 0562 850251).

Disabled Living Foundation, 380-384 Harrow Road, London W9 2HU (tel: 01-289 6111).

Kings Fund, 126 Albert Street, London NW1 7NF (tel: 01-267 6111).

Spastics Society, 12 Park Crescent, London W1N 4EQ (tel: 01-636 5020).

Audio Tapes, Films and Videotapes

Since 1981 many videos, audio tapes and some films have been produced — by the media and by voluntary and statutory organisations. A selection of those appropriate for people with a mental handicap are included here together with a list of suppliers with addresses.

Annotated lists of films, videos, and hire charges can be obtained directly from the distributors.

The governing bodies of sport and Sports Councils can recommend films and videotapes on specific sports

AUDIO TAPES

The following instructional audio tapes for use with people with a mental handicap stress the value of music in promoting physical activity. They aim at encouraging socialisation, co-ordination and concentration.

Chair-based activities (2 tapes). Tape 1: for more severely multiply handicapped people; Tape 2: for a wide ability range, including the ambulant.

Floor-based activities (1 tape). For people whose mental and physical disabilities are such that work can only be done on a one-to-one basis. An introductory talk provides some understanding of the principles upon which the work is based.

Let's have a go (3 tapes). Progressive tapes primarily for ambulant people who are ready to work with a leader in small groups. Tapes 2 and 3 include a little partner work and conclude with very simple folk dances.

Music movement and voice (1 tape). Appropriate for a fairly wide ability range who are ambulant and able to co-operate with a leader in small groups.

Teaching guidelines (1 tape). A practical tape for leaders wanting to understand basic teaching skills. These skills are relevant to the presentation of physical activities in general but the illustrations used are taken from the above tapes in which music provides the stimulus for activity.

All the above tapes are available from: Miss Barbara Norrice, 1 Irving Road, Norwich, Norfolk, NR4 6RA.

Tape tranquility, by David Sun, Music for relaxation or any situation where a group needs to experience quietness. No. C204, New World Cassettes.

FILMS AND VIDEOS

Able to fish, colour/sound, film 23, 32, and 35 mins and video (VHS). Three films showing how sea, coarse and game fishing can be made available to disabled persons of all ages; includes designs of special tackle. National Anglers' Council Committee for Disabled Anglers.

Adventure playgrounds for handicapped children, 16mm colour, sound. Film only. Central Film Library.

Aquatic breathing (in preparation). Concord Video and Film Council.

Building bridges, 16 mm colour/sound and video (VHS and Betamax) 30 mins. Movement for mentally handicapped people, Concord Video and Film Council.

Challenger, 16mm colour/sound, 8 mins film only, 1983. Trimaran adapted for sailing by disabled people. Being further developed by the Seamanship Foundation. Concord Video and Film Council.

Development of movement play in early childhood, VHS and Betamax (sale only). Alan Harris Electronics Services.

Explorations, 16 mm black and white, 29 mins. Film based on movement training. Concord Video and Film Council.

The fun gap, 16 mm colour/sound film and video (VHS), 26 mins, 1981 made in New Zealand for IYDP. For loan from New Zealand High Commission.

Give me a boat, 16mm colour/sound film, 35 min and video (VHS and Betamax). Shows groups of physically and mentally handicapped people enjoying barge holidays and day trips. Concord Video and Film Council.

Give us the chance, 16mm colour/sound, 36 mins, 1982, film and video (VHS and Betamax). Sport and physical recreation for mentally handicapped children and adults. Concord Video and Film Council.

The Halliwick method, 35 mm video. Concord Video and Film Council.

It's fun to care, video (VHS), 35 mins. Records the work of student nurses and staff attending a workshop on using music and movement in developing the potential of people with severe learning difficulties. It is presented in three parts. **Part 1** — Floor-based activities involving body contact are used to establish relationships and to assist relaxation. Students work with each other and then with clients who are severely multiply handicapped **Part 2** — Students perform chair-based activities which lead into simple circle dances. **Part 3** — An appreciation of the aesthetic quality of a parachute is developed while performing a range of folk dances and old time dances. These are activities which can be used to help people enjoy working together even when some have severe disabilities both mental and physical. Miss Barbara Norrice, 1 Irving Road, Norwich, Norfolk, NR4 6 RA.

In touch, 16 mm black and white/sound film and video, 30 mins. Movement for mentally handicapped children. Concord Video and Film Council.

It's a new world, 16mm colour/sound, film only, 1977. Deals with teaching disabled people to swim. National Audio-Visual Aids Library.

It's ability that counts, 16mm sound, 33 mins, 1975. Cinexa Film production. Sport for physically handicapped people highlighting the first International Multi-disabled Sports; includes sequences filmed at schools for disabled children.

A matter of confidence, 16 mm colour/sound, 28 mins, film and video (VHS and Betamax). Movement experience in play in an infants school. Concord Video and Film Council.

Mini-Olympics (picture show and commentary 1979), 20 mins. Slides can be hired from J O'Brien, Havering Training Centre, Spilsby Road, Harold Hill, Romford, Essex. Please give alternative dates when writing for slides. Details of equipment required and method of showing slides will be provided.

Moving and lifting a disabled person, 12 mm colour/sound and video (VHS and Betamax). Concord Video and Film Council.

New games, featured for seven minutes on Thames TV's 'Ace' Broadcast 2.12.80, (VHS or Betamax), hire only. Thames TV.

Not just a spectator, colour/sound film, 35 mins and video (VHS or Betamax), 1974. Shows a wide range of activities and sports for people with different disabilities. Concord Video and Film Council.

Parachute and ribbon activities, colour, 30 mins (VHS). COPE Foundation (Cork Polio General and Aftercare Association).

Riding for the disabled, 16mm and super 8mm film loops, colour/silent, 14 mins, film only. Riding for the Disabled Association.

Riding towards freedom, colour/sound film, 35 mins, and video (VHS), 1973. Explains some of the limitations and frustrations of disability (physical and mental). Riding for the Disabled Association.

Physical activities for severely mentally handicapped adults, video (VHS and Betamax), colour. AVA Centre, University of East Anglia, University Plain, Norwich, Norfolk (sale only).

The right to choose, colour/sound film, 35 mins, or video (VHS). Shows individual adult riders who, despite severe physical damage, have learned to ride with varying degrees of independence and accomplishment. Riding for the Disabled Association.

A sense of movement, 16mm colour/sound, 40 mins and video (VHS and Betamax). Movement for severely retarded children. Concord Video and Film Council.

Special Olympics, 16mm colour/sound, 23 mins, film only. Shows how mentally handicapped people can overcome their disability and enjoy sporting activities. Concord Video and Film Council.

The spirit of Stoke Mandeville, 20 mins, colour/sound film and video (VHS) 1982. British Paraplegic Sports Society.

A sporting chance, video (VHS) 30 mins, 1985. Greater London Association for Disabled People.

Swimming for disabled people, slide programmes, 40 mins, 3 programmes. 35 slides each. Purchase only. Concord Video and Film Council.

Twenty-one years on, 16 mm colour/sound film, 25 mins and video (VHS and Betamax). Riding for the Disabled Association.

Water free, 16 mm colour/sound, 35 mins, or video (VHS). Shows methods of coaching disabled people to swim and dive. Concord Video and Film Council.

Water safety, video and film, 16mm colour/sound, 38 mins. A visual appreciation of the factors affecting the safety of those people who enjoy recreation both in and out of the water, available from: the Royal Society for the Prevention of Accidents.

Note: Although these films are concerned primarily with physi-

Index